■ SECOND EDITION

AUTOMATED STATIC PERIMETRY

Douglas R. Anderson, M.D.

Professor of Ophthalmology
Bascom Palmer Eye Institute
Department of Ophthalmology
University of Miami School of Medicine
Miami, Florida

Vincent Michael Patella, O.D.

Director, New Business Development
Humphrey Systems
Dublin, California

with 187 illustrations

Mosby

St. Louis Baltimore Boston
Carlsbad Chicago Naples New York Philadelphia Portland
London Madrid Mexico City Singapore Sydney Tokyo Toronto Wiesbaden

Mosby
Dedicated to Publishing Excellence

**A Times Mirror
Company**

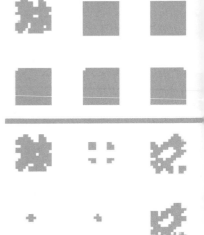

Senior Editor: Laurel Craven
Senior Developmental Editor: Kimberley J. Cox
Project Manager: David Orzechowski
Production Editor: Marian S. Hall
Designer: Carolyn O'Brien
Cover Designer: Maria Bellano
Manager of Production and Manufacturing
   Philadelphia: William A. Winneberger, Jr.

2nd Edition
Copyright © 1999 by Mosby, Inc.

Previous edition copyrighted 1992

Composition by Clarinda Company
Illustrations prepared by Trinity Graphics
Printing/binding by Walsworth Press, Inc.

Mosby, Inc.
11830 Westline Industrial Drive
St. Louis, Missouri 63146

Library of Congress Cataloging-in-Publication Data

Anderson, Douglas R., 1938-
    Automated static perimetry / Douglas R. Anderson, Vincent Michael
Patella.—2nd ed.
        p.   cm.
    Includes bibliographical references and index.
    ISBN 0–8151–4384–2
    1. Perimetry—Automation.   2. Perimetry—Atlases.   I. Patella,
Vincent Michael.   II. Title.
    [DNLM: 1. Perimetry atlases.   2. Visual Fields atlases.   WW
17A546a   1999]
RE79.P4A52   1999
617.7'5—dc21
DNLM/DLC   98–29287
for Library of Congress   CIP

99 00 01 02 03/9 8 7 6 5 4 3 2 1

To all patients who undergo perimetry
May this book help those who perform and interpret the test

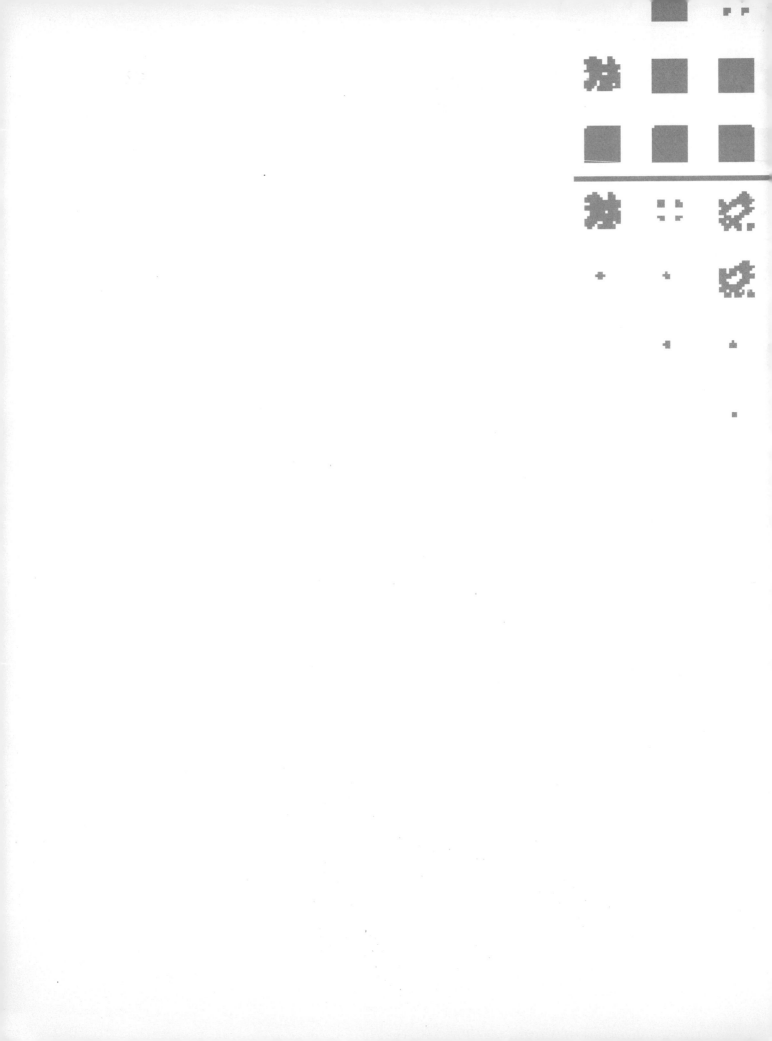

■ PREFACE

Like the first edition, this second edition of *Automated Static Perimetry* is presented in an atlas-like format. The book is intended to be a comprehensive guide to the clinical application of automated perimetry, based on a thorough understanding of fundamental principles. The reader is provided with original sources of scientific information, as well as didactic sources for further reading. Abundant examples illustrate the points made in the text. The principles discussed should apply generally to many current and future commercial instruments. We illustrate them with examples of field tests conducted with the Humphrey perimeter, the instrument with which we are most familiar and which we each use in our practice, and from which we therefore have suitable illustrative examples to offer. Some features we describe may be unique to this instrument. However, we do not intend either to ignore the existence of or to express judgment on the varying capabilities of other instruments. We simply do not pretend to be qualified to address the unique features of other instruments, but hope most of the general principles we discuss will apply to most instrumentation. This edition resembles the previous in this respect. Some obsolete material has been removed, and we hope some concepts are explained more lucidly than before. The new material includes explanation of new testing methods such as SITA and SWAP, the former making the test time shorter without compromise of accuracy and the latter being aimed at the problem of detecting very mild abnormality. The methods of analyzing individual tests are not much changed since the first edition, but the difficult task of judging progression is starting to be more soundly based.

By inviting his co-authorship, the author of the previous edition (DRA) acknowledges the dedicated and considerable contributions of VMP to the art and science of clinical perimetry. We express appreciation that the development team led by Anders Heijl over many years has developed many of the methods described herein. Several people have helped us by providing illustrative material, and these are acknowledged in the figure legends. Others have reviewed sections or chapters, rendering informative advice. These include Boel Bengtsson, Murray Fingeret, Anders Heijl, Chris Johnson, Byron Lam, Jonny Olsson, Michael Siatkowski, Remo Susanna, and Michael Wall. We are very grateful for the help they have given us.

Douglas R. Anderson
Vincent Michael Patella

■ CONTENTS

10 **Alternate and Supplemental Techniques, 301**

PART THREE   TECHNIQUE

11 **Administering the Visual Field Test, 317**

APPENDICES

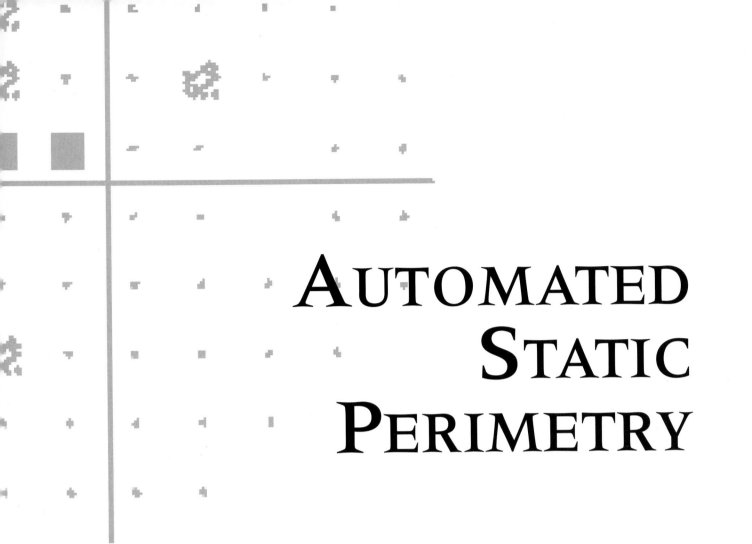

AUTOMATED
STATIC
PERIMETRY

PART ONE

BASICS

CHAPTER 1

Introductory concepts

ANATOMY AND FUNCTION OF THE EYE

The wall of the eye is made up of three layers. The outer layer consists of the *cornea,* which is clear, and the *sclera,* which is white. The region where the cornea and sclera join is called the *limbus.* The middle layer is the *uveal tract,* which has three parts—*iris, ciliary body,* and *choroid.* The iris has an opening, the *pupil,* and the root of the iris inserts into the ciliary body. The ciliary body lies within the anterior-most part of the sclera and contains the ciliary muscle, which is responsible for changing the shape of the *lens.* This allows the eye to focus on objects at varying distances, or to "accommodate." The ciliary body also produces aqueous humor. The third part of the uveal tract is the choroid, which lies under the retina and provides nutrition to the outer retina.

The innermost layer of the ocular wall is the *retina.* It receives and detects the light that has been focused into an image by the cornea and lens. Visual impulses are transmitted from the retina to the brain by the *optic nerve.*

Within the eye, the lens lies directly behind the pupil. It is suspended from the ciliary body by the *zonular ligament.* As noted previously, the lens shape (accommodation) is controlled by the ciliary body muscles, which pull on the lens through the ligament. The *anterior chamber,* filled with aqueous humor, is located in front of the iris and lens. Behind the lens is the *vitreous cavity,* which is filled with vitreous humor.

To reach the retina, light must pass through several normally transparent structures:

The cornea, which begins to focus the light by virtue of its curvature;

The anterior chamber, which is filled with aqueous humor;

The pupil, which can vary in size;

The lens, which completes the process of focusing the light; and

The vitreous humor.

If any of the structures in the optical pathway (cornea, anterior chamber, lens, or vitreous) is altered, blocking or scattering the light rays, or if focusing is imperfect, visual function will be disturbed. When analyzing the cause of visual dysfunction, these "preretinal factors" should be kept in mind, as should possible disturbances in the retina and the neural "visual pathway."

With the exception of Figure 1-2, drawings in this chapter are by Leona M. Allison.

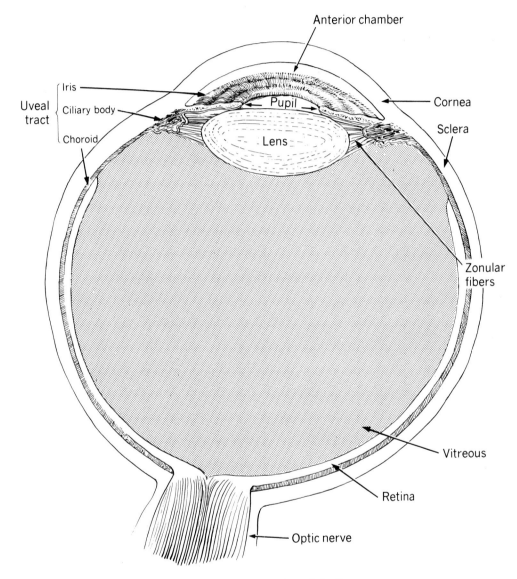

Anterior chamber

Iris

Uveal
tract

Ciliary body

Choroid

Pupil

Cornea

Lens

Sclera

Zonular
fibers

Vitreous

Retina

Optic nerve

FIG. 1-1. Cross-section of the Eye.

VISUAL FIELD

With our eyes directed forward, we pay attention to the details of the object at which we are looking. While looking at an object, we are able to detect the presence of other objects above, below, and to the sides of the object of regard, even though we may not be able to discern the details of the peripheral objects or even know what they are.

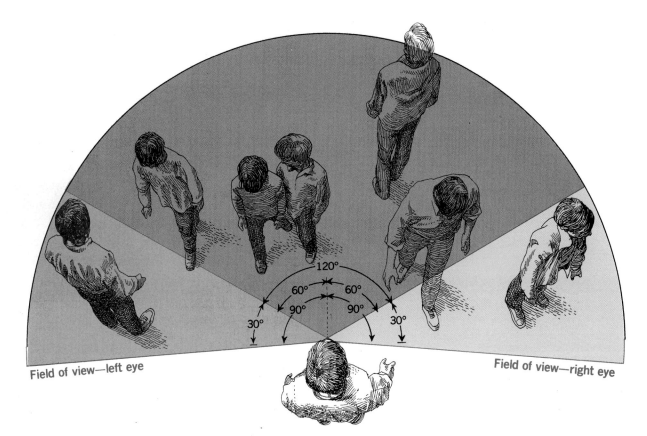

FIG. 1-2. Fields of Vision of the Right and Left Eyes. Note that the visual fields of the two eyes overlap. There is a broad area where objects are seen by both eyes, but to the extreme right or extreme left objects are seen by only one eye. In this way, the field of view with both eyes is greater than with either eye alone. (Illustration by George E. Schwenk.)

CORRESPONDENCE OF THE RETINA AND VISUAL FIELD

Every point in the retina corresponds to a certain direction in the visual field. For example, the fovea (centered at the back of the eye) corresponds to the point on which gaze is fixed, the point of fixation. The fovea is centered in the macula, a part of the retina specialized for such things as sharp vision and color discrimination. This area of the retina can discern detail, allowing one to read very small letters, and also has the highest sensitivity for detecting the stimuli used for visual field testing. Points in the peripheral retina, near the ciliary body, correspond to points in the peripheral visual field.

Because the image formed by the optics of the eye is upside down and backward, just as in a camera, the image is reversed; thus the nasal retina sees objects in the temporal visual field and vice versa. Points in the upper (superior) retina correspond to objects in the lower (inferior) visual field and vice versa.

From all points in the retina, visual information is converted to nervous impulses. These are collected by nerve fibers that course along the inner surface of the retina toward a spot 10 to 15 degrees on the nasal side of the fovea, a little above the horizontal meridian that passes through the fovea. Here the nerve fibers converge to form the optic nerve, which exits from the back of the eye and courses toward the brain. At the spot at which these nerve fibers bundle together, called the optic nerve head or optic disc, an opening in the retina allows the exit of the nerve fibers into the optic nerve. Because light cannot be detected where there is an opening in the retina, a corresponding region exists in the visual field, 10 to 15 degrees from fixation, where stimuli are not seen. This location in the visual field is called the physiologic scotoma or physiologic "blind spot." Because the optic nerve exits from the nasal side of the eye, the blind spot is in the temporal portion of the visual field.

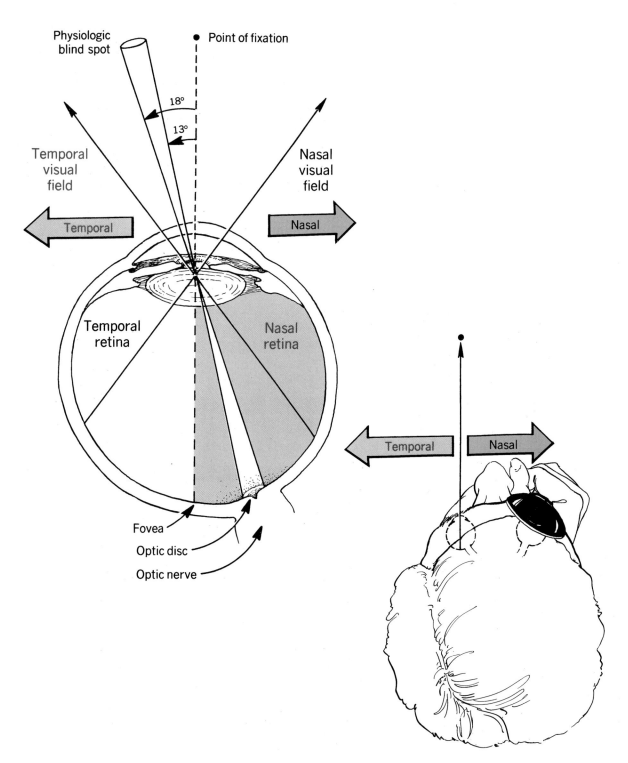

FIG. 1-3. Diagram of the Left Eye. The eye is seen from above to show the relationship between horizontal retinal location and visual field location.

BOUNDARIES OF THE VISUAL FIELD

The boundaries of the field of vision, measured in degrees from the point of fixation (the object at which the eye is directed), are approximately as follows: 60 degrees superiorly (above), 75 degrees inferiorly (below), 100 degrees temporally (to the right for the right eye, to the left for the left eye), and 60 degrees nasally (to the left for the right eye, to the right for the left eye). The extreme boundary of the visual field can be determined by bringing a large object around from behind the head of an individual who is looking straight ahead and asking when the object first becomes visible. If a disease state has contracted the peripheral boundary of the visual field, it may be necessary to bring the object very far around before it can be seen.

FIG. 1-4. Limits of the Typical Visual Field. A, Upward and downward. **B,** Temporal and nasal. **C,** Plot of the limits for the right eye. Note that the field normally is plotted on the field diagram "as the patient sees it," with the border of the visual field to the patient's right side plotted to the right on the field diagram.

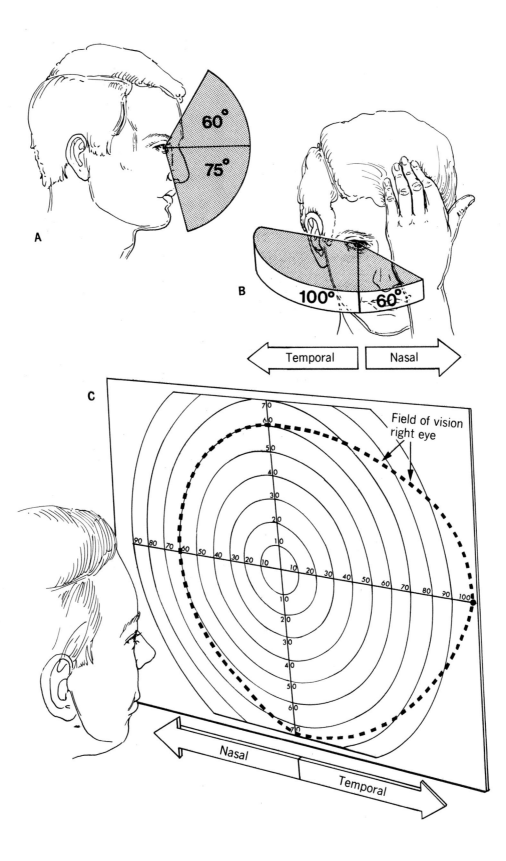

A

B

Temporal   Nasal

C

Field of vision
right eye

Nasal   Temporal

9

CHAPTER 2

The basis of quantitative perimetry

The physiology (psychophysics) of vision and the theoretical bases for instrument design are presented here to the degree that they might be of interest to the clinician in everyday practice. Readers who wish to study the theoretical aspects of perimetry in further detail may wish to consult the additional reading sources given at the end of the chapter.

VISUAL CHARACTERISTICS WITHIN THE VISUAL FIELD

Determining the outermost boundary of the visual field may be considered one aspect of testing the visual field, but it is not the aspect that is of greatest diagnostic importance. More important is the fact that every point within the boundary has certain characteristics of visual function.

For example, the ability to discern details (i.e., visual acuity) is greatest at the point of fixation. Clinically, we ask the patient to look directly at letters so that we can determine the visual acuity at the point of fixation (Fig. 2-1, *A*).

If we wished, we could determine the visual acuity at all other points in the visual field by having the patient fix his gaze on a certain spot, placing a letter chart at selected locations (e.g., 10 degrees to the nasal side), and determining the smallest letter that can be identified correctly (Fig. 2-1, *B*). We could do this for many points scattered throughout the visual field (e.g., 10 degrees temporally, 10 degrees superiorly, 20 degrees nasally, 30 degrees nasally) and thereby document or quantify the functional ability (or visual acuity) in each region of the field of vision in that individual. In a normal visual field, acuity is best at the point of fixation and progressively worse at locations further from fixation.

Acuity away from the fovea can be measured for the purpose of visual field testing,[1-3] but in traditional clinical perimetry we do not quantify the functional ability in various regions within the visual field in terms of acuity. Instead, we quantify functional ability in terms of the weakest spot of light (visual stimulus) that can be seen at representative locations in the field. In standard automated perimetry the stimuli typically consist of projected white spots, the size and intensity of which can be adjusted.

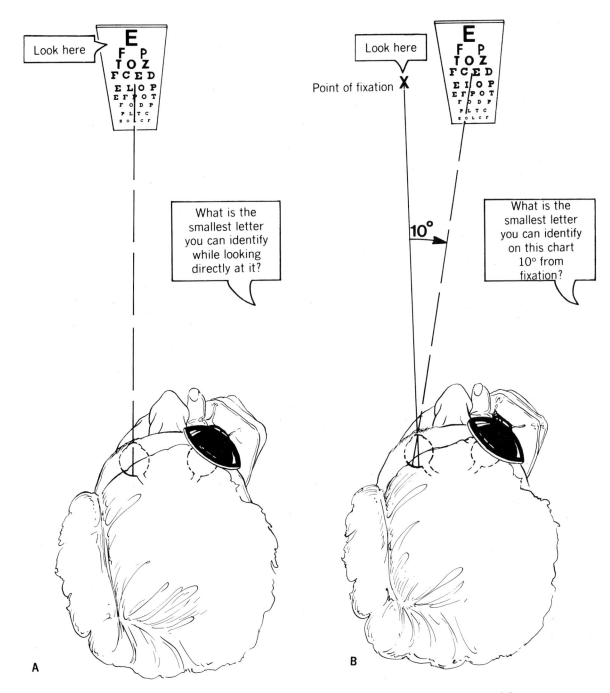

FIG. 2-1. Determining Visual Acuity. A, Usual method for testing at the point of fixation. **B,** Hypothetical method for testing at 10 degrees from the point of fixation.

In quantitative testing of the visual field, special attention is paid to three factors that influence the visibility of a white spot:

1. **Apparent size (diameter or area) of the spot.** The apparent size depends on the real size of the spot and its distance from the eye. Thus a 3-mm spot 1 meter from the eye is equivalent to a 6-mm spot 2 meters from the eye or a 1-mm spot that is 0.33 meter from the eye. With the tangent screen, which

> Visibility depends on stimulus size, stimulus intensity, background intensity and other variables.

can be used at varying distances, both the size of the spot and the distance are considered. With perimeters, the distance is fixed (33 cm for the original Humphrey Field Analyzer [HFA-I], and 30 cm for the HFA-II model and the Goldmann perimeter), and relative visibility relates only to the real size of the spot.

2. **Luminous intensity of the spot.** In a reciprocal relationship two spots may be roughly equivalent visual stimuli if one is 0.5 log-unit more intense but half the diameter (one fourth the area) of the other. The exact equivalency relationship of size and intensity is different in different parts of the visual field (see section on stimulus size and spatial summation later in the chapter).

3. **Background illumination.** The background light intensity has two effects on stimulus visibility. First, a white stimulus of a certain intensity will be less visible against a background of a similar intensity than against a dark one. For this reason, the visual phenomenon tested by perimetry is sometimes called differential light sensitivity, because with a fixed stimulus size the visibility relates to the differential, or contrast, between the stimulus intensity and that of the surrounding region or background. Second, the background intensity also determines the degree of light or dark adaptation of the retina (photopic, mesopic, or scotopic), which influences whether dim stimuli are seen.

Visibility also is affected by such variables as the color of the stimulus, any movement of the stimulus, the duration of the stimulus, the attentiveness of the person tested, and the refractive state of the eye. Throughout most of the visual field, a moving stimulus is somewhat more visible than a nonmoving one, and this may be more evident in defective regions of the field (Riddoch phenomenon). The duration of a stimulus is important for a brief flash (e.g., 1/100 second vs. 2/100 second), but duration has little effect on visibility after a certain critical time; after approximately 1/3 second, a stimulus does not become more visible if it is sustained longer.

UNITS OF LIGHT INTENSITY

The maximum luminosity (intensity) of white stimuli projected by past and current models of the Humphrey perimeter is 10,000 apostilbs* (asb). For comparison, the Goldmann perimeter and the original Octopus perimeter each had a maximum stimulus intensity of 1000 asb.

---

*The apostilb (asb) is the European unit of luminance that has been used in quantitative clinical perimetry for decades. It is equal to 0.1 millilambert, the traditional measurement favored in the United States. The apostilb corresponds to 1 lumen of total emittance per square meter of an illuminated surface, or $1/\pi$ lumens per steradian per square meter of a perfect Lambertian surface. There are several other measurement systems for intensity of light. To achieve international standardization, the currently preferred unit is the candela per square meter (cd/m^2), or the nit, in which the candela is 1 lumen per steradian. To convert asb to cd/m^2, divide by π (3.14159) or multiply by $1/\pi$ (0.31831). Thus a 10,000-asb intensity corresponds to 3183 cd/m^2.

The decibel represents attenuation of the maximal stimulus of the particular perimeter.

When a light stimulus of submaximal intensity is desired, the intensity of the projected spot is reduced by neutral-density filters. For convenience, the attenuation of light is expressed in logarithmic units, or, more commonly, in tenths of log-units, which are called decibels (dB). By convention, the perimeter's nominal maximal intensity stimulus is assigned a value of 0 dB, which means that there is no attenuation of the stimulus. A 10-dB stimulus is simply 10 dB (1 log-unit, or a factor of 10) less intense than the maximal intensity. A 20-dB stimulus is 2 log-units less intense than the maximum (i.e., 1/100 as intense), and a 30-dB stimulus is 1/1000 as intense as the maximum intensity stimulus.

In the Humphrey system, a 40-dB stimulus, which is 1/10,000 of the maximum, or 1 asb, is approximately the least intense stimulus that can be seen foveally by trained young observers. Thus, for practical purposes, the useful intensity range for white light testing is from 0 to 40 dB. The instrument is capable of presenting stimuli even less intense than 40 dB, but few humans are capable of seeing them.

A logarithmic scale (represented by decibels) is used because sensation relates to factors (e.g., a doubling of intensity) rather than addition of intensity; as a result, a change of a certain number of decibels has the same significance across the instrument's whole intensity range. Thus, a decrease of 1 dB always represents more or less a 25% increase in intensity; a 2-dB increase represents about a 60% increase; and a 3-dB increase always represents a 100% increase (doubling the intensity). The clinical importance of this can be illustrated by thinking about the presentation of a stimulus of 1 asb (40 dB). If this stimulus is not seen, then it might be reasonable to present the next stimulus at 2 asb (37 dB); a doubling of its intensity is represented by a 3-dB decrease. Apply this to a case in which the patient has failed to see a 1000-asb (10-dB) stimulus. Increasing the intensity by 1 asb to present a 1001-asb stimulus would make the stimulus only 0.1% more intense. This hardly affects visibility, but doubling the intensity—equivalent to increasing it from 1 asb to 2 asb—increases the stimulus to 2000 asb (or 7 dB, a 3-dB change from 10 dB). A 3-dB change always represents approximately a factor of two change in intensity, and from the point of view of visual field loss, a 3-dB decrease in measured threshold value always means that the eye has lost approximately half of its sensitivity.

In the clinical arena, there are four principles to remember:

1. The conversion from apostilbs to decibels is logarithmic, not a simple multiplication factor.
2. A decibel is 0.1 log-unit (deci = tenth)—no more, no less.
3. Apostilbs and candelas per square meter are absolute units of luminous intensity; thus a 316-asb intensity on one instrument is the same as a 316-asb intensity on another.
4. In contrast, log-units and decibels are relative units; they represent a certain attenuation from the maximum stimulus intensity on a particular instrument, and the maximum intensity is always 0 dB. For example, on the Goldmann perimeter the maximum stimulus is 1000 asb and a 5-dB attenuation results in 316 asb. On the Humphrey perimeter, with a 10,000-asb maximal luminous intensity (0dB), a 5-dB stimulus is a 5-dB attenuation of the

maximal stimulus, or 3160 asb (10 times as much light as the 5-dB attenuation of the maximum stimulus of the Goldmann perimeter). Thus a 15-dB stimulus on one instrument is not the same intensity as a 15-dB stimulus on another, but 15 dB does represent the same *percentage* reduction from maximum intensity in both instruments.

THRESHOLD SENSITIVITY IN TERMS OF STIMULUS INTENSITY

Every point within a patient's visual field has its own threshold of visual sensitivity. If the background intensity of a perimeter is fixed and a standard stimulus size used, the threshold is defined as the intensity that is visible just marginally. A stimulus cannot be seen if it is weaker (less intense) than the threshold stimulus—that is, if it is an infrathreshold (or subliminal*) stimulus. Also visible at each location are all test stimuli that are stronger (more intense) than the threshold stimulus. Such stimuli are suprathreshold (or supraliminal) stimuli.

Visual field testing—the topic of this book—involves exploring the differential light sensitivity throughout the field of vision, not simply making a determination of the extreme outside boundary of the visual field. The term "static threshold perimetry" refers to the process of estimating the threshold sensitivity by determining which in a series of stimulus intensities are suprathreshold and which are infrathreshold. The term "static suprathreshold testing" refers to the process of determining whether a stimulus that should be suprathreshold is in fact visible—a strategy commonly used as a screening test. Both types of testing differ from "kinetic threshold perimetry," in which a stimulus is moved from a region where it is not visible (infrathreshold) into a region where it is visible (suprathreshold). The boundary between regions of invisibility and visibility is the isopter, a line connecting all points at which the stimulus is a threshold stimulus.

> Visual field testing determines vision throughout the field, not just the outer boundary of vision.

When static threshold perimetry is performed at numerous locations, the results may be reported as threshold sensitivity values (in decibels) printed on a map of the visual field (Fig. 2-2, *bottom*). To aid in perceiving a diagnostic pattern at a glance, as a prelude to studying the numeric values in detail, a greyscale also is provided (Fig. 2-2, *top*). Each grey level represents a certain small range of threshold sensitivity values (e.g., 21 to 25 dB).†

Not all locations marked with a greyscale symbol are tested. Untested locations may be assigned presumed threshold values (calculated by interpolation from neighboring points that were tested) to shade in the greyscale plot and make the pattern of field loss easier to appreciate. The greyscale provides a quick impression of the individual's visual field and serves to show the configuration and depth of any regions with less visual sensitivity than others.

---

*More common in European usage; from the Latin word (limen, liminis) for connecting timber or support of a doorway (i.e., the threshold, or the limit).

†The boundary between the grey levels is equivalent to the isopter of kinetic perimetry. For example, consider the boundary between the grey level for 21 to 25 dB and the grey level for 26 to 30 dB. The boundary encloses all the points where the 26-dB stimulus is seen, and it can be thought of as the isopter for the 26-dB stimulus.

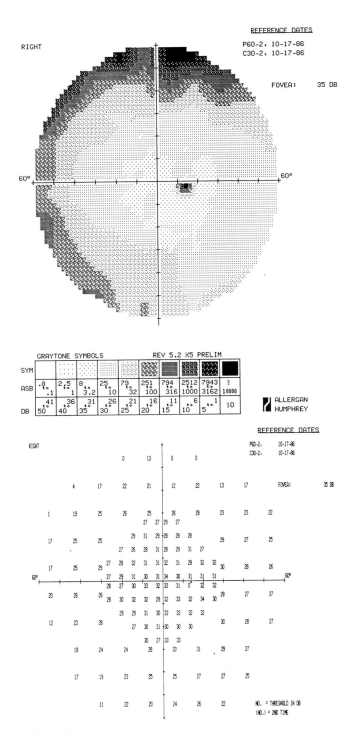

FIG. 2-2. Greyscale and Numeric Printouts of Automated Static Threshold Perimetry. This normal field of a right eye was tested to 60 degrees in a pattern of 144 points that was more closely spaced within the central 30 degrees. The lighter shades of grey indicate higher sensitivity, and the darker shades, less light sensitivity. The numeric values are in decibels of sensitivity at the test locations. The absolute edge of the visual field is reached superiorly and nasally, but temporally the field extends beyond the tested area. Visual sensitivity is best at the center and diminishes toward the edge. The upper field tends to be slightly less sensitive than the lower field, and the temporal periphery (30 to 60 degrees) is more sensitive than the nasal periphery.

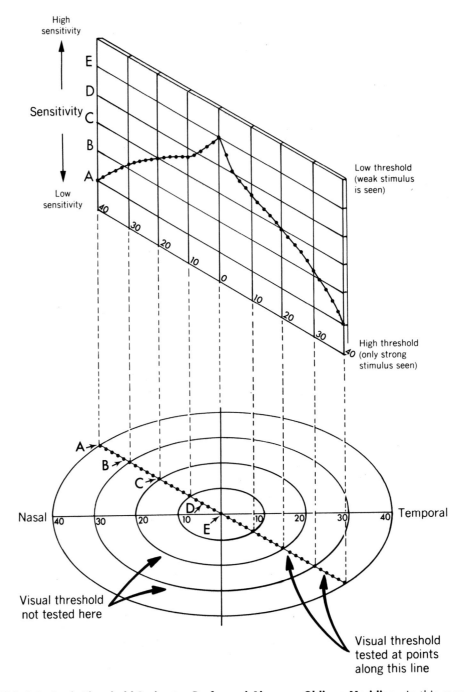

FIG. 2-3. Static Threshold Perimetry Performed Along an Oblique Meridian. In this case, perimetry is performed from the upper nasal quadrant, through the point of fixation, into the lower temporal quadrant. The points where threshold was tested are indicated on the field diagram, and the thresholds at some of these points are indicated by letters *A, B, C, D,* and *E.* The results are also indicated on the graph, which shows greatest sensitivity at the point of fixation. Although currently this "static cut" is rarely used in clinical practice, it illustrates the principle that visual sensitivity is greatest at the center.

Threshold intensity values are more meaningful when compared with the range of normal values. The percentile of deviation within the range of normal values may be shown symbolically in shades of grey (see Chapter 6). Such a representation is helpful because the range of normal values is smaller at some locations in the field than at others, and subtle abnormalities at such locations are highlighted. Conversely, larger deviations at locations with a wide normal range are appropriately de-emphasized.

FREQUENCY-OF-SEEING CURVE AND SHORT-TERM FLUCTUATIONS

As explained at the beginning of the chapter, the visibility of a stimulus depends on such features as its intensity, the background against which it is presented, its size, its color, whether it is moving, and the length of time it is presented. If a given defined stimulus is not visible, one of these factors can be adjusted until it becomes visible. In automated perimetry, luminous intensity is adjusted.

At the boundary between visibility and invisibility, the patient's responses often are uncertain or inconsistent, indicating that a borderline stimulus sometimes is seen and sometimes is not seen. When a stimulus intensity is within this region of uncertain visibility, its intensity can be adjusted slightly to a level at which the patient will respond 25% of the time. At a slightly greater intensity (e.g., 0.5 dB more intense), the patient may respond 50% of the time; at an intensity raised slightly more he may respond 75% of the time. A graph can be made of the percentage frequency that the stimulus is seen according to its intensity; this is called a frequency-of-seeing curve. If the visual responses are determined with such care, the threshold sensitivity is defined as the stimulus intensity at which the patient responds 50% of the time (Fig. 2-4).

> Frequency of seeing: probability of seeing stimuli over a range of intensities

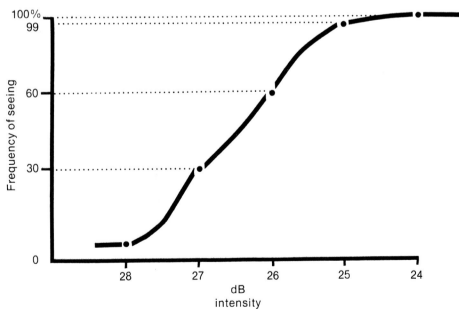

FIG. 2-4. Frequency-of-Seeing Curve. There is a range of stimulus intensities over which the stimulus is seen with varying frequency; this range represents a zone of "uncertainty."

Although such precise, time-consuming measurements of the frequency of seeing may be made in scientific psychophysical studies, clinical perimetry usually has other goals and constraints. Diagnostically, the geographic pattern of visual field loss is important, and threshold sensitivity determined within 2 to 4 dB of accuracy is sufficient for clinical decisions. Thus, clinical perimetry usually involves threshold estimates at many visual field locations, blanketing an area of interest rather than a precise measurement of just a few parts of the visual field, as might be determined in a laboratory environment.

In clinical perimetry, threshold sensitivity is estimated by presenting a series of stimulus intensities 2, 3, or 4 dB apart. Each stimulus intensity is presented only once or twice. The threshold sensitivity estimate is recorded as the weakest stimulus seen (Humphrey perimeter), or the average of the weakest stimulus seen and the strongest not seen (Octopus). The threshold sensitivity estimate that finally is recorded is subject to error because it depends on whether the patient happens to respond to any borderline stimulus that is presented (e.g., the steps of intensity may be 2 or 3 dB apart, not 0.5 dB). To determine threshold sensitivity more accurately, one may estimate the threshold many times with smaller intensity steps and calculate the average value.

| Short-Term Fluctuation: intratest variability |

If the threshold sensitivity is determined at the same point a second or third time, slightly different estimates of threshold intensity are obtained because of test-retest variability (Fig. 2-5). The standard deviation of these replicate threshold estimates is called the short-term fluctuation (SF). Because of the physiologic frequency-of-seeing curve, there always is some minimum short-term fluctuation. Several factors can increase this test-retest variability. First, locations with reduced sensitivity have a broader frequency-of-seeing curve and thus show increased measurement variability. Second, a patient may give frankly unreliable responses because of inattention or make inconsistent decisions about responding to dim stimuli that are barely visible. Third, fatigue may shift the patient's overall visual sensitivity over the course of a test session. The fatigue effect is more noticeable in abnormal regions of the visual field.

Test-retest variability may be affected throughout the visual field because of inattentiveness or inconsistency of patient responses. It may be affected only in certain regions that are abnormal and have a broader frequency-of-seeing curve. In hopes that it might be a useful clinical gauge of patient reliability, the presence of an abnormality, or both, a global index of the test-retest variability is calculated in some test strategies from duplicate threshold measurements and expressed as the SF index. By definition, the SF at a point is the standard deviation around the mean of replicate measurements. The global SF index represents the field as a whole, calculated as the square root of the average variance.

The global short-term fluctuation is estimated by measuring the threshold twice at a preselected sample of locations, typically 10. A standard deviation (SD) estimate is calculated from each duplicate measurement, and these SD estimates are pooled as the square root of the average variance estimate. This is the root

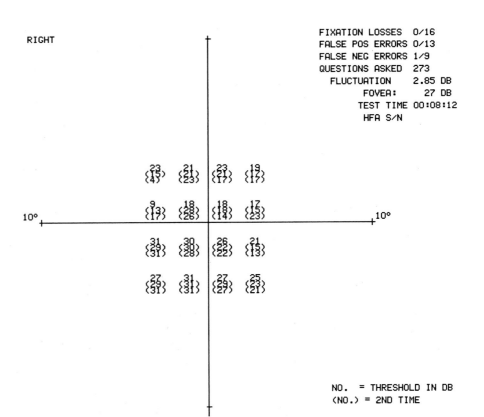

RIGHT

FIXATION LOSSES 0/16
FALSE POS ERRORS 0/13
FALSE NEG ERRORS 1/9
QUESTIONS ASKED 273
FLUCTUATION 2.85 DB
FOVEA: 27 DB
TEST TIME 00:08:12
HFA S/N

NO. = THRESHOLD IN DB
(NO.) = 2ND TIME

FIG. 2-5. Demonstration of Short-Term Fluctuation. In the original macula program of the Humphrey perimeter, a grid of 16 points 2 degrees apart is tested, with threshold sensitivity determined three times at each location. Sensitivity is expressed in decibels (dB). Note that test-retest variability is greater at points with low sensitivity than at points with high sensitivity.

mean square (RMS) of the SD estimates. The formula for the Octopus[4-6] simplifies to:

$$\sqrt{\frac{\sum_{j=1}^{n} (X_{j2} - X_{j1})^2}{2n}}$$

where X_{j1} and X_{j2} are the two threshold measurements at point j, and n is the number of points tested in duplicate (n equaled 10 in the standard Octopus Program 32 when it was introduced, but it can include all points in the Octopus G1 program). The SF index for the Humphrey perimeter is similar and is based on 10 duplicate measurements, but each value is weighted according to location (see Chapter 6).

Clinical use of the global short-term fluctuation index is limited by the accuracy with which it can be measured in a reasonable amount of time. In fact, in a reliable visual field test, the SF at a particular location may be more accurately estimated from the usual slope of the frequency-of-seeing curve at the determined threshold value than from duplicate measurements. Regardless, an estimate of the global SF index based on duplicate threshold measurements at only 10 locations is

19

less reliable than an estimate based on repeated testing of all points.[4] Moreover, test-retest variability is not the same at all locations of a visual field that has both normal and abnormal regions, and a single value cannot represent all of them. Clinical use of the SF index is discussed as it arises in context later in the book.

LONG-TERM FLUCTUATION

The clinician must understand both short-term fluctuation and long-term fluctuation, and the difference between them. The terminology is confusing, but the concepts are both simple and important.

Short-term fluctuation, as defined in the preceding section, represents the variability of threshold sensitivity measurements repeated at the same location in the same test session. Long-term fluctuation is the variability in threshold determination between two sessions, beyond the amount that can be attributed to measurement variability (short-term fluctuation) or to learning effects. Long-term fluctuation represents an actual change in threshold sensitivity.

The fact that long-term fluctuation occurs simply means that people see better on some days than on others, at least to a small degree, which perhaps is dependent on an individual's state of alertness or on biochemical changes that affect neural reactivity. Among the factors known to affect the physiologic state of visual sensitivity are exercise and certain drugs.[7-9] The existence of long-term fluctuation means that if sensitivity was measured at a location many times during a session to obtain an accurate average threshold value, and the procedure was repeated on another day, a different average result would be obtained, and the difference would be statistically significant. A homogeneous component within long-term fluctuation affects sensitivity equally at all locations. Added to this is a heterogeneous component, so that some locations are affected more than others.

Long-term fluctuation is not quantified in clinical perimetry, but its occurrence must be taken into consideration when interpreting a series of visual field examinations over time. Some degree of change in threshold sensitivity, when compared with a previous occasion (see Chapter 9), may result from this physiologic fluctuation in visual status, adding to measurement variation (short-term fluctuation).[10-22] These changes must be distinguished from changes caused by the progression of disease.

| Long-Term Fluctuation: genuine physiologic variation of vision |

SUBJECTIVE STIMULUS BRIGHTNESS

If a stimulus intensity is near the patient's threshold, it is perceived as quite dim—in fact, it is barely visible. When the stimulus is more intense, it appears brighter and is easier to see with certainty. If it is even more intense, it appears quite bright and even easier to see. The apparent degree of brightness of a suprathreshold stimulus is related to how much more intense it is than the threshold stimulus. There are two practical implications.

First, many patients report that most of the stimuli presented during threshold testing are quite dim. Watching for dim stimuli makes the test difficult. Feeling uncertain about whether some stimuli are real creates fear in patients that they have made mistakes. Invisible or nearly invisible stimuli cause concern that they are losing vision because they have more difficulty seeing the test stimuli.

Before the first test begins, therefore, all new patients should be instructed to expect to see only about half of the stimuli, and they should be told that the stimuli that they do see often will be quite dim. Patients should understand that whenever they see a stimulus, the computer is programmed to make the next stimulus dimmer, until the stimulus no longer can be seen. They should understand that it is natural to be unsure about the dim stimuli, and that the test result is not invalidated by an occasional erroneous response. Because the instrument is attempting to work at the limit of seeing, it also is natural that many stimuli will be too dim to see. *Failure to educate the patient about this issue before the first test experience can only add to the patient's apprehension, and may cause enough confusion to reduce the validity of the results. Some patients may be unwilling to submit to future follow-up testing simply because of such unnecessary anxiety.*

Second, the same stimulus will appear brighter and richer in normal regions of the visual field than in abnormal regions. This fact is used in comparison testing by confrontation (see Chapter 10). Thus a stimulus can appear less bright (and of different coloration) in a region where sensitivity is reduced because the intensity of the stimulus exceeds the threshold stimulus value by a lesser amount than it does in the normal portion of the visual field.

BACKGROUND INTENSITY

The intensity of a perimeter's background illumination affects visual threshold. Most significantly, it determines the state of the light- versus dark-adapted retina. The dark-adapted retina can perceive very weak stimuli, but the improvement in sensitivity with dark adaptation is not the same at every point on the retina. The hill of vision becomes flatter with dark adaptation, and the relative peak of sensitivity at the fovea is lost. Indeed, with profound dark adaptation, the fovea (packed with cones) does not gain as much sensitivity as the surrounding region (richer in rods), and in essence a physiologic relative central scotoma* is produced. (This scotopic central scotoma is what makes it easier to see very dim stars when eccentrically fixating on them versus looking directly at them.) However, in most clinical circumstances the visual field test is not performed under dark-adapted (scotopic) conditions, so this scotoma typically is not present.

The visibility of a stimulus is not simply a matter of its luminous intensity; it also is affected by its contrast with the background illumination. This is no more or less mysterious than the familiar observation that slide projectors work well in dark rooms and not so well in well-lit rooms. The image produced by the projector is of the exact same intensity, but it is seen more clearly when it is shown in contrast to a dark background.

---

*A scotoma is a region in which there is less sensitivity than in the surrounding region. A scotoma that includes the point of fixation is a central scotoma.

The contrast of an object under view (a stimulus) with its background is in fact the governing factor for visibility under strongly photopic conditions; however, the absolute intensity of the stimulus becomes progressively more important than its contrast to the background as retinal adaptation moves toward the mesopic and scotopic ranges. When threshold visibility strictly is a matter of contrast, the mathematical representation of threshold stimulus intensity is a constant if expressed as the contrast ratio (known as the Weber fraction) of the stimulus intensity to the background intensity (Weber's law).

There are theoretical advantages if perimetry is performed with a background sufficiently intense to have Weber's law operating. First, increasing or decreasing the pupil area has little effect on stimulus contrast because both background and stimulus are affected equally. Second, small changes in background intensity do not change the visibility of a stimulus if its intensity changes by an equal percentage. Goldmann took advantage of this principle to improve the reliability of his perimeter. It has only one light bulb, which supplies both the stimulus and the background lighting, and if the bulb varies in intensity (e.g., from variations in electric voltage), both the stimulus and the background intensities are affected equally; contrast, and thus stimulus visibility, stays more or less constant.

Given the strongest light source that was practical at the time, and wanting to preserve as large a range of strong stimuli as possible, Goldmann chose a standard background level—31.6 asb (10.1 cd/m^2)—that is just barely intense enough to place the test conditions into the region where Weber's law operates; this standard later was adopted for the Humphrey perimeter as well. At this intensity, most young eyes with large pupils and clear media operate under Weber's law, but older eyes with small pupils and hazy media may not. Some data suggest that 100 trolands* of retinal illumination (which occurs when a 25-asb background is viewed through clear media and a 4-mm pupillary diameter) may be enough to ensure photopic adaptation. Other data show that a 100-asb background may be necessary (especially if the pupil is smaller). The measured threshold value will be unaffected by a change in pupil size only if the retina is sufficiently light adapted at both pupil sizes.

At the light level used in clinical perimetry (31.6 asb), Weber's law may not always hold; as it begins to fail, the threshold stimulus intensity more closely relates to its ratio with the square root of the background intensity (Rose-de Vries law[23,24]) than to its direct ratio with the background intensity. This explains why a small pupil has some effect on retinal sensitivity under the conditions of clinical perimetry. In theory, the effect of pupil size should be less with the background of 31.6 asb (10.1 cd/m^2) used in the Humphrey and Goldmann perimeters than with lower levels of background illumination.

Because of the marginally photopic conditions of clinical perimetry, Weber's law cannot be used to calculate precisely the equivalence of stimuli presented on two perimeters with different background intensities. This is not the only limitation

---

*Troland refers to light reaching the retina through a 1-mm^2 pupillary area from a source that is 1 candela per square meter.

> Under photopic conditions, visibility depends on contrast (Weber's law).

encountered in the comparison of perimeters. A variation in color temperature of the illumination, for example, could in principle have slight effects, so to be rigorous, the relationship of stimuli of different makes and models of perimeters needs to be determined empirically.[25] However, conversion factors still may vary with pupil size, disease, and test conditions.

CONTRAST SENSITIVITY AND VEILING GLARE

Media opacity scatters light and reduces contrast of retinal image, and hence visibility, of perimetric stimuli.

Veiling glare is produced when the ocular media are not fully transparent and thus scatter some of the transmitted light. Such light scatter increases physiologically with age and is most noticeable in a developing cataract. It is not the contrast between the actual object and the actual background that determines the threshold visibility of something an individual is trying to see. Rather, it is the apparent contrast in the *retinal image* that determines whether the object is discernible. If light from more luminous objects in the field of vision is scattered out of its path toward the retina, the image of the object is less intense. At the same time, the deviated light is scattered across the whole field of view, to some degree increasing the background intensity ("veiling glare"). Darker regions in the scene under observation become more intense, whereas the more luminous regions fade. The contrast between any two locations in the field is reduced, which makes details more difficult to discern.

During perimetry, light scatter by the lens reduces the intensity of the image of the stimulus on the retina while increasing by a minuscule amount the background intensity. Of the various effects of cataract, this reduction in stimulus intensity by virtue of scattering light from the beam focused onto the retina[26,27] has more impact on making the perimetric stimulus difficult to see than does defocusing of the image (see following section) or absorption of light by lens pigments[28-30] (which removes light from both the stimulus and the background). Cataracts vary in severity, as well as in the proportion of absorption, blur, and scatter. Therefore, they have a range of differing effects on visual thresholds measured by perimetry in both normal and glaucomatous eyes.[30-34]

Scatter from cataract has more effect on perimetry than blur or light absorption.

In principle, it may one day be possible to determine quantitatively whether a progressive deterioration of the visual field is solely a result of a change in lens scattering properties or a combination of glaucomatous damage superimposed on changing lens clarity. For this determination, hypothetically, one might use an objective measurement of lens scatter[35] (except that front scatter and back scatter might be different[36]), a clinical test of veiling glare, or a statistical estimate derived from change at an undiseased region of the visual field.

REFRACTIVE ERROR AND RETINAL BLUR

The differential light sensitivity measured in clinical perimetry relates to the luminous intensity of a white spot with sharply focused edges compared with the luminous intensity of the background. It is a special case of the general phenomenon of contrast sensitivity, in which contrast detection depends on the space between lighter and darker regions (spatial frequency).

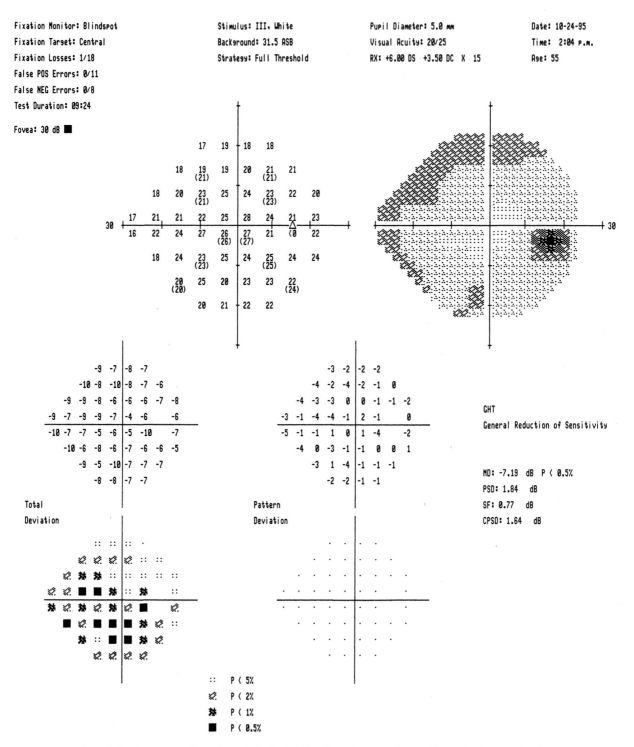

Fixation Monitor: Blindspot
Fixation Target: Central
Fixation Losses: 1/18
False POS Errors: 0/11
False NEG Errors: 0/8
Test Duration: 09:24

Fovea: 30 dB ■

Stimulus: III, White
Background: 31.5 ASB
Strategy: Full Threshold

Pupil Diameter: 5.0 mm
Visual Acuity: 20/25
RX: +6.00 DS +3.50 DC X 15

Date: 10-24-95
Time: 2:04 p.m.
Age: 55

```
              17   19 | 18   18
         18   19   19   20   21   21
             (21)           (21)
         18   20   23   25   24   23   22   20
                 (21)           (23)
      17   21   21   22   25   28   24   21   23
30 +  16   22   24   27   26   27   21  (0   22  + 30
                     (26) (27)         △
         18   24   23   25   24   25   24   24
                 (23)           (25)
              20   25   20   23   23   22
             (20)                   (24)
              20   21 | 22   22
```

GHT
General Reduction of Sensitivity

```
        -9  -7 |-8  -7                    -3  -2 |-2  -2
    -10 -8 -10|-8  -7  -6               -4  -2  -4 |-2  -1   0
  -9  -9  -8  -6 |-6  -6  -7  -8       -4  -3  -3   0 | 0  -1  -1  -2
 -9  -7  -9  -9 |-7  -4  -6      -6    -3  -1  -4  -4 |-1   2  -1       0
-10 -7  -7  -5  -6 |-5 -10      -7    -5  -1  -1   1 | 0   1  -4      -2
  -10 -6  -8  -6 |-7  -6  -6  -5       -4   0  -3  -1 |-1   0   0   1
     -9  -5 -10|-7  -7  -7                -3   1  -4 |-1  -1  -1
        -8  -8 |-7  -7                    -2  -2 |-1  -1
```

MD: -7.19 dB P < 0.5%
PSD: 1.84 dB
SF: 0.77 dB
CPSD: 1.64 dB

Total
Deviation

Pattern
Deviation

```
         ::  :: |::  ·              ·  ·  | ·  ·
      ⊠  ⊠  ⊠ |⊠  ::  ::          ·  ·  | ·  ·  ·
    ⊠  ⊠  ⊠ |::  ::  ::  ::      ·  ·  ·  | ·  ·  ·  ·
  ⊠  ⊠  ■  ■ |⊠  ::  ⊠      ::  ·  ·  ·  · | ·  ·  ·      ·
  ⊠  ⊠  ⊠  ⊠ |⊠  ⊠  ■      ⊠  ·  ·  ·  · | ·  ·  ·      ·
    ■  ⊠  ■  ■ |■  ⊠  ⊠  ::      ·  ·  ·  · | ·  ·  ·  ·
      ⊠  ::  ■ |■  ⊠  ⊠          ·  ·  · | ·  ·  ·
         ⊠  ⊠ |⊠  ⊠              ·  ·  | ·  ·
```

:: P < 5%
⊠ P < 2%
⊠ P < 1%
■ P < 0.5%

FIG. 2-6. Demonstration of the Effect of Refractive Blur. In this case, the patient was mistakenly tested with a +6.00-D sphere in place. The foveal threshold is depressed to an abnormal level, and the field is generally reduced in sensitivity by 5 to 6 dB, as reflected in the Total Deviation plots, the MD global index, and the Glaucoma Hemifield Test result. Compare with Figure 2-7.

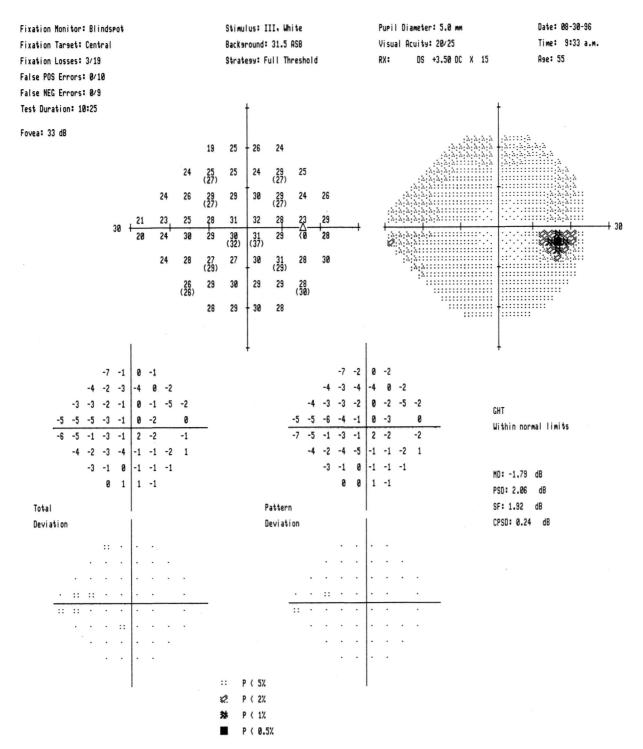

Fixation Monitor: Blindspot

Fixation Target: Central

Fixation Losses: 3/19

False POS Errors: 0/10

False NEG Errors: 0/9

Test Duration: 10:25

Fovea: 33 dB

Stimulus: III, White

Background: 31.5 ASB

Strategy: Full Threshold

Pupil Diameter: 5.0 mm

Visual Acuity: 20/25

RX: DS +3.50 DC X 15

Date: 08-30-96

Time: 9:33 a.m.

Age: 55

FIG. 2-7. Visual Field without the Inadvertent Use of a +6.00-D Spherical Correction (same patient as in Figure 2-6). The greyscale has a lighter shade, and the other parameters are normal.

When the retinal image is blurred, the edge of the stimulus is no longer sharp. In effect, the high spatial frequency components of the stimulus, represented by its sharp edges, are removed. Small stimuli, which have only high spatial frequencies, may become undetectable. Large stimuli with the same degree of blur may retain visibility because their low spatial frequency components are less affected by the blur. Thus, visibility of a size-III stimulus, 0.43 degree wide, does not demand as sharp a focus as the 1 minute of arc resolution required to see a 20/20 Snellen letter.

The visibility of a stimulus of any size is optimal when it is well focused on the retina. Blur spreads the available light energy over a larger retinal area, and although spatial summation effects (see following section on stimulus size and spatial summation) compensate somewhat, the general effect of increasing blur is to depress threshold sensitivity. When testing within the central 30 degrees, it is standard practice to fully correct the patient's refractive error and to include a presbyopic addition when needed. Outside of 30 degrees, refractive correction generally is not used for at least four reasons. First, the holder for the trial lens blocks peripheral vision and produces an area of artifactual loss in the test result. Second, standard trial lenses are too small to allow testing outside the central field. Third, blur is believed to have less of an effect in the periphery, perhaps because of greater spatial summation; thus, precise refractive correction is considered to be less important. Fourth, normative data are mostly nonexistent outside the central 30 degrees, making a meticulous testing approach less rewarding diagnostically. In the peripheral visual field, the topography of any loss is more interpretable than the exact threshold values.

Because there is a price to be paid for using corrective lenses, mostly in terms of the artifacts that the trial lens holder can induce even in central field tests, it is reasonable to ask how much blur can be tolerated before the use of trial lenses is necessary. Blur affects small stimuli much more than large ones, and this is among the reasons that most automated perimeters use the middle-sized Goldmann III stimulus. At least four papers have quantified blur effects on thresholds obtained using size-III stimuli in Octopus and Humphrey perimeters.[37-40] The reports are not in exact agreement, but it is safe to say that usually each diopter (D) of refractive blur will depress the entire hill of vision by a little more than 1 dB when using a size-III stimulus (Figs. 2-6 and 2-7). Thus, it is reasonable to ignore refractive errors of 1 D or less when using size-III or larger stimuli and simply to make note of the known amount of refractive blur. Note well: this recommendation applies to size-III stimuli; a size-I stimulus is another matter altogether and requires more meticulous refractive correction.

Visibility of size-III stimulus is reduced 1 dB for 1 diopter of blur. Size-I stimulus is more affected by refraction error.

STIMULUS SIZE AND SPATIAL SUMMATION

Consider two objects, one larger than the other. If the intensity of the larger object is reduced until it is just about as visible as the more intense smaller one, we have quantified part of the visibility relationship between size and intensity, known as the phenomenon of spatial summation. However, spatial summation works differently in different parts of the retina; if we shift our gaze so that the two objects are seen in a different part of the peripheral visual field, we probably will find that one object is seen more easily than the other.

Two equally visible stimuli are related by the formula

$$A^k \times I = C,$$

where A is the area of the stimulus, I is the luminous intensity, and C is a constant representing visual perception at that location. The value for the exponent k varies with retinal position from 0.55 to 0.9. In developing his perimeter, Goldmann wished to establish a fixed table roughly equating larger, less intense stimuli with smaller, more intense ones. Because it was impractical to have the table vary with retinal position, he chose a compromise k value of 0.8. With this k value, doubling the stimulus diameter has the same effect on visibility as increasing intensity by 0.5 log-unit (5 dB). It therefore made sense for Goldmann to build into his perimeter stimulus sizes that increased in diameter by factors of two, as shown in Table 2-1.

Goldmann knew that the shape of the stimuli in his perimeter varied from perfectly round to elliptical, depending on where in the field they were projected. Thus, the angular subtense values given in Table 2-1 are averages. The Humphrey and Octopus perimeters use Goldmann's stimulus sizes (appropriately corrected for the bowl radius to maintain the same angular size) and use either roman or arabic numerals 1 to 5 to designate the stimulus size.

In addition to varying with retinal position, the relationship between size and intensity also depends on the following: (1) there is increasing spatial summation with dark adaptation (which depends on background illumination); (2) differences exist among individuals; (3) the value of the exponent k varies slightly with the size of the stimulus; and (4) the equivalence in diseased visual regions may be different from that seen in normal retinal regions. This variability of the area-intensity relationship means that Goldmann's stated equivalence between two stimuli is only an approximation. For example, the III-2e (0.43 degree, 100 asb), II-3e (0.21 degree, 316 asb), and I-4e (0.11 degree, 1000 asb) stimuli of the Goldmann perimeter are indeed roughly equivalent but are not precise substitutes for one another under all conditions and in all retinal locations. When considering only the central 30-degree field of current automated perimetry, the increase from size III to size V corresponds in normal fields to less than the 10-dB intensity increase that would be predicted from the Goldmann formulation, which is an average estimate for normal points in the whole field (periphery included).[41]

Table 2-1. Goldmann's stimulus sizes

Size	Angular subtense (degrees)	Stimulus area on 30-cm bowl (mm²)
0	0.05	1/16
I	0.11	1/4
II	0.22	1
III	0.43	4
IV	0.86	16
V	1.72	64

TEMPORAL SUMMATION AND STIMULUS DURATION

By means of a phenomenon called temporal summation, the visual system integrates a light stimulus over time so that an initially unseen stimulus may become visible with time. Therefore, a brief static stimulus presented for 0.002 second is approximately twice as visible as one presented for 0.001 second. However, after a certain exposure time, temporal summation is complete, and if the stimulus has not become visible, it can be left on indefinitely without becoming visible. For example, if a stimulus is presented for 1 second and is not seen, it will not become visible regardless of how long it continues. Although the limits of temporal summation depend on several factors (e.g., background illumination, target size), it can be said roughly that the amount of temporal summation begins to decline after 0.06 second. Summation is largely complete by 0.1 second but under some conditions there may be additional summation to 0.5 or even 1 second. Automated perimeters take advantage of temporal summation to maximize their effective intensity ranges, and thus tend to use stimulus durations of about 0.1 (Octopus) or 0.2 second (Humphrey). With such exposure times, after which temporal summation essentially is complete, small variations in shutter duration have little effect. Use of a stimulation duration of 0.2 second or less tends to stabilize gaze because it does not allow enough response time for the patient to move his eyes to look at the stimulus after the patient believes it has been seen.

> Temporal summation is nearly complete in 0.1 second. Stimuli 0.2 second or shorter disappear before the patient can shift gaze.

LEARNING EFFECTS

Automated threshold perimetry demands a certain level of skill and attention from patients. Many patients with normal visual fields and some who already have field loss can produce reliable and stable perimetric test results during their first test. Most patients with glaucomatous visual field loss, however, must be allowed a practice testing session before they can produce reliable and stable results.[42-44]

Learning effects generally are smaller in the most central portion of the field than in more peripheral sections.[42-46] Fields with moderate loss are more likely to improve with experience than those with minimal or extensive loss; and highly disturbed points within the field tend to improve less than ones that are nearly normal.[42,47] Interestingly, perimetric testing skill appears to be somewhat specific to the particular task at hand; thus, improvements in Short-Wavelength Automated Perimetry (SWAP) perimetric performance (see chronic perimetry later in this chapter) occur as familiarity with the test increases, regardless of previous experience with standard white-on-white testing.[48]

In general, central threshold field tests produced by a patient in need of further training typically look nonspecifically depressed in the periphery but more or less consistent and in line with other clinical signs in the center. On a practical basis, it is unlikely that a reliable and normal-looking threshold visual field result could be produced accidentally. Thus, if a patient's first visual field test looks entirely normal and its reliability indices are within acceptable limits, the test probably can be accepted as valid. If the first test does not look both normal and reliable, then a confirmatory second test should be scheduled.

> After experience, threshold improves at normal points (especially near the edge), which highlights abnormal points, where threshold does not improve.

FATIGUE EFFECTS

Early automated threshold testing protocols frequently took as long as half an hour to complete for each eye. Test times were cut in half in the mid 1980s, and in half again in 1997.[49] Nevertheless, healthy young perimetric subjects frequently show at least some fatigue effects in their visual field results, and elderly patients—even when experienced—can find perimetry challenging and tiring.

Fatigue typically causes depression of threshold sensitivity, especially in the periphery of the central field,[50,51] and can produce results quite similar to those produced by learning effects. Lid artifacts and nonspecific depressions increasingly appear as the patient tires. Because it is especially evident at abnormal points in glaucomatous visual fields,[52,53] fatigue may be thought of as a stress test for glaucoma. Thus, longer protocols show deeper and larger glaucomatous visual field defects than shorter tests, but this apparent advantage is offset by increased artifacts, greater intersubject variability, and decreased patient compliance.

One remedy for fatigue effects is to tell patients that they may pause the test when they feel tired by holding down the patient response button. Alternatively, the perimetrist should enforce a short rest in those patients who clearly are tiring in the middle of a test. Third, the test time can be shortened by thresholding fewer points or by using shortened thresholding strategies, such as Fastpac or the newer Swedish Interactive Thresholding Algorithm (SITA).

The best way to manage fatigue is to consider the diagnostic needs and tailor the testing to the capabilities of each patient. Threshold testing protocols for patients with glaucoma are available on the Humphrey perimeter, ranging from 15 minutes (30-2 Full Threshold) down to 3 minutes (24-2 SITA Fast). Although there is some compromise in diagnostic information associated with use of a test with fewer test points or a less accurate thresholding strategy, using a shorter test is better than forcing patients to struggle through procedures that simply are too long for them. The authors find that the SITA Standard strategy with either the 30-2 or 24-2 protocol offers the best diagnostic performance for most patients, with SITA Fast being reserved for those needing an even shorter test (see Chapter 5).

> Of three ways to minimize fatigue artifact, the best is to tailor test selection.

KINETIC AND STATIC STIMULI

As the stimulus moves across the retina, a type of temporospatial summation occurs that makes kinetic stimuli somewhat more visible than static ones. This may be particularly striking in disease conditions, in which large, intense objects are not seen until they move (see Riddoch phenomenon, Chapter 3). However, if a stimulus is moved slowly enough in kinetic perimetry, the threshold intensities for kinetic and static stimuli are very similar.

CHROMATIC PERIMETRY

Some advantages may be realized by testing a subset of the visual system rather than the system as a whole. An advantage may be gained if one subset of ganglion cells is affected earlier or more severely than another subset, and a test is devised to recognize an abnormality of the preferentially affected portion of the visual apparatus. An advantage also may be derived simply from reducing the redundancy of responsiveness to the stimulus. To explain the latter, consider that a white stimulus stimulates three types of cones in addition to the rods. Consider a mosaic of ganglion cells that responds to red stimuli and another mosaic that responds to blue stimuli. If (arbitrarily) 10% of red ganglion cells are missing and 10% of blue ganglion cells also are missing, but the locations do not overlap, a white stimulus at any location is seen. However, if a red stimulus is used, it may detect a region where red ganglion cells are missing even though blue ganglion cells are present. Thus, there are theoretical advantages to stimuli that test an isolated subset of ganglion cells, even if all subpopulations of ganglion cells are affected equally by the disease, but at independently scattered locations. There may be no advantage if the disease has affected ganglion cell axons of all types in a bundle that serves a given retinal location.

Since the early days of perimetry, colored stimuli (particularly red stimuli) have been used empirically; but clinicians have debated whether colors are simply represented as dim stimuli or whether they permit the subject to take hue into account in addition to visibility, and whether stimulus detection or recognition of color is the more useful diagnostic endpoint. The last decade has seen a more focused approach, based on psychophysical principles, including the testing of the blue cones, or perhaps more accurately, the testing of the ganglion cells responding to blue stimuli in isolation, with possibly less redundancy of function, so that visual loss is detected at an earlier stage in the disease process.

The perimetric method currently being used in some clinics is blue-yellow perimetry, or Short-Wavelength Automated Perimetry (SWAP). SWAP evolved as an idea in the 1980s at the San Diego, Davis, and Berkeley campuses of the University of California.[54-65] The technique uses an intense yellow background and blue stimuli to isolate the blue cone system for testing. The green and red cone pigments are bleached by the intense yellow background, whereas the blue cones are much less affected. Thus, the sensitivities of the green and red systems are markedly reduced, whereas the blue system is left largely unaffected and thus fully sensitive to the test stimuli. The wavelength spectrum of the blue stimulus is also chosen to be near the peak response wavelength of blue cones. Although green cones also react to this wavelength, they are approximately 15 dB—1.5 log-units—less sensitive than the blue cones because of the intense yellow adapting background. This 15-dB sensitivity difference is called the *isolation* of the blue system from the green system and represents the amount of blue cone sensitivity loss that may be recorded before the green cones begin to contribute to the patient's response. Clinical application of this technique is discussed in Chapter 8.

It is useful to contemplate what the patient might perceive during SWAP testing. The blue cone system is considerably slower than that of the other cones, and it has a much lower visual acuity—about 20/200. As a result, SWAP stimuli are fuzzy and indistinct, and they often seem to appear and disappear sluggishly—as if drops of blue paint were falling onto the testing screen. The testing experience is quite different from what patients may be used to in standard testing, and therefore it is important to tell them about these differences and to demonstrate them, so that patients know what to expect.

The blue system's low visual acuity may have some unexpected benefits. First, uncorrected refractive error probably has less of an effect on the thresholds of a visual system that already is operating at the 20/200 level, especially because a size-V stimulus is standard. Second, refractive blur may well improve the isolation of the blue cones because the blur has a greater depressive effect on the response of the green cones than on the response of the blue system (Chris Johnson, Ph.D., personal communication, 1995).

SWAP testing is, perhaps, the most carefully evaluated new diagnostic method ever introduced in ophthalmology.[54-65] Nevertheless, many questions remain that only will be answered with broader clinical experience.

OTHER TYPES OF PERIMETRY

This book addresses standard light sense perimetry, in which white or colored stimuli are projected on a uniformly illuminated background. Light sense perimetry generally is accepted and used extensively throughout the world. Clinical standards have been developed for the administration and interpretation of tests, and therapeutic options have been laid out based on light sense findings.

Other visual functions also may be measured throughout the visual field, either to detect a preferentially affected type of visual function or to overcome redundancy of the systems that respond to the test stimuli. Such a redundancy of ganglion cell domains occurs not only with respect to color, but presumably in connection with many other characteristics of visual stimuli. Perimeters have been built that quantify peripheral visual response to flickering stimuli, acuity targets, small movements, varying gratings, and random motion. All these are legitimate measures of visual function, and any may turn out to be as useful as—or perhaps more useful than—the current clinical standard of light sense perimetry to white or colored stimuli. To date, however, none has been shown to be clearly superior to the current method, and thus, none has displaced it as the clinical standard. High-pass resolution ring targets[66] have been used in one commercial instrument, but the method has not been widely accepted and available. More recently, frequency doubling perimetry is undergoing evaluation.[67] This method is based on the frequency doubling illusion, in which large rapidly flickering gratings are presented in the peripheral vision. An illusion is seen in healthy parts of the retina in which twice as many bars are perceived as actually exist. In abnormal parts of the field, the illusion is present only if the bars are at higher-than-normal contrast levels. Frequency doubling perimetry is available in a portable table-top instrument, which may lead to easy acceptance for use in settings primarily devoted to disease detection. However, its potential usefulness in disease management is not yet determined.

REFERENCES
1. Phelps CD: Acuity perimetry and glaucoma, *Trans Am Ophthalmol Soc* 82:753-791, 1984.
2. Blondeau P, Phelps CD: Peripheral acuity in normal subjects, *Doc Ophthalmol Proc Ser* 42:511-520, 1985.

3. Phelps CD, Blondeau P, Carney B: Acuity perimetry: A sensitive test for the detection of glaucomatous optic nerve damage, *Doc Ophthalmol Proc Ser* 42:359-363, 1985.
4. Bebie H, Fankhauser F, Spahr J: Static perimetry: Accuracy and fluctuations, *Acta Ophthalmol* 54:339-348, 1976.
5. Flammer J, Drance SM, Augustiny L, Fankhauser A: Quantification of glaucomatous visual field defects with automated perimetry, *Invest Ophthalmol Vis Sci* 26:176-181, 1985.
6. Flammer J: The concept of visual field indices, *Graefes Arch Klin Exp Ophthalmol* 224:389-392, 1986.
7. Flammer J, Drance SM: Effect of acetazolamide on the differential threshold, *Arch Ophthalmol* 101:1378-1380, 1983.
8. Koskela PU, Airaksinen PJ, Tuulonen A: The effect of jogging on visual field indices, *Acta Ophthalmol* 68:91-93, 1990.
9. Wild JM, Betts TA, Ross K, Kenwood C: Influence of antihistamines on central visual field assessment. In Heijl A, editor: *Perimetry update: 1988/89 Proceedings of the VIIIth international perimetric society meeting, Vancouver, May 9-12, 1988, p 439.* Berkeley, 1989, Kugler Publications.
10. Bebie H, Fankhauser F, Spahr J: Static perimetry: Accuracy and fluctuations, *Acta Ophthalmol* 54:339-348, 1976.
11. Flammer J, Drance SM, Schulzer M: The estimation and testing of the components of long-term fluctuation of the differential light threshold, *Doc Ophthalmol Proc Ser* 35:383-389, 1983.
12. Flammer J, Drance SM, Zulauf M: Differential light threshold. Short- and long-term fluctuations in patients with glaucoma, normal controls, and patients with suspected glaucoma, *Arch Ophthalmol* 102:704-706, 1984.
13. Flammer J, Drance SM, Fankhauser F, Augustiny L: Differential light threshold in automated static perimetry. Factors influencing short-term fluctuation, *Arch Ophthalmol* 102:876-879, 1984.
14. Flammer J, Drance SM, Schulzer M: Covariates of the long-term fluctuation of the differential light threshold, *Arch Ophthalmol* 102:880-882, 1984.
15. Lewis RA, Johnson CA, Keltner JL, Labermeier PK: Variability of quantitative automated perimetry in normal observers, *Ophthalmology* 93:878-881, 1986.
16. Parrish RK, Schiffman J, Anderson DR: Static and kinetic visual field testing. Reproducibility in normal volunteers, *Arch Ophthalmol* 102:1497-1502, 1984.
17. Ross DF, Fishman GA, Gilbert LD, Anderson RJ: Variability of visual field measurements in normal subjects and patients with retinitis pigmentosa, *Arch Ophthalmol* 102:1004-1010, 1984.
18. Brenton RS, Argus WA: Fluctuations on the Humphrey and Octopus perimeters, *Invest Ophthalmol Vis Sci* 28:767-771, 1987.
19. Heijl A, Lindgren G, Olsson J: Normal variability of static perimetric threshold values across the central visual field, *Arch Ophthalmol* 105:1544-1549, 1987.
20. Flammer J: Fluctuations in the visual field. In Drance SM, Anderson DR, editors: *Automatic perimetry in glaucoma. A practical guide,* p 161, Orlando, 1985, Grune & Stratton.
21. Wilensky JT, Joondeph BC: Variation in visual field measurements with an automated perimeter, *Am J Ophthalmol* 97:328-331, 1984.
22. Katz J, Sommer A: A longitudinal study of the age-adjusted variability of automated visual fields, *Arch Ophthalmol* 105:1083-1086, 1987.
23. Fankhauser F: Problems related to the design of automatic perimeters. I. The optimal choice of experimental variables, *Doc Ophthalmol* 47:89-138, 1979.
24. Tate GW, Jr: The physiological basis for perimetry. In Drance SM, Anderson DR, editors. *Automated perimetry in glaucoma. A practical guide,* p 1, Orlando, 1985, Grune & Stratton.
25. Anderson DR, Feuer WJ, Alward WLM, Skuta GL: Threshold equivalence between perimeters, *Am J Ophthalmol* 107:493-505, 1989.
26. Heuer DK, Anderson DR, Knighton RW, et al: The influence of simulated light scattering on automated perimetric threshold measurements, *Arch Ophthalmol* 106:1247-1251, 1988.
27. Wood JM, Wild JM, Crews SJ: Induced intraocular light scatter and the sensitivity gradient of the normal visual field, *Graefes Arch Clin Exp Ophthalmol* 225:369-373, 1987.
28. Heuer DK, Anderson DR, Feuer WJ, Gressel MG: The influence of decreased retinal illumination on automatic perimetric threshold, *Am J Ophthalmol* 108:643-650, 1989.

29. Klewin KM, Radius RL: Background illumination and automated perimetry, *Arch Ophthalmol* 104:395-397, 1986.

30. Lam BL, Alward WL, Kolder HE. Effect of cataract on automated perimetry, *Ophthalmology* 98:1066-1070, 1991.

31. Budenz DL, Feuer WJ, Anderson DR: The effect of simulated cataract on the glaucomatous visual field, *Ophthalmology* 100:511-517, 1993.

32. Stewart WC, Rogers GM, Crinkley CMC, Carlson AN: Effect of cataract extraction on automated fields in chronic open-angle glaucoma, *Arch Ophthalmol* 113:875-879, 1995.

33. Smith SD, Katz, Quigley H: Effect of cataract extraction on the results of automated perimetry in glaucoma, *Arch Ophthalmol* 115:1515-1519, 1997.

34. Chen P, Budenz DL: Effect of cataract extraction on the glaucomatous visual field, *Am J Ophthalmol* 125:325-333, 1998.

35. Guthauser U, Flammer J: Quantifying visual field damage caused by cataract, *Am J Ophthalmol* 106:480-484, 1988.

36. Dengler-Harles M, Wild JM, Searle AET, Crews SJ: The relationship between backward and forward intraocular light scatter. In Mills RP, Heijl A: *Perimetry Update 1990/91, Proceedings of the IXth International Perimetric Society Meeting, 1990*, pp 577-582, Amsterdam/New York, 1990, Kugler Publications.

37. Goldstick BJ, Weinreb RN: The effect of refractive error on automated global analysis program G-1, *Am J Ophthalmol* 104:229-232, 1987.

38. Heuer DK, Anderson DR, Feuer WJ, Gressel MG: The influence of refraction accuracy on automated perimetric threshold measurements, *Ophthalmology* 94:1550-1553, 1987.

39. Weinreb RN, Perlman JP: The effect of refractive correction on automated perimetric thresholds, *Am J Ophthalmol* 101:706-709, 1986.

40. Herse PR: Factors influencing normal perimetric thresholds obtained using the Humphrey Field Analyzer, *Invest Ophthalmol Vis Sci* 33:611-617, 1992.

41. Choplin NT, Sherwood MB, Spaeth GL: The effect of stimulus size on the measured threshold values in automated perimetry, *Ophthalmology* 97:371-374, 1990.

42. Heijl A, Bengtsson B: The effect of perimetric experience in patients with glaucoma, *Arch Ophthalmol* 114:19-22, 1996.

43. Werner EB, Krupin T, Adelson A, Feitl ME: Effect of patient experience on the results of automated perimetry in glaucoma suspect patients, *Ophthalmology* 97:838, 1990.

44. Wild JM, Dengler-Harles M, Searle AE et al: The influence of the learning effect on automated perimetry in patients with suspected glaucoma, *Acta Ophthalmol* [Copenh] 67:537-545, 1989.

45. Heijl A, Lindgren G, Olsson J: The effect of perimetric experience in normal subjects, *Arch Ophthalmol* 107:81-86, 1989.

46. Wood JM, Wild JM, Hussey MK, Crews SJ: Serial examination of the normal visual field using Octopus automated projection perimetry. Evidence for a learning effect, *Acta Ophthalmol* [Copenh] 65:326-333, 1987.

47. Kulze JC, Stewart WC, Sutherland SE: Factors associated with a learning effect in glaucoma patients using automated perimetry, *Acta Ophthalmol* [Copenh] 68:681-686, 1990.

48. Wild JM, Moss ID: Baseline alterations in blue-on-yellow normal perimetric sensitivity, *Graefes Arch Clin Exp Ophthalmol* 234:141-149, 1996.

49. Bengtsson B, Olsson J, Heijl A, Rootzén H: A new generation of algorithms for computerized perimetry: SITA. *Acta Ophthalmol Scand* 75:368-375, 1997.

50. Hudson C, Wild JM, O'Neill EC: Fatigue effects during a single session of automated static threshold perimetry, *Invest Ophthalmol Vis Sci* 35:268-280, 1994.

51. Heijl A: Time changes of contrast thresholds during automatic perimetry, *Acta Ophthalmol* (KBH) 55:696-708, 1977.

52. Heijl A, Drance SM: Changes in differential threshold in patients with glaucoma during prolonged perimetry, *Br J Ophthalmol* 67:512-516, 1983.

53. Fujimoto N, Adachi-Usami E: Fatigue effect within 10 degrees visual field in automated perimetry, *Ann Ophthalmol* 25:142-144, 1993.

54. Johnson CA, Adams AJ, Casson EJ, Brandt JD: Blue-on-yellow perimetry can predict the development of glaucomatous field loss, *Arch Ophthalmol* 111:645-650, 1993.

55. Sample PA, Taylor JDN, Martinez GA et al: Short-wavelength color visual fields in glaucoma suspects at risk, *Am J Ophthalmol* 115:225-233, 1993.
56. Johnson CA, Adams AJ, Casson EJ, Brandt JD: Progression of early glaucomatous visual field loss as detected by blue-on-yellow and standard white-on-white perimetry, *Arch Ophthalmol* 111:651-656, 1993.
57. Sample PA, Weinreb RN: Progressive color visual field loss in glaucoma, *Invest Ophthalmol Vis Sci* 33:2068-2071, 1992.
58. Johnson CA, Brandt JD, Khong AM, Adams AJ: Short-wavelength automated perimetry in low-, medium-, and high-risk ocular hypertensive eyes, *Arch Ophthalmol* 113:70-76, 1995.
59. Keltner JL, Johnson CA: Short-wavelength automated perimetry in neuro-ophthalmologic disorders, *Arch Ophthalmol* 113:475-481, 1995.
60. Sample PA, Martinez GA, Weinreb RN: Short-wavelength automated perimetry without lens density testing, *Am J Ophthalmol* 18:632-641, 1994.
61. Wild JM, Moss ID, Whitaker D, O'Neill EC: The statistical interpretation of blue-on-yellow visual field loss. *Invest Ophthalmol Vis Sci* 36:1398-1410, 1995.
62. Heron G, Adams AJ, Husted R: Foveal and non-foveal measures of short wavelength sensitive pathways in glaucoma and ocular hypertension, *Ophthalmic Physiol Opt* 7:403-404, 1987.
63. Heron G, Adams AJ, Husted R: Central visual fields for short wavelength sensitive pathways in glaucoma and ocular hypertension, *Invest Ophthalmol Vis Sci* 29:64-72, 1988.
64. Sample PA, Weinreb RN, Boynton RM: Acquired dyschromatopsia in glaucoma, *Surv Ophthalmol* 31:54-64, 1986.
65. Hamill TR, Post RB, Johnson CA, Keltner JL: Correlation of color vision deficits and observable changes in the optic disc in a population of ocular hypertensives, *Arch Ophthalmol* 102:1637-1639, 1984.
66. Frisen L: High-pass resolution targets in peripheral vision, *Ophthalmology* 94:1104-1108, 1987.
67. Johnson CA, Samuel SJ: Screening for glaucomatous visual field loss with frequency-doubling perimetry, *Invest Ophthalmol Vis Sci* 38:413-425, 1997.

ADDITIONAL READING

Aulhorn E, Harms H: Early visual field defects in glaucoma. In Leydhecker W, editor: *Glaucoma: Tutzing symposium,* Basel, 1967, S Karger, pp 151-186. (Lucid presentation of the underlying considerations in perimetry, with glaucoma as the example.)

Aulhorn E, Harms H: Visual perimetry. In Jameson D, Hurvich LM, editors: *Visual psychophysics: Handbook of sensory physiology,* vol 7, no 4, New York, 1972, Springer-Verlag, pp 102-145. (Authoritative encyclopedia of information about the psychophysical basis of perimetry.)

Bebie H, Fankhauser F, Spahr J: Static perimetry: Strategies, *Acta Ophthalmol* [Copenh] 54:325-338, 1976. (The beginnings of Octopus perimetry.)

Fankhauser F: Problems related to the design of automatic perimeters, *Doc Ophthalmol* 47:89-139, 1979.

Fankhauser F, Jenni A: Programs SARGON and DELTA: Two new principles for automated analysis of the visual field, *Graefes Arch Klin Exp Ophthalmol* 216:41-48, 1981.

Fankhauser F, Koch P, Roulier A: On automation of perimetry, *Graefes Archiv Klin Exp Ophthalmol* 184:126-150, 1972. (Concepts that evolved into Octopus perimetry.)

Fankhauser F, Spahr J, Bebie H: Some aspects of the automation of perimetry, *Surv Ophthalmol* 22:131-141, 1977.

Greve EL: Single and multiple stimulus static perimetry in glaucoma: The two phases of perimetry, *Doc Ophthalmol* 36:21-355, 1973. (A major thesis on many details of modern perimetry.)

Haberlin H, Jenni A, Fankhauser F et al: Researches on adaptive high resolution programming for automatic perimeter: Principles and preliminary results, *Int Ophthalmol* 2:1-9, 1980.

Heijl A: Computer test logics for automatic perimetry, *Acta Ophthalmol* 55:837-853, 1977.

Heijl A, Krakau CET: An automatic static perimeter, design and pilot study, *Acta Ophthalmol* 53:293-310, 1975.

Johnson C, Keltner JL: Principles and techniques of the examination of the visual sensory system. In Miller NR, Newman NJ: *Walsh and Hoyt's clinical neuro-ophthalmology, p 153, vol 1,* Baltimore, 1998, Williams & Wilkins.

National Research Council, Committee on Vision, Assembly of Behavioral and Social Sciences: First interprofessional standard for visual field testing: Report of Working Group 39. *Adv Ophthalmol* 40:173-224, 1980. (Detailed discussion of variables that influence clinical visual field testing and their standardization.)

Tate GW, Jr: The physiological basis for perimetry. In Drance SM, Anderson DR, editors: *Automatic perimetry in glaucoma. A practical guide,* p 1, Orlando, 1985, Grune & Stratton. (A recent review with extensive list of original references.)

Tate GW Jr, Lynn JR: *Principles of quantitative perimetry: testing and interpreting the visual field,* New York, 1977, Grune & Stratton. (This general clinical visual field textbook concentrates on the physiology and psychophysics underlying visual field testing, and the technique of performing visual fields.)

CHAPTER 3

Topographic classification of visual field defects

ANATOMIC BASIS

All field defects can be classified as prechiasmal, chiasmal, or postchiasmal depending on the anatomic location of the disease that produced the visual abnormality. Therefore mapping the pattern of visual loss enables a topographical diagnosis.

Approximately one half of the nerve fibers from each eye cross at the optic chiasm to the opposite side of the brain in such a manner that impulses derived from objects to the right side of the field of vision are received by the left visual cortex and objects to the left are received by the right visual cortex. Thus a stimulus in the right (temporal) visual field of the right eye is seen by the nasal retina of the right eye, and nerves carrying these impulses cross at the chiasm to the left side of the brain. However, objects to the left of fixation seen by the right eye in its nasal visual field stimulate points in the temporal retina of the right eye, and nerves carrying these impulses from the temporal retina (Fig. 3-1) do not cross the chiasm but remain on the right side of the brain. The point dividing the nasal and temporal halves of the retina is the fovea (represented by fixation), not the optic nerve head (represented by the physiologic blind spot).

In this chapter the characteristics of field defects are discussed in relation to the location of the lesion in the visual pathway. The greyscale representation of quantitative threshold perimetry is presented to illustrate the character of these field defects. The darker shades of grey indicate regions with less light sensitivity.

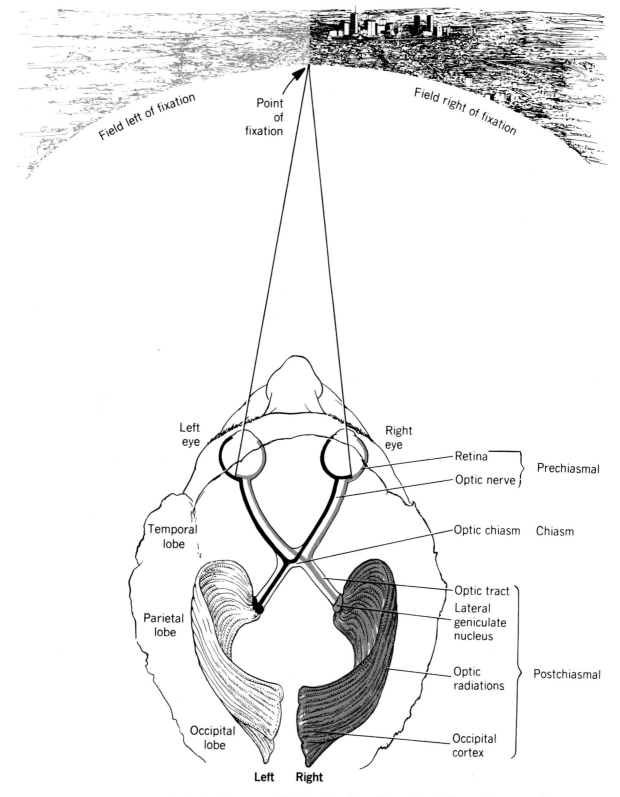

FIG. 3-1. Anatomic Basis of Topographic Classification. The optics of the eye (cornea and lens; see Fig. 1-1) focus an image on the retina. The retina converts the light to nervous impulses that are processed and conducted ultimately to the occipital (or visual) cortex.

PRECHIASMAL DEFECTS

Prechiasmal lesions include preretinal abnormalities in the refractive properties and clarity of the ocular media (cornea, lens, and vitreous), as well as diseases affecting the retina and optic nerve. Glaucoma, a disease characterized by intraocular pressure damaging the optic nerve, is one example of a prechiasmal lesion.

Prechiasmal lesions produce visual field defects with the following characteristics:

1. The defect may occur in one eye only, but often the disease affects both retinas or optic nerves, in which case both eyes will have visual field defects. If there is a visual field defect in one eye only, and the other eye has no defect at all, the lesion must be prechiasmal. **If there is no preretinal or retinal lesion (almost any of which would be evident during examination of the eye), an optic nerve lesion must cause the uniocular field defect.**

> Uniocular field defects are prechiasmal.

2. The defect may or may not extend uninterrupted across the vertical meridian. The diagnostic importance of this fact is that a defect resulting from a postchiasmal lesion does *not* cross the vertical meridian. Therefore **if a defect crosses the vertical midline uninterrupted, the lesion is not postchiasmal, but must be prechiasmal (or combined chiasmal and prechiasmal).**

3. If a defect in the nasal visual field results from a lesion of the optic nerve (or the retinal nerve fiber layer), it may end abruptly with a straight horizontal border nasal to fixation (i.e., a nasal step or a scotoma with a flat horizontal edge). However, if it results from a lesion in the temporal retina or choroid, it may extend across the horizontal meridian uninterrupted. **If a defect has a sharp horizontal border nasally, it undoubtedly is the result of a prechiasmal lesion.** If it does not have a horizontal nasal border, it may or may not be caused by a prechiasmal lesion.

4. Although they share the typical features mentioned, a variety of scotomas and depressions are produced by prechiasmal lesions.

5. A prechiasmal visual field defect may be associated with any of the following:
   a. Reduced visual acuity (e.g., either a generalized depression resulting from media opacities or a central scotoma resulting from macular or optic nerve disease);
   b. Abnormal pupil reaction (afferent pupillary defect), which also may occur with lesions of the optic chiasm and tract; in bilateral prechiasmal lesions, there may be a relative afferent pupillary defect if the involvement of the two eyes is unequal, as in unequal glaucoma;
   c. Abnormality evident by ophthalmoscopy: retinal lesion, optic disc lesion, or optic atrophy;
   d. Abnormal color vision.

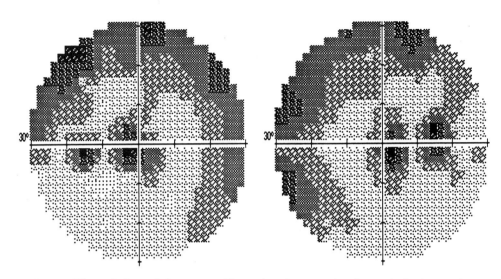

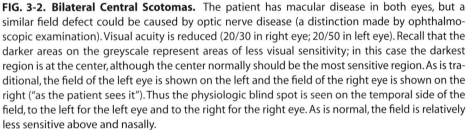

FIG. 3-2. Bilateral Central Scotomas. The patient has macular disease in both eyes, but a similar field defect could be caused by optic nerve disease (a distinction made by ophthalmoscopic examination). Visual acuity is reduced (20/30 in right eye; 20/50 in left eye). Recall that the darker areas on the greyscale represent areas of less visual sensitivity; in this case the darkest region is at the center, although the center normally should be the most sensitive region. As is traditional, the field of the left eye is shown on the left and the field of the right eye is shown on the right ("as the patient sees it"). Thus the physiologic blind spot is seen on the temporal side of the field, to the left for the left eye and to the right for the right eye. As is normal, the field is relatively less sensitive above and nasally.

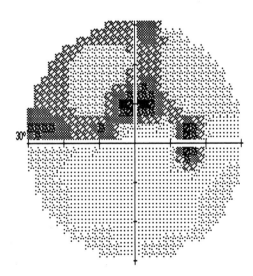

FIG. 3-3. Nerve Fiber Bundle Defect (Glaucoma). The right eye has an arcuate defect that crosses the vertical midline uninterrupted but ends abruptly at the nasal horizontal meridian. Glaucoma is a common cause of nerve fiber bundle defects (see Chapter 4), but giant drusen of the optic nerve (pseudopapilledema), anterior ischemic optic neuropathy, and branch retinal vessel occlusions are among other causes of field defects with these features.

Some features of prechiasmal field defects are affected by the location of the lesion:
1. Preretinal optical media
2. Outer retina and choroid
3. Inner retina and optic nerve

The prechiasmal causes of field defects can be conveniently subdivided into three "territories":

1. **Preretinal factors** (see Chapter 1). Abnormalities in the optical pathways may defocus the image, scatter the light, or block the light. The result is a generalized visual depression, often with flattening of the slope of the hill of vision. Infrequently, a localized opacity in the media may produce a shadow on the retina, resulting in a localized reduction of visual sensitivity.

2. **Lesions of the outer retina and choroid.** Lesions in these areas can produce a variety of defects that may not have any specific or characteristic features. These defects do not respect the vertical or nasal horizontal meridians but correspond to the portions of the retina involved.

3. **The retinal nerve fiber layer and optic nerve.** Typical field defects include central or centrocecal scotomas, paracentral or arcuate defects in the Bjerrum region (as if emanating from the blind spot), scotomas or localized depressions that respect the nasal horizontal meridian, and wedge-shaped defects with the apex pointed at the blind spot (not hemianopic wedges with the apex pointed at fixation).

CHIASMAL DEFECTS

Lesions affecting the chiasm—for example, pituitary adenomas and other tumors—produce visual field defects in the temporal fields of both eyes (bitemporal hemianopia*). The field defect ends abruptly at the vertical meridian if only the chiasm is affected. Often, one or both optic nerves are affected by the same tumor that presses on the chiasm, in which case characteristics of a prechiasmal (optic nerve) lesion may be present in addition to the temporal hemianopia.

With chiasmal lesions the visual acuity is normal unless the optic nerve also is involved.

---

*Hemianopia is defective vision within half of the visual field. Temporal hemianopia is defective vision confined to the temporal half of the field. Bitemporal hemianopia is temporal hemianopia in both eyes.

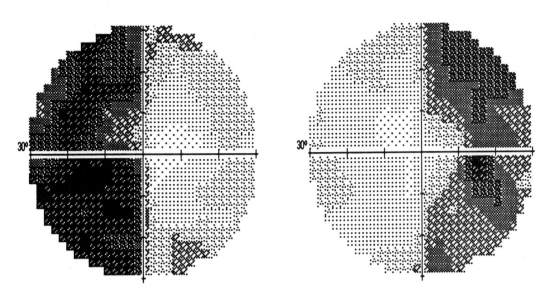

FIG. 3-4. Bitemporal Hemianopia. The defective vision is in the temporal field of each eye, ending abruptly at the vertical meridian. As is usually the case, it is not of the same severity in both eyes. Typically the superior field is more affected than the inferior field, although not in this case.

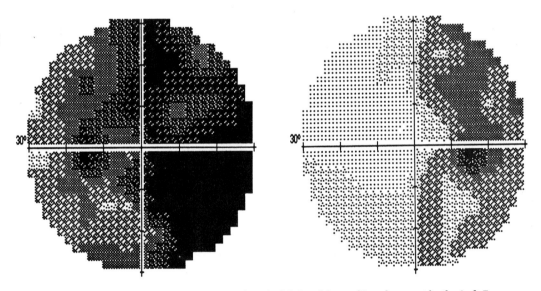

FIG. 3-5. Bitemporal Hemianopia Associated with Prechiasmal Involvement in the Left Eye. The right eye has a temporal hemianopia with 20/15 visual acuity. The field defect in the left eye crosses the vertical midline, with the acuity reduced to 20/50. Such a combination of findings, producing a "junctional scotoma," would be caused by a tumor compressing both the chiasm and the left optic nerve at their junction.

POSTCHIASMAL DEFECTS

> Postchiasmal lesions affect the right half or the left half of the field in both eyes.

Lesions affecting the postchiasmal visual pathway produce visual field defects in both eyes, but the two eyes may not be affected equally. The field defects are limited to half the field (hemianopia) and end abruptly at the vertical midline (the vertical meridian may be slanted if the head is tilted slightly during field testing).

The hemianopic defects are homonymous. In homonymous hemianopia, the defects of the two eyes are both to the right or both to the left. Therefore the defect is nasal in one eye and temporal in the other.

When the lesion is in the occipital cortex (usually vascular), the defects tend to be identical (congruous); however, lesions in most other locations (e.g., optic tract or temporal lobe), which usually are tumors, typically produce incongruous defects. Lesions affecting the optic radiations usually produce semicongruous defects, that is, congruity increases with more posterior location. Inferior fibers serving the upper field loop forward into the temporal lobe so that the temporal lobe lesions typically produce a superior "pie-in-the-sky"-shaped defect. Parietal lobe lesions tend to produce defects that are denser in the inferior field. When a hemianopia spreads and deepens to complete visual loss in one hemifield, it no longer can be determined whether the defect was congruous or incongruous as it evolved. It is misleading to think of a complete hemianopia as either congruous or incongruous.

Associated findings are sometimes important to a diagnosis when there is homonymous hemianopia:

1. With postchiasmal lesions, the visual acuity is unaffected, except when optic tract lesions are accompanied by chiasmal or optic nerve damage or when there is postchiasmal involvement on both sides (bilateral occipital lobe infarction).

2. Pupillary reactions usually are normal (unlike the partial or total afferent pupillary defect with prechiasmal lesions), except that there may be a hemianopic pupil with a reduced reaction to light on the involved side of the visual field with optic tract lesions. This occurs only with optic tract lesions and not with lesions behind the lateral geniculate body.

3. Results of ophthalmoscopy typically are normal, with two exceptions: (1) there may be papilledema associated with a brain tumor and (2) in the rare instance in which the hemianopia is caused by an optic tract or lateral geniculate body lesion, the optic disc is pale and in a "bow tie"-shaped region in the eye on the opposite side of the lesion, whereas the disc of the eye on the same side shows temporal pallor.

4. Opticokinetic nystagmus may be abnormal toward the involved side with postchiasmal lesions, specifically those of the parietal lobe.

5. Associated neurologic abnormalities, including the inability to perform well on visual field testing, reflect the position of the brain affected and are expected, except with occipital lobe lesions. Typically with temporal lobe or parietal lobe lesions, it is the neurologic symptom rather than the visual symptom that causes the patient to seek medical attention.

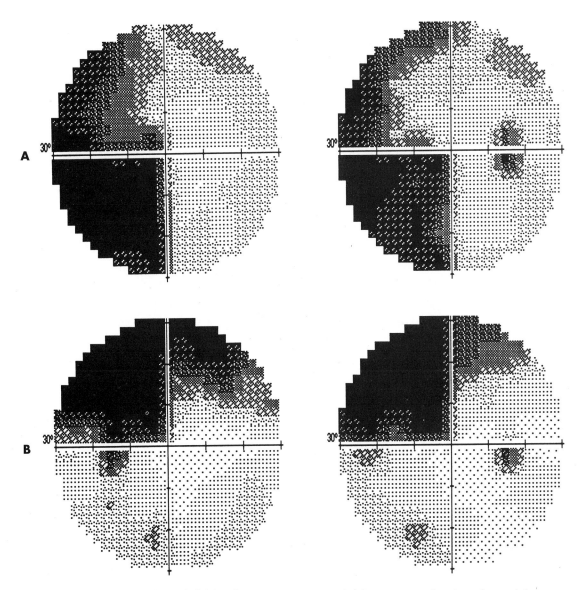

FIG. 3-6. Postchiasmal Field Defects. A, Incongruous left homonymous hemianopia, as might be produced by a tumor of the right parietal lobe. The defect ends abruptly at the vertical midline (making it a hemianopia), the left half of the field is affected in both eyes (making it homony-mous), and the defect is not of equal extent and severity in both eyes (making it incongruous). Lesions of the temporal lobe tend to produce similar wedge-shaped ("pie-in-the-sky") defects, ending at the vertical midline in the upper field. **B,** Congruous homonymous hemianopia, typical of occipital lobe lesions, often the result of vascular occlusion.

STATO-KINETIC DISSOCIATION (RIDDOCH PHENOMENON)

With a hemianopic field defect, a test stimulus may be visible if it is moving but may not be visible while stationary, as if there were a much greater abnormality of visual threshold with static stimuli than with kinetic stimuli. Thus the defect may be represented much more extensively in the printout of static threshold perimetry than is evident in kinetic perimetry, if both have been performed. This marked difference in visibility between moving and nonmoving stimuli within an abnormal region of the visual field is known as the Riddoch phenomenon, after the British neurologist George Riddoch (1888-1947). Although most typical of occipital lobe lesions, the phenomenon is demonstrable in defects caused by lesions throughout the sensory visual system.

Accurate representation of the stato-kinetic dissociation requires that the same stimuli be compared. For example, the kinetic I2e, I4e, and III4e isopters of the Goldmann perimeter might be compared on the Humphrey Field Analyzer by single intensity suprathreshold screening with a 20-dB size-I, 10-dB size-I, and 10-dB size-III stimulus, respectively. Currently, this phenomenon typically is recognized during confrontation field testing or with the use of a tangent screen.

ADDITIONAL READING

For those seeking more details on the topographic approach to visual field diagnosis, especially as relevant to neurologic conditions, considerable information can be found in the following books. The emphasis is on defining the typical field defect of various conditions, and inversely, the lesions that cause particular types of defects.

Budenz DL, Siatkowski RM: Nonglaucomatous optic nerve disorders, chiasmal visual field loss, and retrochiasmal visual field loss. In Budenz DL: *Atlas of Visual Fields,* p 195, Philadelphia, 1997, Lippincott-Raven Publishers.

Burde RM, Savino PJ, Trobe JD: *Clinical decisions in neuro-ophthalmology,* p 1, St. Louis, 1985, Mosby-Year Book.

Duane TD, editor: *Clinical ophthalmology,* vol 2, New York, 1976, Harper & Row.

Glaser JS, editor: *Neuro-ophthalmology,* ed 2, Philadelphia, 1990, JB Lippincott.

Harrington DO, Drake MV: *The visual fields: A textbook and atlas of clinical perimetry,* ed 6, St. Louis, 1990, Mosby-Year Book.

Johnson C, Keltner JL: Principles and techniques of the examination of the visual sensory system. In Miller NR, Newman NJ: *Walsh and Hoyt's clinical neuro-ophthalmology, p 153,* Baltimore, 1998, Williams & Wilkins.

Mills RP: Diseases of the optic nerve, optic chiasm, and the retrochiasmal visual pathways. In Werner EB: *Manual of visual fields, p 157,* New York, 1991, Churchill Livingstone.

Scott G: *Traquair's clinical perimetry,* ed 7, London, 1957, Henry Kimpton.

Traquair HM: *An introduction to clinical perimetry,* ed 6, St. Louis, 1949, Mosby-Year Book.

Wirtschafter JD: Anatomic basis and differential diagnosis of field defects. In Walsh TJ, editor: *Visual fields. Examination and interpretation,* p 39, ed 2, Ophthalmology monographs 3, San Francisco, 1996, American Academy of Ophthalmology.

CHAPTER 4

Visual field loss in glaucoma

Glaucoma is an example of a prechiasmal cause of visual field loss. It is the most common reason for performing a visual field test in most clinical practices and thus is the subject of this separate chapter.

LOCAL AND DIFFUSE LOSS

In glaucoma, axons (nerve fibers) of the optic nerve are damaged, and visual function is diminished or lost in the retinal area served by the damaged axons. The most recognizable type of damage begins as localized injury to one or more bundles of axons that serve particular regions of the retina. In such cases, visual sensitivity may at first be reduced only in some locations, proceeding to dense visual loss in some regions with retention of normal sensitivity in others (Fig. 4-1). Eventually, in the full course of progressive disease, all regions of the visual field become involved (Fig. 4-2). Later the eye ultimately proceeds to lose all vision.

The rate at which most or all of the visual field becomes affected is variable. At times, the initially affected region loses all visual sensation so that no perimetric stimulus is visible, while other regions remain entirely normal, at least for the moment. In other cases, nearly all regions of the visual field are affected to some degree, while the initially involved region remains only mildly or moderately defective. The manner in which such diffuse involvement of the visual field can be manifest in glaucoma has been described by a number of observers.[1-13] Very rarely, glaucoma diffusely affects all regions of the field to an exactly equal degree in the earliest stage, but the disease does not progress very far before affecting some regions noticeably more than others. Examples of all these variations are shown at the end of this chapter.

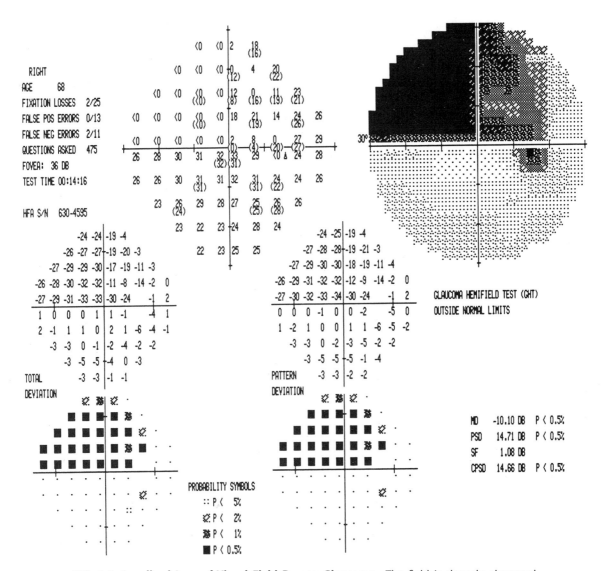

FIG. 4-1. Localized Loss of Visual Field Due to Glaucoma. The field is densely abnormal above fixation and on the nasal side, but most locations have normal sensitivity (right eye).

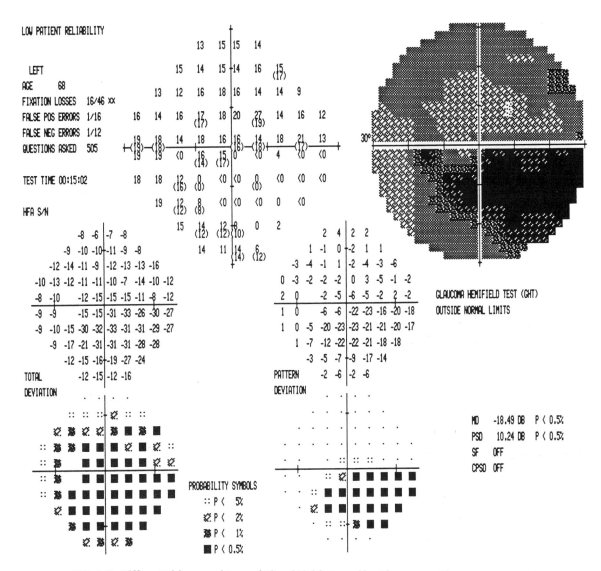

LOW PATIENT RELIABILITY

LEFT

AGE   68
FIXATION LOSSES   16/46 xx
FALSE POS ERRORS 1/16
FALSE NEG ERRORS 1/12
QUESTIONS ASKED   505

TEST TIME 00:15:02

HFA S/N

```
                13  15 | 15  14
            15  14  15 +14  16  (15)
                                (17)
        13  12  16  18  16  14  14   9
    16  14  16  17  18  20  27  14  16  12
               (17)        (19)
 19   18  14  18  16  16  14  18  21  13
(19) (18)          (16) (18)    (17)
 19   19     <0  16  15  <0   4  <0  <0
               (14)(17)
    18  18  12   8  <0  <0   8  <0  <0  <0
           (16) (0)        (0)
        19  12   8  <0  <0  <0   0  <0
           (12) (8)
        15  14  12  8   0   2
           (12)(12)(10)
            14  11  14   6
               (14) (12)
```

```
    -8  -6 |-7  -8                         2   4  2  2
  -9 -10 -10|-11 -9 -8                   1  -1  0 -2  1  1
-12 -14 -11 -9 |-12 -13 -13 -16       -3 -4 -1  1 -2 -4 -3 -6
-10 -13 -12 -11 -11|-10 -7 -14 -10 -12  0 -3 -2 -2 -2  0  3 -5 -1 -2
 -8 -10    -12 -15|-15 -15 -11 -8 -12   2  0    -2 -5 -6 -5 -2  2 -2
 -9  -9    -15 -15|-31 -33 -26 -30 -27  1  0    -6 -6 -22 -23 -16 -20 -18
 -9 -10 -15 -30 -32|-33 -31 -31 -29 -27 1  0 -5 -20 -23 -23 -21 -21 -20 -17
    -9 -17 -21 -31|-31 -31 -28 -28       1 -7 -12 -22 -22 -21 -18 -18
    -12 -15 -16|-19 -27 -24              -3 -5 -7 -9 -17 -14

TOTAL    -12 -15|-12 -16          PATTERN   -2 -6|-2 -6
DEVIATION                         DEVIATION
```

GLAUCOMA HEMIFIELD TEST (GHT)

OUTSIDE NORMAL LIMITS

MD   -18.49 DB   P < 0.5%
PSD   10.24 DB   P < 0.5%
SF   OFF
CPSD   OFF

PROBABILITY SYMBOLS

:: P < 5%
⚹ P < 2%
▨ P < 1%
■ P < 0.5%

FIG. 4-2. Diffuse, Widespread Loss of Visual Field Caused by Glaucoma. There are no normal locations, but the lower nasal and inferior arcuate regions are much more densely abnormal (left eye).

Detectable localized field defects probably are associated with loss of fewer ganglion cells than is detectable generalized loss.

The localized nature of typical glaucomatous visual field loss and the rarity of uniform diffuse involvement have important diagnostic consequences. First, detection of mild localized disease is possible for two reasons:

1. Threshold sensitivity values at various locations are compared not only to a range of normal values, but also to the threshold sensitivities of their neighbors and those at other locations in the field. Mild but *unequal* deviation of threshold sensitivity values is recognized as abnormal with more certainty than is simple, fairly equal deviation from normal values.

2. The broader the defective region, the larger the total number of optic nerve axons that must be damaged for the thresholds to be recognizably depressed. Very localized damage may be recognized when only a small percentage of the nerve fibers are destroyed. For example, a bundle of axons may be destroyed completely and produce an unmistakable dense scotoma at a small group of points but still represent loss of less than 5% of the total number of axons in the optic nerve.

Second, the pattern of localized loss helps reduce the diagnostic possibilities that must be considered. Arcuate scotomas and nasal steps, for example, are characteristic features of glaucoma. These patterns of field loss, typical of anterior prechiasmal disease, are mimicked by other, less common causes of nerve fiber bundle defects. However, they differ from hemianopia, which is characteristic of more posterior parts of the visual pathway, and from the generalized depression that is characteristic of several common, more anterior conditions.

Third, glaucoma can be recognized despite the presence of other disease. Many people with glaucoma also have mild cataract or other conditions that cause nonspecific diffuse disturbance of visual sensation. If glaucoma produces localized loss, its presence will not be hidden by the superimposed effect of another condition that adds an additional depression that is equal at all locations.

ANATOMIC BASIS OF NERVE FIBER BUNDLE PATTERN

As discussed in Chapter 1, each location in the retina corresponds to a certain direction in the visual field; for example, a specific location on the inferior retina corresponds to a location in the superior visual field. The nasal retina represents the temporal visual field. The fovea represents the point of fixation and thus separates the nasal from the temporal side.

The optic nerve exit is nasal to the fovea and is centered slightly above the horizontal meridian. Therefore the physiologic blind spot is in the temporal visual field and is centered somewhat below the horizontal meridian. Because the visual field diagram shows the field "as the patient sees it" (Fig. 4-3), the blind spot is to the right of fixation for the right eye and to the left of fixation for the left eye. If there is a region of the retina that does not see, the visual field defect appears in the mirror-image, inverted location of the field.

Nerve fibers pass from every point in the retina to the optic nerve head, or optic disc. The pathway of the nerve fibers affects the character of field defects. From

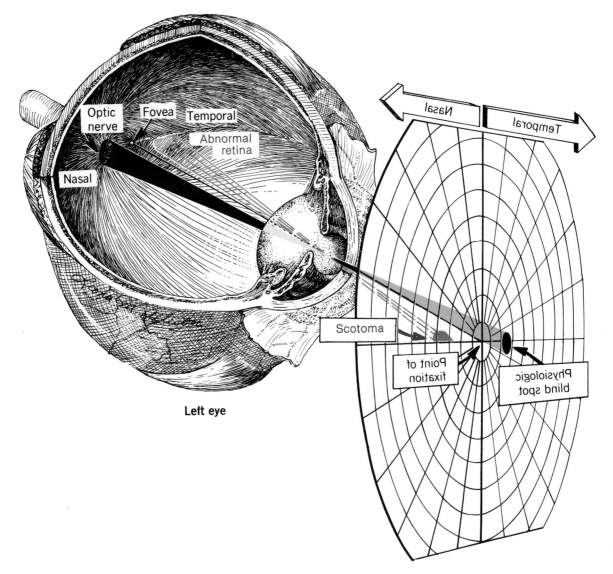

FIG. 4-3. Relationship of the retina to the visual field.

the region nasal to the optic disc, the fibers take a straight course to the nasal sector of the disc. Fibers from the nasal side of the fovea, but temporal to the disc, pass directly toward the temporal margin of the disc; those that originate above or below the horizontal meridian traverse a somewhat curved course. The fibers from the retina temporal to the fovea extend in an arcuate pathway around the fovea to pass into the upper and lower poles of the optic disc. If the retina is divided by an imaginary horizontal line on the temporal side of the fovea, fibers from above the line arc around the fovea superiorly and enter the upper pole of the disc. Similarly, fibers from below the line arc inferiorly around the fovea to enter the inferior pole of the disc.

In glaucoma, when bundles of nerve fibers are damaged at the optic disc, the region of the visual field supplied by these fibers loses its visual sensitivity. The result is either a scotoma or a localized depression. Typically the first nerve fiber bundles affected in glaucoma are those entering the upper or lower pole of the optic disc. Because of this, in keeping with the now classic descriptions of glaucomatous field defects,[4,14] paracentral scotomas appear (and may coalesce into a curved, nerve fiber bundle defect) within the so-called Bjerrum region,* an arcuate zone that begins at the blind spot and expands nasally around the point of fixation; or there is a depression in the nasal field of vision; or both (Fig. 4-4). The disease is unlikely to affect only a very small region that includes only one test point in the visual field examination. Typically a patch is abnormal, with a slight reduction of sensitivity and inconsistent responses. Therefore, a cluster of points is abnormal; however, on repeat testing an overlapping, slightly different cluster of points has abnormal sensitivity.[15-20] Usually, but not always, the upper portion of the field is more affected than the lower half. When loss in the inferior field dominates, and especially if the defective area encroaches on the point of fixation (see Fig. 4-8), the patient is more symptomatic because the loss interferes with reading and ambulation more than loss in the superior field does. Least commonly, localized loss of tissue on the nasal side of the optic disc may produce a "temporal wedge"—a wedge-shaped region of reduced sensitivity with its apex at the physiologic blind spot.[21]

---

*So named because Jannik Petersen Bjerrum (1851-1920), who devised the tangent screen, first stated that glaucomatous field defects tend to occur in an arcuate region that emerges from the blind spot and widens as it circles around to the nasal side of the fovea. (Bjerrum J. Om en tilfjelse til den saedvanlige synsfelfundersogelse samt om synsfeltet ved glaukom, Nordisk Ophthalmologisk Tidsskrift II:141-185, 1989.)

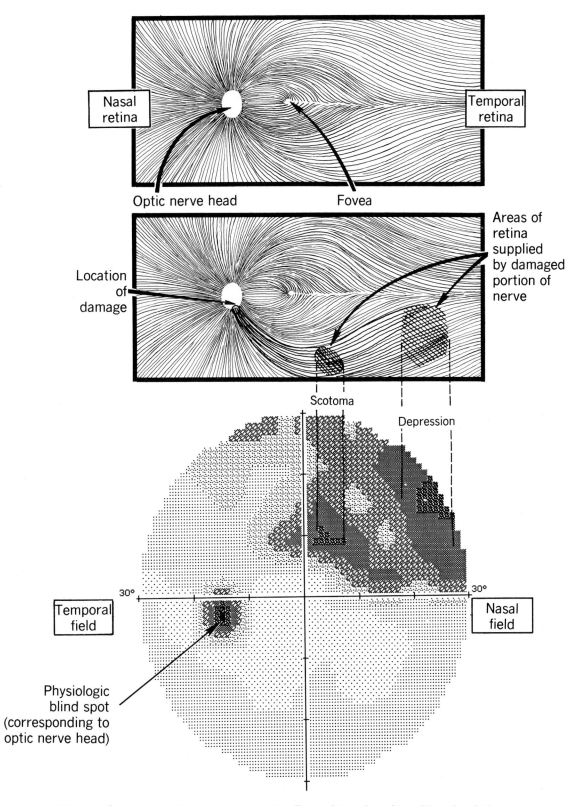

FIG. 4-4. Glaucomatous Damage to Nerve Bundles and Location of Resulting Visual Abnormalities. Damage at the lower pole of the optic disc causes abnormalities in the visual field as shown (left eye).

51

HEMIFIELD ASYMMETRY AND NASAL STEPS

The degree of damage at the upper pole of the optic disc usually differs from the degree of damage at the corresponding sector of the lower pole. Therefore the threshold visual sensitivities at locations in the upper and lower hemifields are likely to deviate from normal values unequally. Thus to recognize the presence of mild, localized glaucomatous visual field loss, it often is useful to compare corresponding parts of the upper and lower hemifields by visual inspection or by statistical means (see Chapter 6).

The asymmetry often is particularly striking when the row or cluster of points just above the horizontal nasal meridian is compared with a row or a cluster of points just below the nasal horizontal meridian. Points that are immediately adjacent across the nasal horizontal meridian may have very different sensitivities because in the temporal retina the region just above the horizontal meridian sends its nerve fibers to the upper pole of the disc, and the region just below the horizontal meridian sends nerve fibers to the lower pole of the disc (Fig. 4-5).

This asymmetry across the nasal horizontal meridian has been revealed classically in kinetic perimetry by moving the stimulus toward the center just above and below the nasal horizontal meridian. The isopter position is different above and below the horizontal meridian; this produces the "nasal step" described by Bjerrum and Rønne.[22] Diagnostically, in kinetic or static perimetry, a striking difference in the extent and density of the defect above and below the horizontal nasal meridian places the lesion in the prechiasmal nerve fiber pathway of the inner retina or of the optic nerve. Lesions damaging the outer retinal layers produce field defects corresponding to the patch of retina involved, and it would be an unlikely coincidence for a boundary of the lesion to coincide with the horizontal meridian. Similarly, there is no reason for the generalized depression from preretinal conditions or for the hemianopias from chiasmal lesions and postchiasmal lesions to respect the horizontal meridian. Thus, in cases of undiagnosed visual loss, attention to the nasal horizontal meridian is helpful in localizing the lesion (topographical diagnosis).

In the present context, if glaucoma already is suspected, attention to the nasal horizontal meridian also is one means of recognizing very early glaucomatous optic nerve loss. Very slight damage to one pole of the disc may produce a subtle but recognizable difference in sensitivity above and below the nasal horizontal meridian, even if the threshold values are within the normal range in both locations. An equivalent degree of generalized loss would be difficult to recognize as abnormal or to distinguish from the effects of age, cataract, and other preretinal factors. Thus it is fortunate that any unevenness in the depression, as is likely to occur in glaucoma, produces a nasal step, asymmetry between the upper and lower hemifields, or other evidence of localized field loss. Glaucoma is the most common cause of field defects with nasal steps, but other, less common diseases affecting the optic nerve head may cause an identical field defect.

Asymmetry of field loss above and below the horizontal meridian facilitates detection and diagnosis in glaucoma.

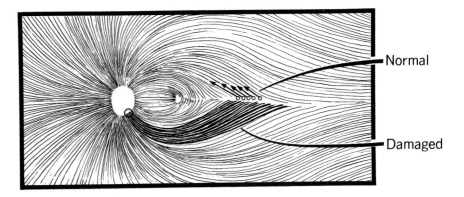

Normal

Damaged

FIG. 4-5. Basis of the Nasal Step. When a bundle of nerve fibers that enters the bottom of the optic disc is damaged in glaucoma—or in other diseases affecting the optic nerve head—a scotoma or depression may result in the upper nasal visual field. However, the immediately adjacent region is supplied by fully functioning nerve fibers that enter the undamaged upper part of the optic disc. Thus there may be a sharply demarcated discrepancy in the sensitivity of locations just above and below the horizontal meridian on the nasal side of the field.

POINT OF FIXATION

Although a central island of vision typically is preserved until late in the course of glaucomatous optic nerve damage, visual function at the point of fixation may be affected either by diffuse loss of axons (generalized depression of the field) or by a localized field defect impinging on the point of fixation. In such cases, tests of central acuity, color vision, and contrast sensitivity may be detectably abnormal. Such mild abnormality at or around the point of fixation is common, sometimes early in the course of the disease; but it is atypical for a scotoma affecting fixation to predominate. Recognizing that dense defects at or around the point of fixation do sometimes occur in glaucoma, especially in eyes with axial myopia, the examiner nonetheless must be cautious. A person with elevated intraocular pressure also may have macular disease or a compressive lesion of the optic nerve that produces a progressive central scotoma.

> Predominantly foveal and parafoveal loss usually is nonglaucomatous, except when associated with a myopic optic nerve head configuration.

GENERALIZED DEPRESSION

In some contexts the term "generalized depression" has been used strictly to mean the kind of abnormality produced by cataract, and that all parts of the field are affected equally—or if unequal, with only some flattening of the hill of vision by a graded reduction closer to the center. When the term is used in this strict sense, there is no suggestion of a nerve fiber bundle defect or of some regions affected more than others.

In a less strict usage, any form of visual loss affecting all regions of the visual field could be called "generalized," meaning simply that there is no normal region of the field. However, if some parts of the field are more abnormal than others, we prefer to call the visual loss widespread loss to distinguish it from pure forms of generalized loss. The reason for making the distinction at all is that in the pure form, *generalized loss* usually results from preretinal optical effects that impact all retinal locations or from diseases that affect nonpreferentially all elements in that part of the visual neurosensory system. In *widespread loss,* a pattern of greater loss in a nerve fiber loss distribution typically may be recognized in glaucoma, or, as another example, a central scotoma caused by a compressive lesion of the optic nerve may be recognized. Most diseases that are not preretinal affect particular regions of the visual field preferentially.

In advanced cases of glaucoma affecting most regions of the visual field, it is not important to distinguish whether the defect was first localized and later became widespread, or whether it initially was generalized before some locations became more advanced than others. In the end, the visual fields look the same. There is no entirely normal region, and diagnostic features are revealed by a pattern of locations that have greater loss than others.

However, we dwell on a careful description of the few early cases of glaucoma in which the axon damage is mild and diffuse, but a greater loss in some locations than in others has not yet become evident. We dwell on such cases, not because they are frequent in glaucoma, but because they present a diagnostic challenge. It is difficult to diagnose early glaucomatous damage that produces a uniform depression of the field for two fundamental reasons:

> Purely generalized loss usually results from pre-retinal optical effects.

1. **The visual depression is mild.** If axons are lost diffusely in glaucoma, the visual impact is very small at first. The threshold values may not fall outside the normal range until a large proportion of axons are lost.[23-25] Nearly always, by the time the diffuse threshold decline is distinctly abnormal, some locations are more affected than others, and localized defects begin to emerge.

2. **It is nonspecific.** Patients with widespread, mild visual depression also may have preretinal conditions (e.g., a small pupil or mild cataract) that accompany age. Similarly, a generalized depression may occur in eyes that are anatomically outside the normal range (small eyes with hyperopia, large eyes with myopia, or misshapen eyes with astigmatism), in eyes that are frankly anomalous (e.g., microphthalmic or nanophthalmic), or in eyes that have diffuse ocular disease (e.g., uveitis or diabetic retinopathy). Even when such eyes have high intraocular pressure, generalized depression may not represent glaucomatous damage.

Despite these limitations, widespread depression in the early stages of glaucoma sometimes can be detected and recognized as a result of glaucomatous optic nerve damage. First, it may be recognized when static thresholds are compared with a previous field examination of that patient (instead of being compared with the normal range), provided that the visual decline is confirmed on a second occasion and is not the result of other disease or of long-term fluctuations (see Chapters 2, 7, and 9).

Second, the defect also may be recognized as glaucomatous if the visual sensitivities in the two eyes are recognizably different, especially if the eye with the lower sensitivity also has a higher intraocular pressure and larger excavation of the optic nerve (provided that the difference is not explained by amblyopia, anisometropia, asymmetric media opacity, or some other accompanying difference between the two eyes) (see Chapter 7).

A third clue indicating glaucomatous widespread or generalized depression is that, again, certain localized areas probably are affected slightly more than others. This unevenness may be suggested to the attentive clinician by the total deviation and pattern deviation plots, by the pattern standard deviation (PSD) index or by the Glaucoma Hemifield Test (see Chapters 6 and 7). In doubtful cases, when there is no definitive localized component to the field loss, it is wise to remain dubious because cataract and other ocular diseases are far more frequent causes of evenly distributed generalized field loss than glaucoma.

SUMMARY AND EXAMPLES

Nerve fiber bundle defects are the classic and typical glaucomatous defects. They usually are the result of glaucoma, but they may occur with ischemic optic neuropathy or other optic nerve disorders. Central scotomas most often represent optic nerve disease (or macular disease) but rarely may represent glaucoma, especially in eyes with axial myopia. Diffuse loss also occurs in glaucoma, but usually to a greater degree in one region than another, in a nerve fiber bundle pattern. Generalized or widespread depression without exaggerated loss in localized regions most often is the result of cataract or other preretinal factors, but mild widespread loss can be the result of early, diffuse glaucomatous optic nerve damage.

The following examples show a variety of types and stages of glaucomatous field loss. You may wish to read Chapters 5 and 6 for explanations of the various statistical features of the printouts. For more examples and further insights into the spectrum of field defects that occur in glaucoma, see the publications listed in the Additional Reading section.

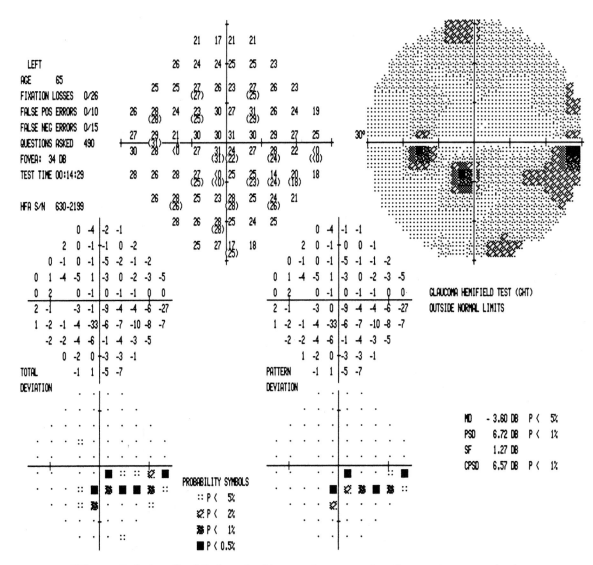

FIG. 4-6. Early Localized Defect. In this case, the grey scale calls attention to an absolute (strongest available stimulus not seen) paracentral scotoma below fixation, as well as an absolute defect at the nasal edge just below the horizontal meridian. The total deviation and pattern deviation plots call attention to the fact that these two absolute defects are part of a broader inferior arcuate area of loss, most of which is too subtle to be appreciated easily on the grey scale. These probability plots also call attention to the fact that the abnormality comes close to the point of fixation from the lower nasal side. The upper half of the field is normal. Although the abnormality is obvious, it is a very localized defect with fewer than 15% of the points involved. The fovea has a normal threshold (34 dB), and the visual acuity is 20/20 (left eye).

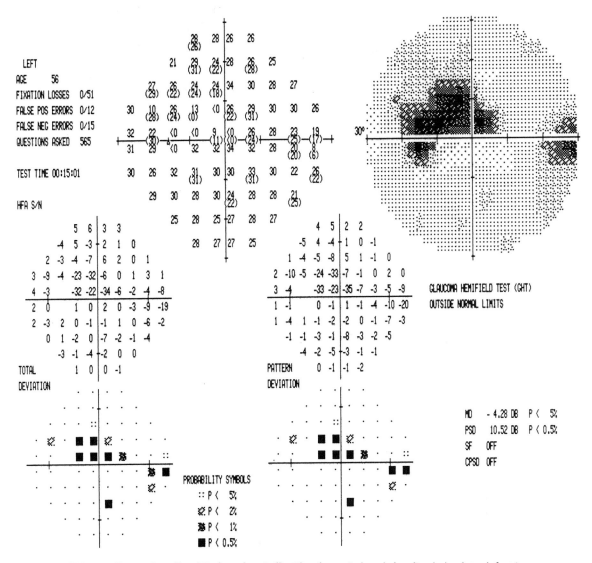

FIG. 4-7. Dense Localized Defect that Splits Fixation. A sharply localized, absolute defect impinges on fixation, but a small number of points is involved. Except for this sharply localized defect and the relative depression at the nasal edge, most of the points are unaffected. Fewer than 15% of the points are abnormal. Visual acuity is 20/15 (left eye).

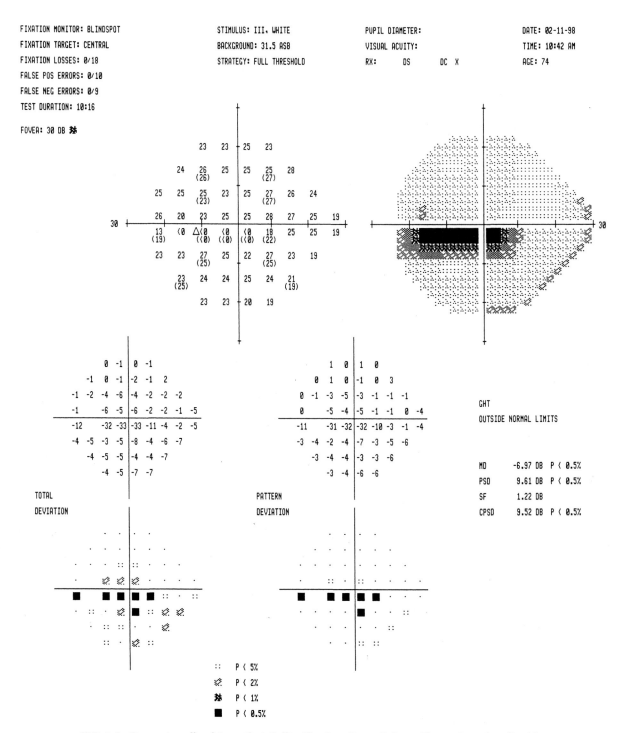

FIXATION MONITOR: BLINDSPOT
FIXATION TARGET: CENTRAL
FIXATION LOSSES: 0/18
FALSE POS ERRORS: 0/10
FALSE NEG ERRORS: 0/9
TEST DURATION: 10:16

FOVEA: 30 DB

STIMULUS: III, WHITE
BACKGROUND: 31.5 ASB
STRATEGY: FULL THRESHOLD

PUPIL DIAMETER:
VISUAL ACUITY:
RX: DS   DC X

DATE: 02-11-98
TIME: 10:42 AM
AGE: 74

TOTAL DEVIATION

PATTERN DEVIATION

GHT
OUTSIDE NORMAL LIMITS

MD   -6.97 DB   P < 0.5%
PSD   9.61 DB   P < 0.5%
SF   1.22 DB
CPSD   9.52 DB   P < 0.5%

:: P < 5%
⊠ P < 2%
▨ P < 1%
■ P < 0.5%

FIG. 4-8. Dense Localized Loss that Splits Fixation From Below. The patient described in Figure 4-7, and even the one described in Figure 4-1, may be asymptomatic. Defects in the inferior field, especially those that come close to the point of fixation, such as the one shown here, will cause considerable annoyance during reading. Broader involvement of the inferior field loss will cause trouble during walking (left eye).

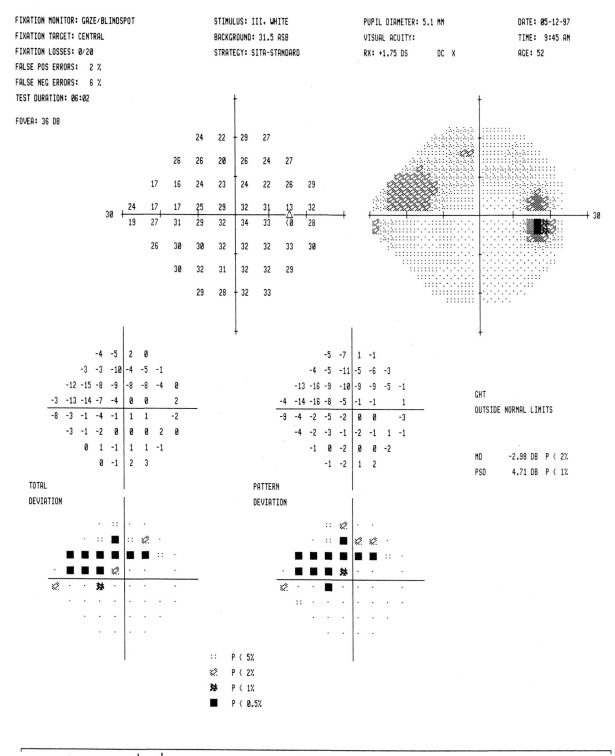

FIXATION MONITOR: GAZE/BLINDSPOT
FIXATION TARGET: CENTRAL
FIXATION LOSSES: 0/20
FALSE POS ERRORS: 2 %
FALSE NEG ERRORS: 6 %
TEST DURATION: 06:02

FOVEA: 36 DB

STIMULUS: III, WHITE
BACKGROUND: 31.5 ASB
STRATEGY: SITA-STANDARD

PUPIL DIAMETER: 5.1 MM
VISUAL ACUITY:
RX: +1.75 DS   DC X

DATE: 05-12-97
TIME: 9:45 AM
AGE: 52

```
              24  22   29  27
          26  26  20   26  24  27
      17  16  24  23   24  22  26  29
  24  17  17  25  29   32  31  13  32
  19  27  31  29  32   34  33  <0  28
      26  30  30  32   32  32  33  30
          30  32  31   32  32  29
              29  28   32  33
```

TOTAL DEVIATION

```
          -4  -5    2   0
       -3  -3 -10   -4  -5  -1
  -12 -15  -8  -9   -8  -8  -4   0
  -3 -13 -14  -7  -4   0   0       2
  -8  -3  -1  -4  -1   1   1      -2
      -3  -1  -2   0   0   0   2   0
           0   1  -1   1   1  -1
               0  -1   2   3
```

PATTERN DEVIATION

```
          -5  -7    1  -1
       -4  -5 -11   -5  -6  -3
  -13 -16  -9 -10   -9  -9  -5  -1
  -4 -14 -16  -8  -5  -1  -1       1
  -9  -4  -2  -5  -2   0   0      -3
      -4  -2  -3  -1  -2  -1   1  -1
          -1   0  -2   0   0  -2
              -1  -2   1   2
```

GHT
OUTSIDE NORMAL LIMITS

MD   -2.98 DB   P < 2%

PSD   4.71 DB   P < 1%

::   P < 5%
⚄   P < 2%
✖   P < 1%
■   P < 0.5%

FIG. 4-9. **Broad, Relative Upper Arcute Scotoma.** Unlike the preceding examples, the field has no locations of absolute loss at which the 0-dB stimulus was not seen. In fact, all locations have threshold values of 15 dB or greater. Although the greyscale shows the mildness of the defect, the probability plots show that the abnormality is statistically strong at more locations than might be suspected from the greyscale alone. The Glaucoma Hemifield Test (GHT) and the PSD index also reflect the localized abnormality of the upper hemifield (SITA-Standard 24-2; right eye).

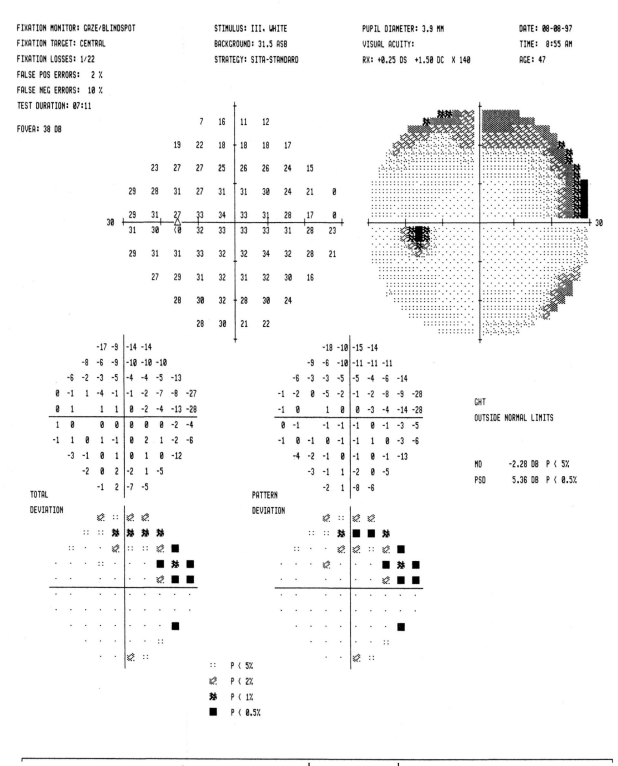

FIXATION MONITOR: GAZE/BLINDSPOT   STIMULUS: III, WHITE   PUPIL DIAMETER: 3.9 MM   DATE: 08-08-97
FIXATION TARGET: CENTRAL   BACKGROUND: 31.5 ASB   VISUAL ACUITY: TIME: 8:55 AM
FIXATION LOSSES: 1/22   STRATEGY: SITA-STANDARD   RX: +0.25 DS +1.50 DC X 140   AGE: 47
FALSE POS ERRORS: 2 %
FALSE NEG ERRORS: 10 %
TEST DURATION: 07:11

FOVEA: 38 DB

```
              7   16 | 11  12
         19   22  18 | 18  18  17
      23  27  27  25 | 26  26  24  15
   29 28  31  27  31 | 31  30  24  21   0
   29 31  27  33  34 | 33  31  28  17   0
30 31 30  <0  32  33 | 33  33  31  28  23
   29 31  31  33  32 | 32  34  32  28  21
      27  29  31  32 | 31  32  30  16
         28  30  32 | 28  30  24
              28  30 | 21  22
```

```
        -17 -9 |-14 -14
     -8  -6 -9 |-10 -10 -10
   -6 -2 -3 -5 | -4  -4  -5 -13
 0 -1  1 -4 -1 | -1  -2  -7  -8 -27
 0  1     1  1 | 0   -2  -4 -13 -28
 1  0     0  0 | 0    0   0  -2  -4
-1  1  0  1 -1 | 0    2   1  -2  -6
   -3 -1  0  1 | 0    1   0 -12
     -2  0  2 |-2    1  -5
         -1  2 |-7  -5

TOTAL
DEVIATION
```

```
         -18 -10 |-15 -14
       -9  -6 -10 |-11 -11 -11
     -6 -3 -3 -5 | -5  -4  -6 -14
  -1 -2  0 -5 -2 | -1  -2  -8  -9 -28
  -1  0     1  0 | 0   -3  -4 -14 -28
   0 -1    -1 -1 | -1   0  -1  -3  -5
  -1  0 -1  0 -1 | -1   1   0  -3  -6
    -4 -2 -1  0 | -1   0  -1 -13
      -3 -1  1 |-2    0  -5
          -2  1 |-8  -6

PATTERN
DEVIATION
```

GHT
OUTSIDE NORMAL LIMITS

MD   -2.28 DB P < 5%
PSD   5.36 DB P < 0.5%

```
 ::  P < 5%
 ▨  P < 2%
 ▩  P < 1%
 ■  P < 0.5%
```

FIG. 4-10. Early Glaucomatous Abnormality at the Upper Nasal Edge of the Central Visual Field. This case illustrates that field loss may not involve the entire hemifield at the onset. The region around fixation is uninvolved, but on close inspection the points above the nasal horizontal meridian may be depressed subtly compared with those just below, as close as 10 degrees from fixation (SITA-Standard 30-2; left eye).

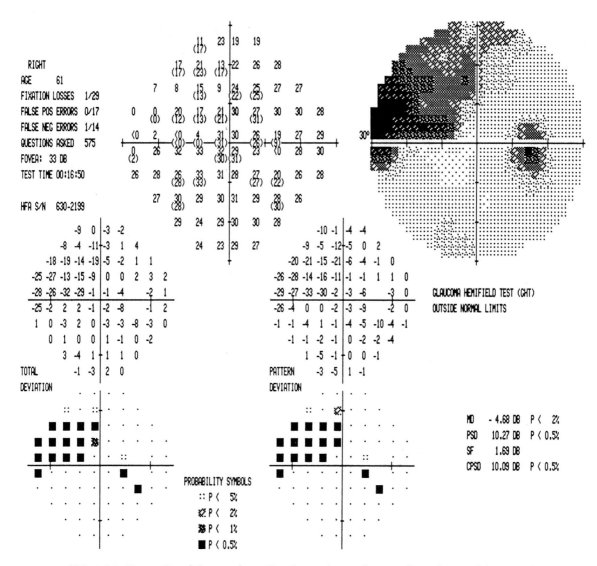

FIG. 4-11. Upper Nasal Depression. The depression is densest along the nasal horizontal meridian, does not approach fixation, and is not connected with the physiologic blind spot. Between 15% and 50% of the points are abnormal.

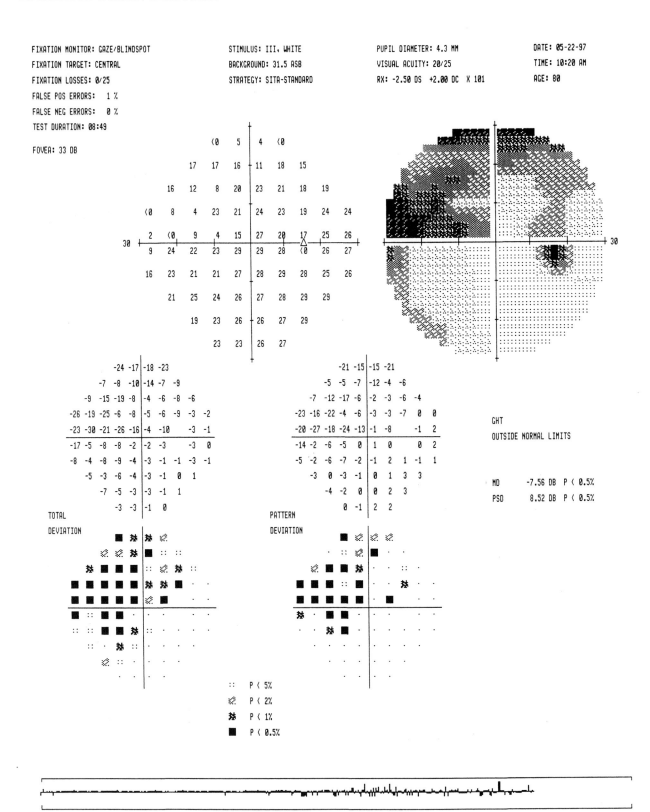

FIXATION MONITOR: GAZE/BLINDSPOT
FIXATION TARGET: CENTRAL
FIXATION LOSSES: 0/25
FALSE POS ERRORS: 1 %
FALSE NEG ERRORS: 0 %
TEST DURATION: 08:49

FOVEA: 33 DB

STIMULUS: III, WHITE
BACKGROUND: 31.5 ASB
STRATEGY: SITA-STANDARD

PUPIL DIAMETER: 4.3 MM
VISUAL ACUITY: 20/25
RX: -2.50 DS +2.00 DC X 101

DATE: 05-22-97
TIME: 10:20 AM
AGE: 80

```
           <0   5  | 4   <0
        17  17  16 |11  18  15
     16  12   8  20|23  21  18  19
  <0   8   4  23  21|24  23  19  24  24
   2  <0   9   4  15|27  20  17△ 25  26
30 ─ 9  24  22  23  29|29  28  <0  26  27 ─ 30
  16  23  21  21  27|28  29  28  25  26
     21  25  24  26|27  28  29  29
        19  23  26 |26  27  29
           23  23  |26  27
```

```
        -24 -17|-18 -23
      -7  -8 -10|-14  -7  -9
   -9 -15 -19  -8|-4  -6  -8  -6
-26 -19 -25  -6  -8|-5  -6  -9  -3  -2
-23 -30 -21 -26 -16|-4 -10      -3  -1
-17  -5  -8  -8  -2|-2  -3      -3   0
 -8  -4  -8  -9  -4|-3  -1  -1  -3  -1
    -5  -3  -6  -4|-3  -1   0   1
      -7  -5  -3|-3  -1   1
         -3  -3|-1   0
```

```
        -21 -15|-15 -21
      -5  -5  -7|-12  -4  -6
   -7 -12 -17  -6|-2  -3  -6  -4
-23 -16 -22  -4  -6|-3  -3  -7   0   0
-20 -27 -18 -24 -13|-1  -8      -1   2
-14  -2  -6  -5   0| 1   0       0   2
 -5  -2  -6  -7  -2|-1   2   1  -1   1
    -3   0  -3  -1| 0   1   3   3
      -4  -2   0| 0   2   3
          0  -1| 2   2
```

TOTAL
DEVIATION

PATTERN
DEVIATION

GHT
OUTSIDE NORMAL LIMITS

MD   -7.56 DB P < 0.5%
PSD   8.52 DB P < 0.5%

```
::  P < 5%
�khatched  P < 2%
▓  P < 1%
■  P < 0.5%
```

FIG. 4-12. Upper Nasal Depression With Fixation Threat. The depressed region in the upper hemifield is more extensive and approaches the point of fixation. The foveal threshold itself is normal (33 dB), and visual acuity is 20/20. The lower nasal quadrant is also abnormal, the extent of which is more evident on the deviation probability plots than on the greyscale (right eye).

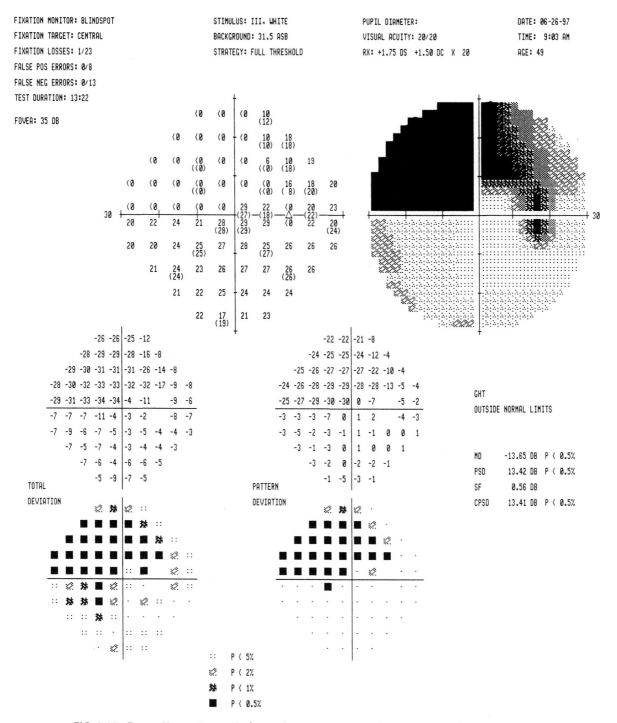

FIG. 4-13. Dense Upper Arcute Defect. The arcuate nature of the defect is evident. Although it comes close to fixation from the nasal side, the foveal threshold is normal (35 dB), and visual acuity is 20/20. Note the characteristic features: the defect clearly emanates from the physiologic blind spot, it becomes broader as it arcs over the point of fixation into the nasal field, and it comes closer to the foveal point from the nasal side than it does from the temporal side. The lower nasal quadrant also is depressed, and more than half the points are abnormal (Full Threshold 30-2; right eye).

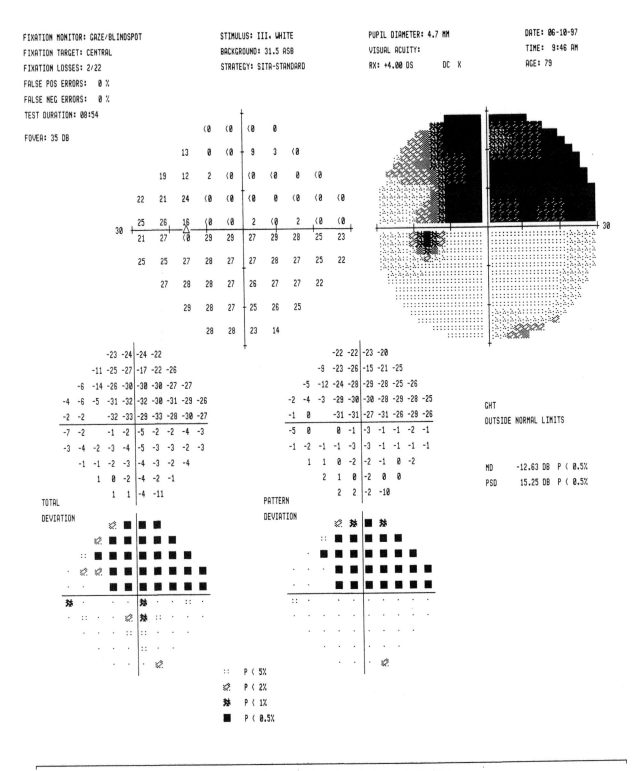

FIG. 4-14. Absolute Altitudinal Defect. The dense defect splits fixation from above. Its arcuate nature still is evident from the peninsula of retained vision extending upward on the temporal side of the physiologic blind spot. Of note is the striking contrast between the absolute visual loss in the upper half of the field and the completely normal lower half of the field. The foveal threshold is normal at 35 dB (SITA-Standard 30-2; left eye).

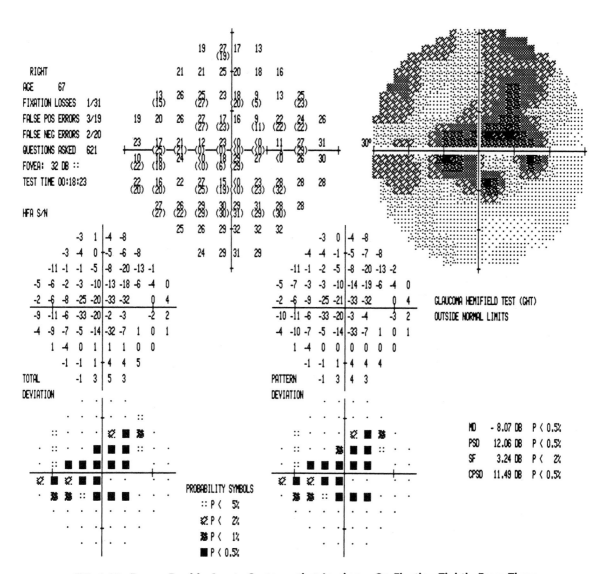

RIGHT

AGE 67

FIXATION LOSSES 1/31

FALSE POS ERRORS 3/19

FALSE NEG ERRORS 2/20

QUESTIONS ASKED 621

FOVEA: 32 DB ::

TEST TIME 00:18:23

HFA S/N

30°

TOTAL DEVIATION

PATTERN DEVIATION

GLAUCOMA HEMIFIELD TEST (GHT)

OUTSIDE NORMAL LIMITS

MD − 8.07 DB P < 0.5%

PSD 12.06 DB P < 0.5%

SF 3.24 DB P < 2%

CPSD 11.49 DB P < 0.5%

PROBABILITY SYMBOLS

:: P < 5%

⌧ P < 2%

▩ P < 1%

■ P < 0.5%

FIG. 4-15. Dense, Double Arcute Scotoma that Impinges On Fixation Tightly From Three Sides. The fovea has a slightly reduced threshold (32 dB), and visual acuity is 20/25. Such early involvement or threat to the fovea, while most of the points remain normal, is unusual in glaucoma, except in patients with axial myopia.

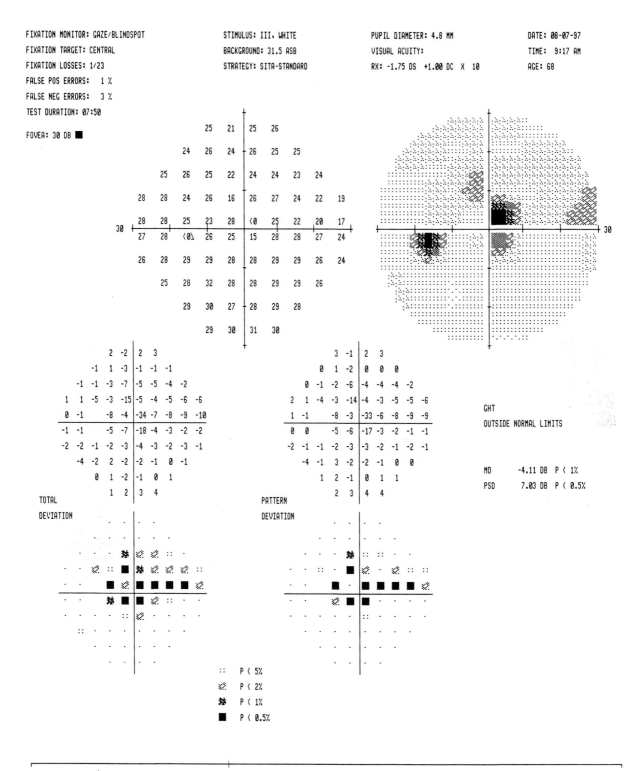

FIG. 4-16. Fixation Threat From Above and Below. The grey scale highlights the dense scotoma above and nasal to fixation. The probability plots show the parafoveal points in the inferior hemifield to be statistically abnormal, and the foveal threshold itself is reduced to 30 dB (SITA-Standard 30-2; left eye).

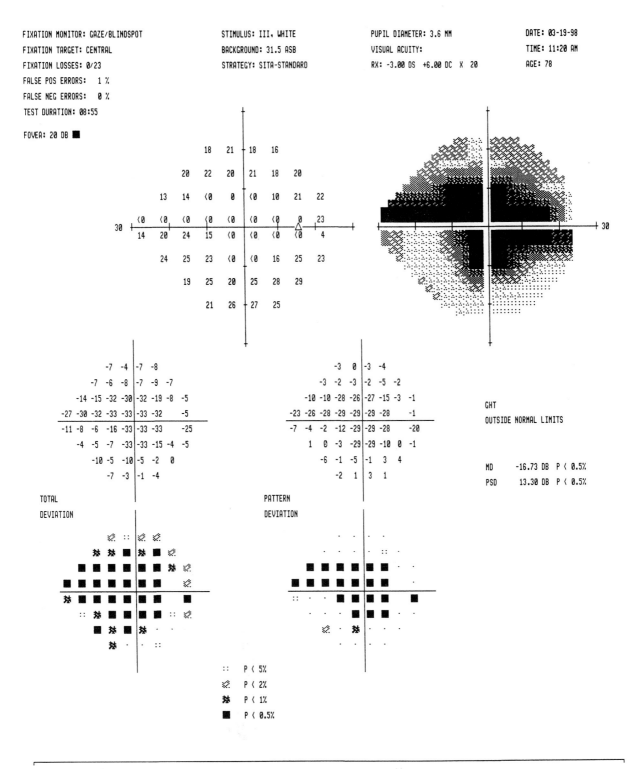

FIG. 4-17. Prominent Central Involvement. The point of fixation is crowded by upper and lower arcuate scotomas, but retains a foveal threshold of 20 dB and a visual acuity of 20/70. Note that the upper defect extends further toward the nasal edge than does the lower defect, producing a nasal step. This feature localizes the disease to the optic nerve or inner retina. It is unlikely that outer retinal disease, such as age-related macular degeneration, would produce a defect that respected the nasal horizontal meridian. Prominent central involvement with relatively less abnormality in the rest of the field is unusual in glaucoma (right eye, SITA-Standard, 24-2).

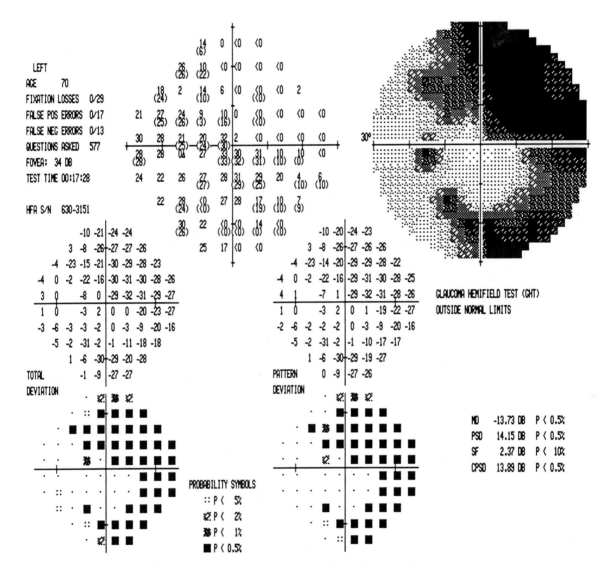

FIG. 4-18. Double Arcute Scotoma with Threatened Fixation. The dense upper nasal depression comes close to fixation, although the foveal threshold is good (34 dB) and visual acuity still is 20/25. The asymmetric involvement of the upper and lower nasal quadrants produces a "nasal step," at which the extent and density of the defect is different above and below the horizontal nasal meridian.

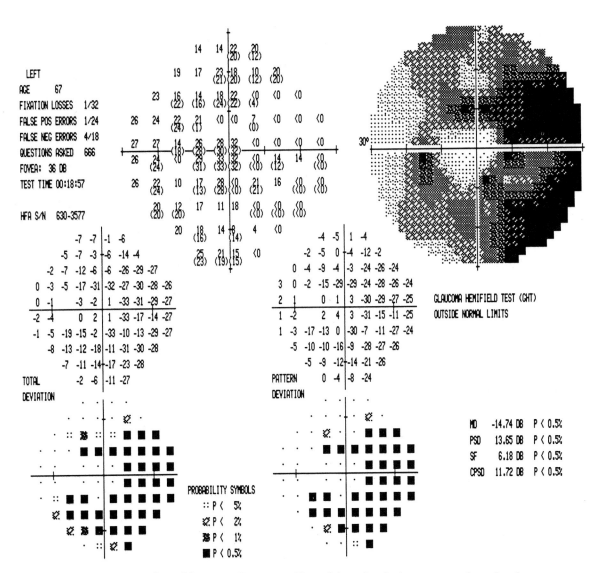

FIG. 4-19. Broad, Double Arcute Scotoma. Most of the points in the arcuate and nasal regions are abnormal, but the points surrounding the center and temporal to the blind spot remain normal. The foveal sensitivity is high (36 dB). There is no nasal step, but it is worth noting again that the defect broadens as it eminates from the blind spot and sweeps nasally, coming closer to fixation and the edge nasally compared to temporally.

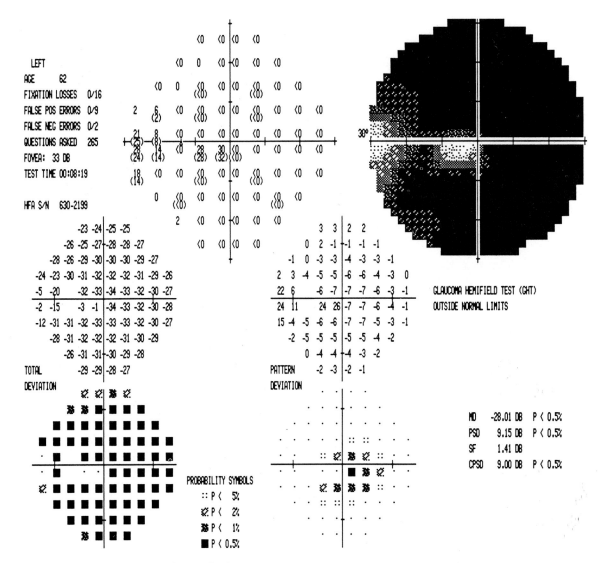

FIG. 4-20. More Advanced Glaucoma. Only a small central island and a temporal island remain, with broad, dense abnormality in both the upper and lower arcuate regions extending nasally from the blind spot. The foveal threshold is good (33 dB, within normal limits for age), and visual acuity is 20/20 (left eye).

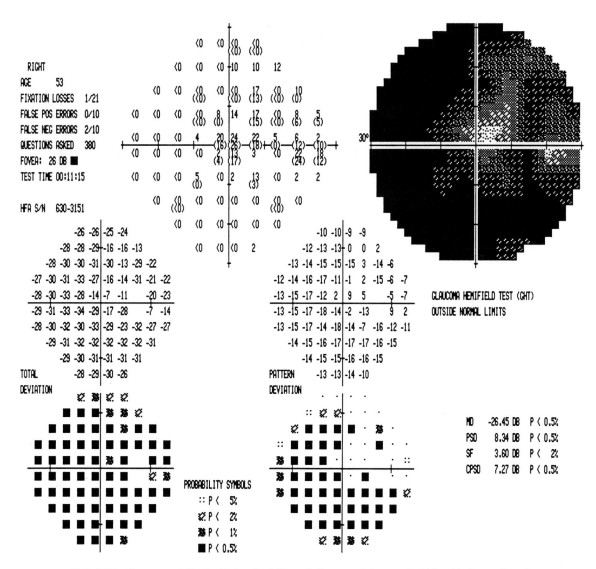

FIG. 4-21. Depressed Central Island. Although the remaining central island is larger than in Figure 4-15, even the best locations are abnormal. The fovea has a depressed sensitivity (26 dB), and visual acuity is 20/50 (right eye).

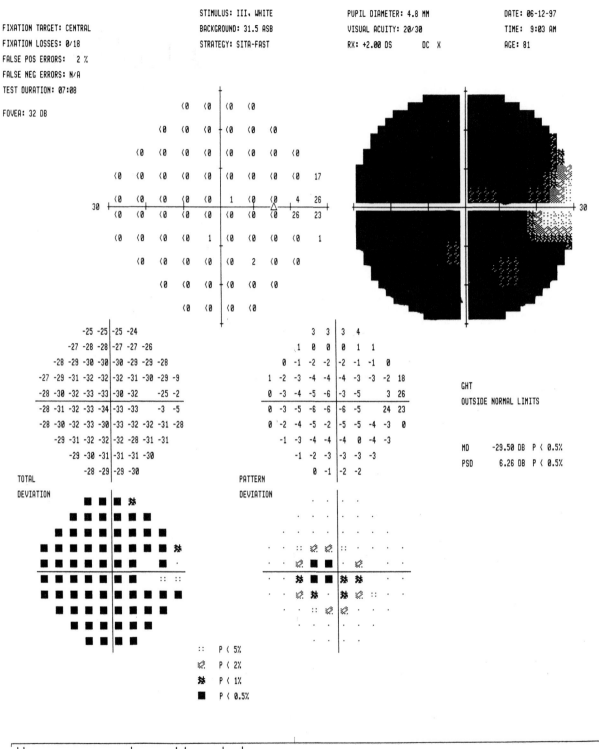

FIXATION TARGET: CENTRAL
FIXATION LOSSES: 0/18
FALSE POS ERRORS: 2 %
FALSE NEG ERRORS: N/A
TEST DURATION: 07:08

FOVEA: 32 DB

STIMULUS: III, WHITE
BACKGROUND: 31.5 ASB
STRATEGY: SITA-FAST

PUPIL DIAMETER: 4.8 MM
VISUAL ACUITY: 20/30
RX: +2.00 DS   DC X

DATE: 06-12-97
TIME: 9:03 AM
AGE: 81

```
                    <0  <0  <0  <0
                <0  <0  <0  <0  <0  <0
            <0  <0  <0  <0  <0  <0  <0  <0
        <0  <0  <0  <0  <0  <0  <0  <0  17
   30   <0  <0  <0  <0  <0  1  <0  <0   4  26
        <0  <0  <0  <0  <0  <0  <0  <0  26  23
        <0  <0  <0  <0  <0  1  <0  <0  <0   1
            <0  <0  <0  <0  <0  2  <0  <0
                <0  <0  <0  <0  <0  <0
                    <0  <0  <0  <0
```

```
   -25 -25 -25 -24                    3   3   3   4
 -27 -28 -28 -27 -27 -26            1   0   0   0   1   1
 -28 -29 -30 -30 -30 -29 -29 -28      0  -1  -2  -2  -2  -1  -1   0
 -27 -29 -31 -32 -32 -32 -31 -30 -29 -9    1  -2  -3  -4  -4  -4  -3  -3  -2  18
 -28 -30 -32 -33 -33 -30 -32     -25 -2    0  -3  -4  -5  -6  -3  -5       3  26
 -28 -31 -32 -33 -34 -33 -33      -3  -5    0  -3  -5  -6  -6  -6  -5      24  23
 -28 -30 -32 -33 -30 -33 -32 -32 -31 -28    0  -2  -4  -5  -2  -5  -5  -4  -3   0
   -29 -31 -32 -32 -32 -28 -31 -31           -1  -3  -4  -4  -4   0  -4  -3
   -29 -30 -31 -31 -31 -30                     -1  -2  -3  -3  -3  -3
      -28 -29 -29 -30                            0  -1  -2  -2
```

TOTAL
DEVIATION

PATTERN
DEVIATION

GHT
OUTSIDE NORMAL LIMITS

MD   -29.50 DB P < 0.5%
PSD   6.26 DB P < 0.5%

```
::   P < 5%
▨    P < 2%
▩    P < 1%
■    P < 0.5%
```

FIG. 4-22. Advanced Glaucoma. A few points with reduced sensitivity remain temporally. This remaining temporal island of vision would not have been detected with a 24-2 pattern. Remarkably, there also is residual vision in a tiny central island smaller than 3 degrees in radius, with a foveal threshold of 32 dB and visual acuity of 20/30; very steady fixation is recorded by the gaze tracker (SITA-Fast 30-2; right eye).

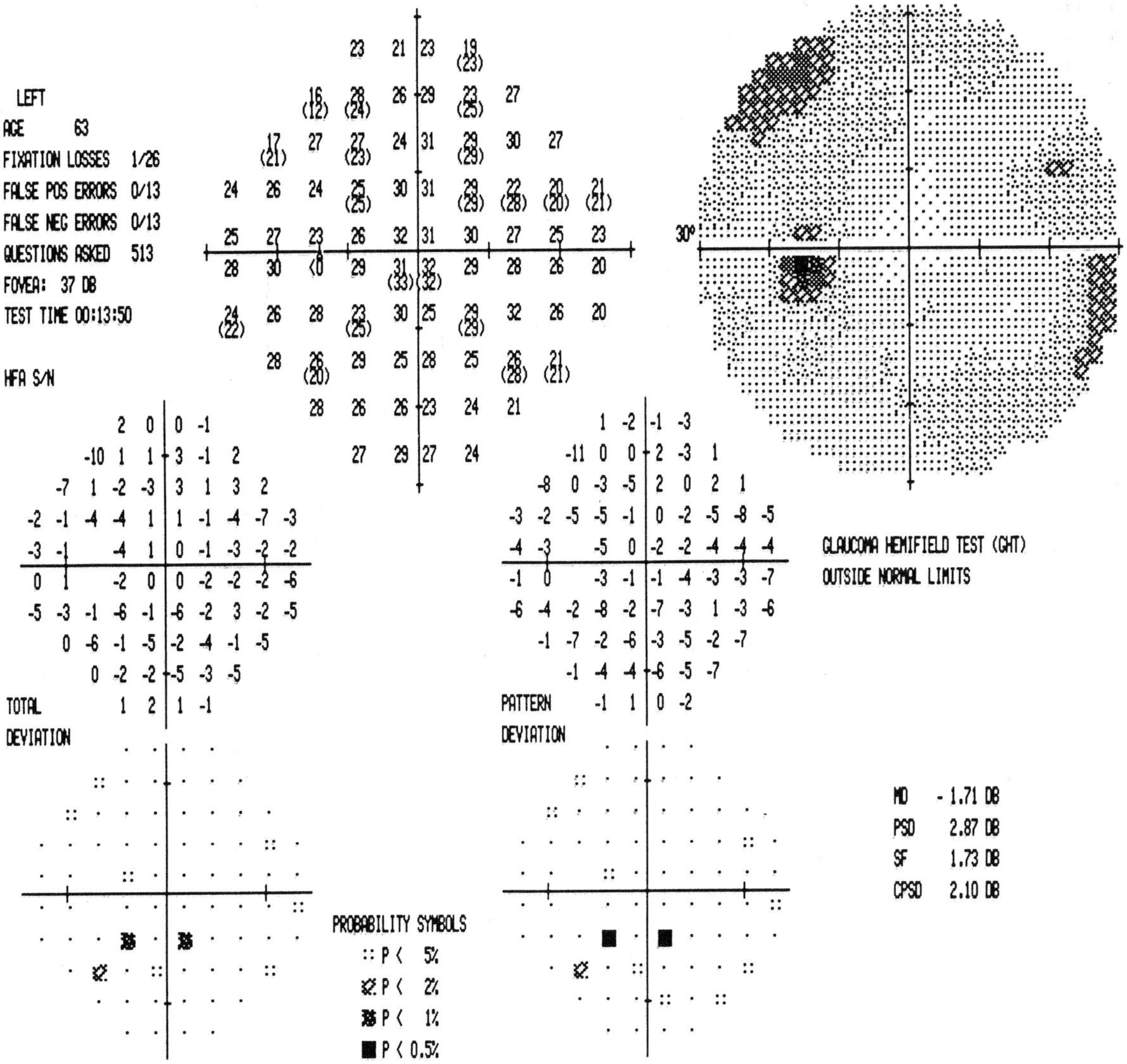

LEFT

AGE 63
FIXATION LOSSES 1/26
FALSE POS ERRORS 0/13
FALSE NEG ERRORS 0/13
QUESTIONS ASKED 513
FOVEA: 37 DB
TEST TIME 00:13:50

HFA S/N

```
                23  21  23  18
                            (23)
          16  28  26  29  23     27
         (12)(24)        (25)
      17    27  27  24  31  28     30  27
     (21)       (23)        (28)
   24  26  24  25  30  31  28  22  20  21
             (25)        (29)(28)(20)(21)
   25  27  23  26  32  31  30  27  25  23
   28  30  (0  29  31  32  28      28  20
                 (33)(32)
   24  26  28  23  30  25  28     32  26  20
  (22)        (25)        (23)
      28  26  29  25  28  25  28      21
         (20)                 (28) (21)
          28  26  26  23  24  21
                27  29  27  24
```

Total Deviation
```
        2   0   0  -1
   -10   1   1   3  -1   2
    -7   1  -2  -3   3   1   3   2
 -2  -1  -4  -4   1   1  -1  -4  -7  -3
 -3  -1      -4   1   0  -1  -3  -2  -2
  0   1      -2   0   0  -2  -2  -2  -6
 -5  -3  -1  -6  -1  -6  -2   3   2  -5
     0  -6  -1  -5  -2  -4  -1  -5
         0  -2  -2  -5  -3  -5
```
TOTAL   1   2   1 -1
DEVIATION

Pattern Deviation
```
        1  -2  -1  -3
   -11   0   0   2  -3   1
    -8   0  -3  -5   2   0   2   1
 -3  -2  -5  -5  -1   0  -2  -5  -8  -5
 -4  -3      -5   0  -2  -2  -4   4   4
 -1   0      -3  -1  -1  -4  -3  -3  -7
 -6  -4  -2  -8  -2  -7  -3   1  -3  -6
    -1  -7  -2  -6  -3  -5  -2  -7
        -1  -4  -4  -6  -5  -7
```
PATTERN   -1   1   0 -2
DEVIATION

GLAUCOMA HEMIFIELD TEST (GHT)
OUTSIDE NORMAL LIMITS

MD   -1.71 DB
PSD   2.87 DB
SF   1.73 DB
CPSD 2.10 DB

PROBABILITY SYMBOLS
:: P < 5%
   P < 2%
   P < 1%
■ P < 0.5%

FIG. 4-23. Early Widespread Loss. Scattered points are abnormal, especially in the lower arcuate region. The abnormality is revealed by the Glaucoma Hemifield Test but not by the CPSD index (left eye). In glaucoma, as a small or large patch of points becomes abnormal, the region typically shows variable threshold values (increased short-term fluctuation). Several such points may appear abnormal on the probability map, and on repeat testing a different selection of points in the same region is suggestively abnormal.[15-20]

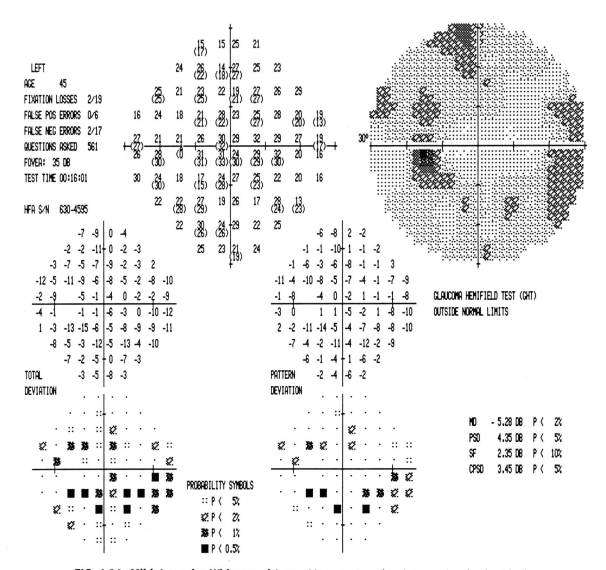

FIG. 4-24. Mild, Irregular Widespread Loss. Many scattered points are involved, with the pattern deviation probability plot revealing an inferior and superior arcuate configuration. The Glaucoma Hemifield Test and CPSD index are abnormal (left eye).

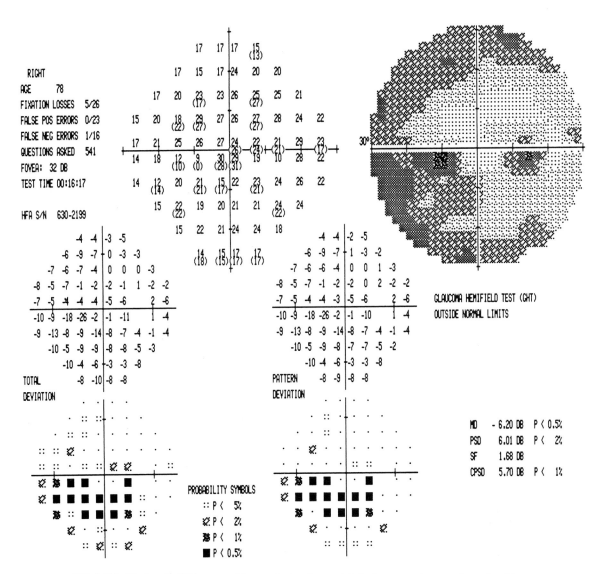

FIG. 4-25. Moderate Widespread Loss. Only a few points in the upper temporal quadrant have normal sensitivity. Although most points are involved, none has an absolute loss (sensitivity reduced to 0 dB). Although the loss is relative (not absolute) and widespread, it is exaggerated in the inferior arcuate and inferior nasal regions, and the CPSD index is abnormal; thus it is not a pure generalized loss of the type that could be attributed to media opacity (right eye).

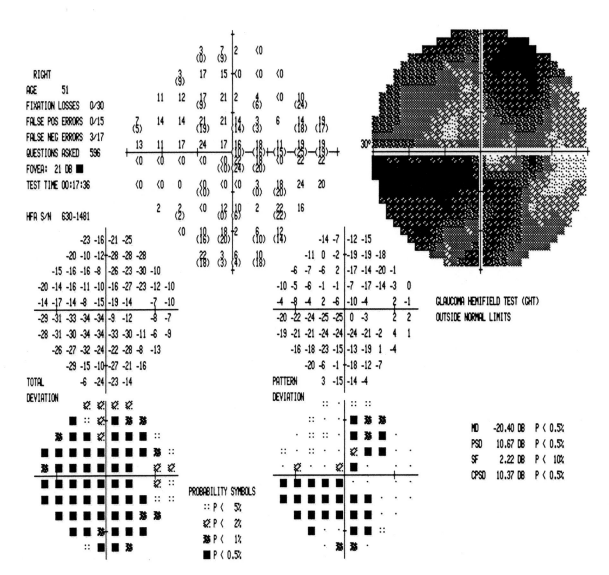

FIG. 4-26. Advanced Widespread Loss. All of the field is depressed, but absolute loss is limited to the lower nasal quadrant. The fovea is involved (21 dB) with visual acuity reduced to 20/80. The ocular media in this patient were completely clear. This example shows how one can arrive at the end-stage (such as in Figs. 4-15 and 4-17) from widespread loss as well as from loss that begins well localized and expands to close in on the point of fixation (right eye).

REFERENCES

1. Airaksinen PJ, Drance SM, Douglas GR et al: Visual field and retinal nerve fiber layer comparisons in glaucoma, *Arch Ophthalmol* 103:205-207, 1985

2. Anctil JL, Anderson DR: Early foveal involvement and generalized depression of the visual field in glaucoma, *Arch Ophthalmol* 102:363-370, 1984.

3. Armaly MF: Ocular pressure and visual fields: A ten-year follow-up study, *Arch Ophthalmol* 81:25, 1969.

4. Aulhorn E, Harms H: Early visual field defects in glaucoma. In Leydhecker W, editor: *Glaucoma Tutzing Symposium,* p 151, Basel, 1967, Karger.

5. Caprioli J, Sears M: Patterns of early visual field loss in open angle glaucoma, *Doc Ophthalmol Proc Ser* 49:307-1315, 1987.

6. Feuer WJ, Anderson DR: Static threshold asymmetry in early glaucomatous visual field loss, *Ophthalmology* 96:1285-1297, 1989.

7. Glowazki A, Flammer J: Is there a difference between glaucoma patients with more diffuse visual field damage? *Doc Ophthalmol Proc Ser* 49:317-320, 1987.

8. Heijl A: Lack of diffuse loss of differential light sensitivity in early glaucoma, *Acta Ophthalmol* 67:353-360, 1989.

9. Katz J, Sommer A: Similarities between the visual fields of ocular hypertensive and normal eyes, *Arch Ophthalmol* 104:1648-1651, 1986.

10. Lichter PR, Standardi CL: Early glaucomatous visual field defects and their significance to clinical ophthalmology, *Doc Ophthalmol Proc Ser* 19:111, 1979.

11. Motolko M, Drance SM, Douglas GR: The early psychophysical disturbances in chronic open-angle glaucoma: A study of visual functions with asymmetric disc cupping, *Arch Ophthalmol* 100:1632, 1982.

12. Pederson JE, Anderson DR: The mode of progressive disc cupping in ocular hypertension and glaucoma, *Arch Ophthalmol* 98:490-495, 1980.

13. Chauhan BC, LeBlanc RP, Shaw AM et al: Repeatable diffuse visual field loss in open-angle glaucoma, *Ophthalmology* 104:532-538, 1997.

14. Drance SM: The glaucomatous visual field, *Br J Ophthalmol* 56:186-200, 1972.

15. Flammer J, Drance SM, Zulauf M: Differential light threshold: Short- and long-term fluctuation in patients with glaucoma, normal controls, and patients with suspected glaucoma, *Arch Ophthalmol* 102:704-706, 1984.

16. Heijl A, Lindgren G, Olsson J, Åsman P: Visual field interpretation with empiric probability maps, *Arch Ophthalmol* 107:204-208, 1988.

17. Holmin C, Krakau CET: Variability of glaucomatous visual field defects in computerized perimetry, *Graefes Arch Klin Exp Ophthalmol* 210:235-250, 1979.

18. Werner EB, Drance SM: Early visual field disturbances in glaucoma, *Arch Ophthalmol* 95:1173-1175, 1977.

19. Werner EB, Drance SM: Increased scatter of responses as a precursor of visual field changes in glaucoma, *Can J Ophthalmol* 12:140-142, 1977.

20. Werner EB, Saheb N, Thomas D: Variability of static visual threshold responses in patients with elevated IOPs. *Arch Ophthalmol* 100:1627-1631, 1982.

21. Werner EB, Beraskow J: Temporal visual field defects in glaucoma, *Can J Ophthalmol* 15:13-14, 1980.

22. Ronne H: Uber das Gesichtfeld beim Glaukom, *Klin Monastsbl Augenheilkd* 47:12-33, 1909.

23. Anderson DR, Knighton RW: Perimetry and acuity perimetry. In Shields MB, Pollack IP, Kolker AE, editors: *Perspectives in glaucoma,* Thorofare, NJ, 1988, Slack Inc.

24. Quigley HA, Addicks EM, Green WR: Optic nerve damage in human glaucoma. III. Quantitative correlation of nerve fiber loss and visual field defect in glaucoma, ischemic neuropathy, papilledema, and toxic neuropathy, *Arch Ophthalmol* 100:135-146, 1982.

25. Quigley HA, Addicks EM, Green WR, Maumenee EA: Optic nerve damage in human glaucoma. II. The site of injury and susceptibility to damage, *Arch Ophthalmol* 99:635-649, 1981.

ADDITIONAL READING

Aulhorn E, Harms H: Early visual field defects in glaucoma. In Leydhecker W, editor: *Glaucoma Tutzing Symposium,* p 151. Basel, 1967, S Karger.

Budenz DL: *Atlas of Visual Fields,* Philadelphia, 1997, Lippincott-Raven Publishers.

Drance SM: The glaucomatous visual field, *Br J Ophthalmol* 56:186-200, 1972.

Harrington DO: The Bjerrum scotoma, *Trans Am Ophthalmol Soc* 62:324, 1964.

Harrington DO: The differential diagnosis of the arcuate scotoma, *Invest Ophthalmol Vis Sci* 8:96, 1969.

Henson DB, Spenceley SE, Bull DR: Spatial classification of glaucomatous visual field loss, Br J Ophthalmol 80:526-531, 1996.

Reed H, Drance SM: *The Essentials of Perimetry, Static and Kinetic,* p 66, ed 2, Oxford, 1972, Oxford University Press.

Traquair HM: The nerve fiber bundle defect, *Trans Ophthalmol Soc UK* 64:1-23, 1944.

PART TWO

OFFICE PERIMETRY

CHAPTER 5

Clinical static perimetry

BASIC GOALS

In general, doctors are interested in two basic issues: diagnosis of disease and monitoring of disease progress. First, is this patient sick and if so, what is the diagnosis? Second, if the patient is sick, is the current clinical management optimal (or at least acceptable), or is there something further that can and should be done? Diagnostic procedures, perimetric or otherwise, typically are aimed at answering these questions, and the choice of procedures must be made within this context. This chapter introduces the most commonplace procedures for automated perimetry.

MAINSTREAM PERIMETRIC PROTOCOLS

The doctor must exercise judgment as to the extent of diagnostic testing that should be performed.

Disease diagnosis frequently requires the exercise of judgment about the extent of testing that should be performed. Diagnosis and management of glaucoma, and of other diseases affecting the visual field, are not exceptions. Were it possible, each glaucoma patient or suspect, for example, might receive complete threshold testing of numerous, closely spaced locations in every part of both the central and the peripheral regions in the visual field. Of course, this is not practical; few patients have the endurance or patience required. Moreover, at some point the associated human and economic costs of increased thoroughness of testing outweigh the incremental diagnostic benefit.

Practitioners have learned to direct their efforts most intently toward testing the central visual field, where most important diagnostic information seems to be located. The tests most frequently used in glaucoma management focus on the central 30 or 24 degrees of the visual field, at locations 6 degrees apart (the 30-2 or the 24-2 pattern), using a white size-III stimulus. Most early disease affects this central region, and early localized defects rarely are so focal in nature that they would escape detection between tested points 6 degrees apart.[1] A different pattern of points (e.g., a blanket of points only 2 degrees apart, covering only the central 10 degrees of the visual field) or a different size stimulus may be used under certain conditions—for example, when following the course of severe disease (see Chapter 8). By virtue of their familiarity and because they offer a baseline experience for interpreting results, the 24-2 and 30-2 size-III threshold tests also have become the most frequently used tests for many purposes besides glaucoma and, all told, have the most established track record. Therefore, before variations are explored, it may be useful to describe in detail the classic central threshold test, with the original "Full Threshold" algorithm applied to the 30-2 pattern of test locations.

THE ORIGINAL, CLASSIC CENTRAL STATIC THRESHOLD TEST

The original standard program of the first model of the Humphrey Field Analyzer (HFA-I)[2-5] is the static threshold determination at locations 6 degrees apart within the central 30 degrees, with the grid spanning the horizontal and vertical meridians. This original Central 30-2 Threshold test used what we now call the Standard Full Threshold testing algorithm; this algorithm is standard on the original HFA and is available on the newer HFA-II, as well.[6] If the fovea test option is on, the classic test begins with the patient gazing at the center of a fixation diamond projected about 10 degrees below the normal fixation spot, which occupies the center of the bowl. A size-III stimulus of sufficient intensity to be seen by most normal people is projected onto the center of the diamond for 0.2 second. The machine waits for a response for an additional 1.8 seconds after the stimulus ends.

If there is no response before the end of the acceptance interval, a stimulus 4 dB more intense is presented. The process is repeated, each time with a stimulus 4 dB more intense, until the patient responds, indicating that the stimulus has become intense enough to be visible, or until the maximum available stimulus has been presented without eliciting a response. If and when a response is obtained, the next stimulus presented is 2 dB less intense. This bracketing, or staircase, process is repeated with stimuli successively 2 dB less intense until the patient fails to respond. The last stimulus responded to is recorded as the foveal threshold.

If the patient does respond to the initial stimulus, a stimulus 4 dB less intense is presented. The process is repeated with stimuli successively 4 dB less intense until the patient finally does not respond within the acceptance interval. The next stimulus presented is then 2 dB more intense. Stimuli successively 2 dB more intense are presented until the patient does respond. The stimulus intensity when the patient responds is recorded as the visual threshold at the fovea.

After the foveal threshold sensitivity has been determined, the patient is instructed to shift his gaze to the fixation target at the center of the bowl. The differential light sensitivity threshold then is determined at the 76 locations that make up the grid covering the central 30 degrees of the visual field, with the same bracketing strategy that was used to determine the foveal threshold.

After 10 responses have been recorded, an adjustment is made in the acceptance interval, which is the average response time of the patient plus 0.85 second. This adjustment slows down the test for slow responders. For fast responders, it speeds up the test, increases alertness, and saves time. The response time is

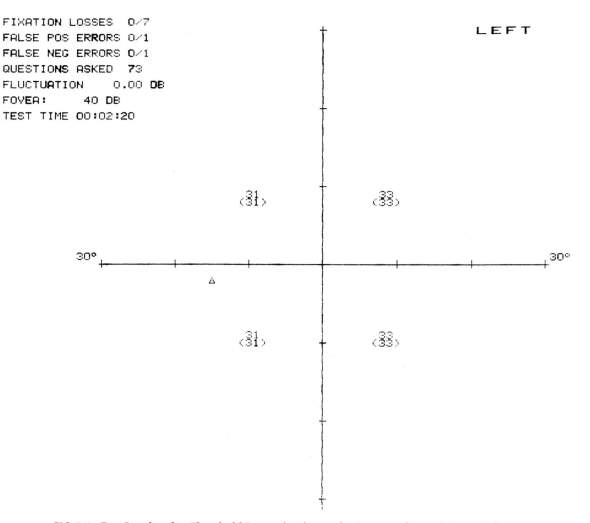

```
FIXATION LOSSES  0/7
FALSE POS ERRORS 0/1
FALSE NEG ERRORS 0/1
QUESTIONS ASKED  73
FLUCTUATION    0.00 DB
FOVEA:      40 DB
TEST TIME 00:02:20
```

LEFT

⟨31⟩   ⟨33⟩

30°   30°

⟨31⟩   ⟨33⟩

FIG. 5-1. Test Results after Threshold Determination at the Fovea and Four Primary Points.
The triangle indicates the blind spot location.

monitored throughout the test, and, based on a running average, the acceptance interval may be lengthened if the patient slows down during the session.

The threshold is determined first at four primary locations, one in each quadrant, symmetrically placed 9 degrees from both the horizontal and vertical meridians (Fig. 5-1). Stimuli are presented in random order at the four primary locations. The initial stimulus intensity is 25 dB, which usually is easily seen at these locations. The intensity of each subsequent stimulus presentation is determined by the patient's response to the stimulus presented most recently at that location. As the criterion for threshold determination is met (the second crossover between seen and unseen stimuli), the threshold sensitivity value is recorded and presented on the screen so that the perimetrist can monitor the progress of the test. At these four primary points, the entire procedure for threshold determination is performed twice.

After the threshold sensitivity has been doubly determined at the four primary locations, the thresholding procedure is undertaken at adjacent points radiating from each of the primary points (Fig. 5-2). To minimize the number of

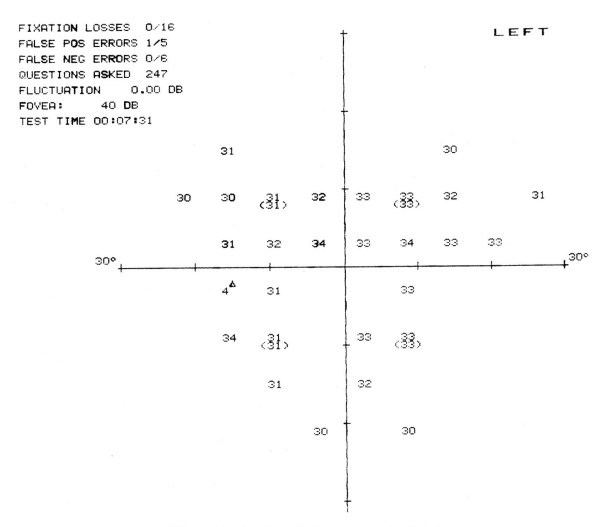

FIG. 5-2. Test Results as Further Locations Are Tested.

presentations required for thresholding and to save time, the initial stimulus used at each location is extrapolated from the threshold sensitivity at nearby points already thresholded. The principle is that points adjacent to normal points tend to be normal, whereas those adjacent to abnormal points tend to be abnormal.

In addition to the four primary points, there are six other locations (Fig. 5-3) where the thresholding procedure always is performed twice, yielding a total of 10 preselected points at which the test-retest difference is used to calculate the measurement error, or short-term fluctuation (SF).

Additional locations, not preselected, undergo duplicate threshold determination whenever the threshold sensitivity value is more than 4 dB different from what might be expected, taking into account the value at the previously thresholded neighboring locations and an adjustment for the relative eccentricity of the locations being compared. These additional double determinations are not included in the calculation of SF because the calculation would be biased by inclusion of points that were selectively double determined because of an aberrant value on the first determination.

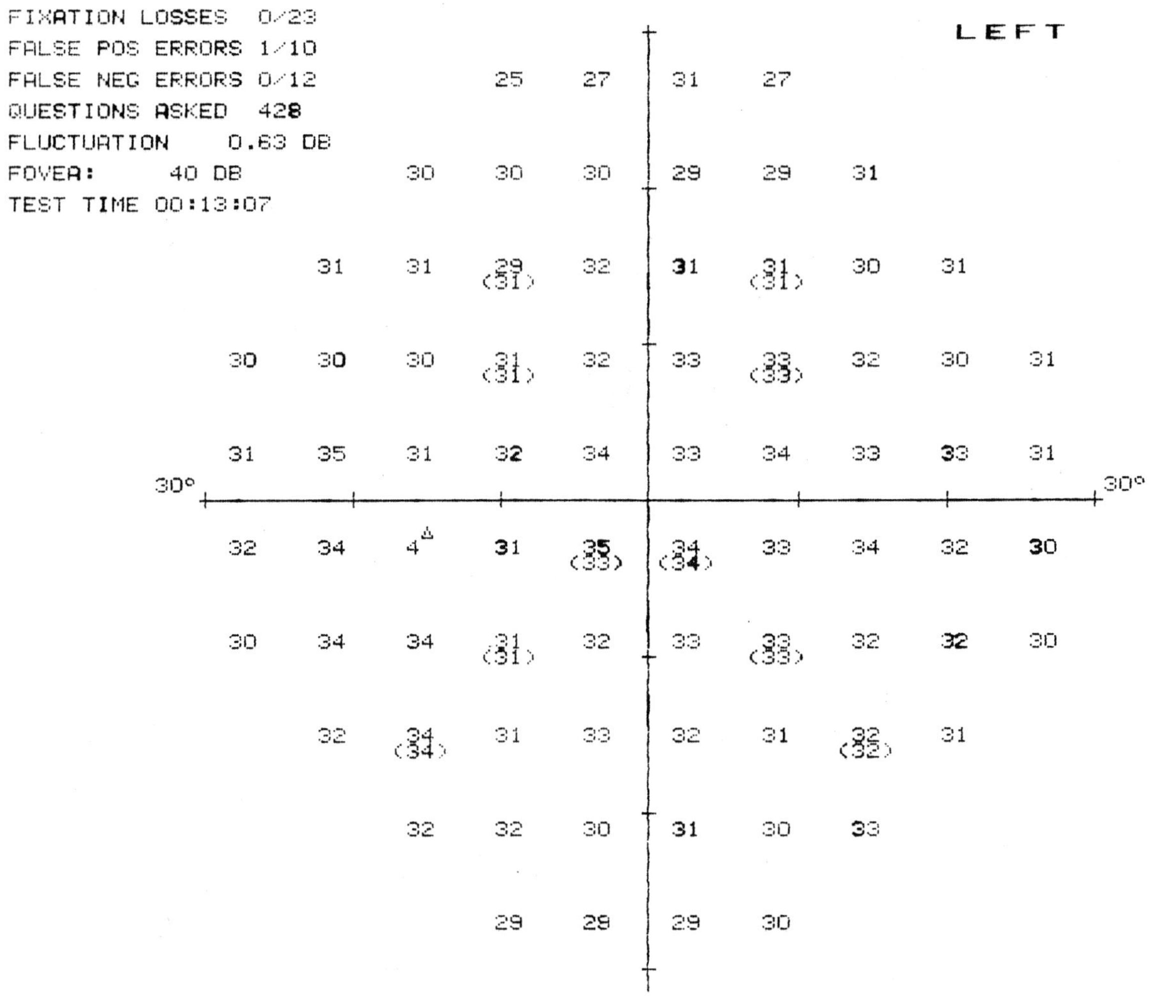

```
FIXATION LOSSES   0/23                                              L E F T
FALSE POS ERRORS 1/10
FALSE NEG ERRORS 0/12              25    27  | 31    27
QUESTIONS ASKED   428
FLUCTUATION      0.63 DB
FOVEA:      40 DB                30    30    30  | 29    29    31
TEST TIME 00:13:07


                          31    31    29    32  | 31    31    30    31
                                     (31)            (31)

                     30    30    30    31    32  | 33    33    32    30    31
                                     (31)            (33)

                     31    35    31    32    34  | 33    34    33    33    31
         30° ─────────────────────────────────────────────────────────── 30°

                     32    34    4△   31    35  | 34    33    34    32    30
                                       (33)  (34)

                     30    34    34    31    32  | 33    33    32    32    30
                                     (31)            (33)

                          32    34    31    33  | 32    31    32    31
                                (34)                        (32)

                                32    32    30  | 31    30    33


                                     29    29  | 29    30
```

FIG. 5-3. Completed Test. The 10 locations at which threshold is double determined are used for calculating the short-term fluctuation (SF) index.

Three types of catch trials: to detect fixation loss, false-positive responses, and false-negative responses.

Throughout the test, three types of catch trials are performed: those to detect loss of fixation, those to detect a tendency for false-positive responses, and those to detect a tendency for false-negative responses. These methods are discussed later in this chapter, and their implications are covered in Chapter 7.

NEWER THRESHOLDING ALGORITHMS

Fastpac

The Fastpac algorithm crosses threshold only once, and has a larger intratest variability than does Full Threshold.

The Full Threshold algorithm just described in detail was used with the original Humphrey perimeter in 1984. Introduced in 1991, the Fastpac strategy changes stimulus intensity in 3-dB steps, either stronger or weaker depending on the initial patient response. When the sequence crosses threshold (i.e., either from seeing to nonseeing or vice versa), testing stops without reversing direction in smaller steps. Threshold is recorded as the last seen stimulus intensity in the sequence. The criterion for measuring the threshold a second time is similar to that of the Full Threshold algorithm. The theoretical best threshold resolution is 3 dB rather than the theoretical 2-dB resolution of the earlier, Standard Full Threshold algorithm. Because the Fastpac algorithm defines threshold on the basis of only a single crossing of threshold, it is somewhat more vulnerable to patient response errors than is the Full Threshold method. Fastpac also has somewhat higher intratest variability (SF). Intertest variability has been reported to be similar to that of Full Threshold. These compromises in exchange for a shorter test time have proved to be acceptable for many clinical needs.[7-11] Fastpac test times are approximately 70% of those of Full Threshold, although in some types of field loss test times may nearly approach those of Full Threshold.

Swedish interactive threshold algorithm (SITA)

The two SITA thresholding strategies run in half the time of the methods they replace with no loss of reproducibility.

The SITA strategy became commercially available in 1997, after a decade of development.[12-21] This strategy permits a more time-efficient estimation of threshold than noninteractive staircase strategies. With the same reliability as the previously established methods, the test time is cut in half. Two versions of SITA have been produced to date: SITA-Standard, which runs in about half the time of the Standard Full Threshold algorithm with the same test-retest reproducibility, and SITA-Fast, which runs in about half the time of Fastpac with the same reproducibility as Fastpac. Because of the rapid real-time computing power required as the test is conducted, the SITA strategies run only on the newer 700 series of Humphrey perimeter (HFA-II).[6]

A number of factors contribute to the time-saving efficiencies of SITA, primarily including (1) detailed visual field modeling; (2) use of an information index to determine threshold endpoints; (3) test pacing that is more responsive to the patient's reaction time; (4) posttest recomputation of threshold values; and (5) reduction of "catch trials" by the use of inferential calculation to determine reliability indices.

Visual field modeling.[22] SITA starts with prior probability models of normal and abnormal visual fields. The model is based on age-corrected values in the normal and glaucomatous populations, frequency-of-seeing curves around threshold values, and correlations between adjacent test points. Based on the patient's responses to the staircase presentations, a Bayesian posterior probability function is adjusted continuously as the test proceeds, and at any moment the peak of the function represents the current threshold estimate that best corresponds to the patient's responses. Threshold estimates under this system are based on the complete pattern of responses to stimuli at a given point (not just the last pair of responses); this approach makes more complete use of available information than earlier methods, and thus reduces the test time needed to achieve a given level of reliability.

Information index. The visual field model also produces an information index that computes, as the test proceeds, how sure the model is of the current threshold estimate. When the information index at a particular test point location reaches a preselected level, testing stops at that location.[23] The information index will quickly approach the selected level at locations where patient responses are internally consistent and also in line with responses at surrounding points. In the absence of such consistency, the index remains low, and testing will continue. This real-time method means that testing stops early if confidence in the threshold determination at a location is high (a time saver), but testing with another staircase is initiated if there still is uncertainty, in principle improving the accuracy of the test result at those locations. However, for practical reasons there is a limit to the amount of testing undertaken at a given location.

The confidence limit selected as the criterion to stop testing at each location determines the balance between accuracy and test time. The limit that is selected is the major difference between SITA Standard and SITA Fast. In SITA Standard, the criterion does not stop the test unless there has been at least one crossover from seeing to nonseeing (or visa versa).[17] At least two crossovers are required if the confidence interval cannot be reduced to the selected limit,[17] so that the threshold determination in such instances is at least as reliable as that obtained with the Full Threshold method.

Reaction time. Earlier testing algorithms made adjustments to test pacing based on patient reaction times, primarily to slow the pace for slow responders. They waited 0.85 second longer for a response than the longest average of 10 consecutive responses to stimuli. In the SITA method,[24] updated averages and standard deviations of the patient's response times are used to determine the interval during which to wait for (and accept) a response before moving to the next stimulus. For quick responders, the pace picks up, and this is technically more feasible because of the faster computer and faster test motors in HFA-II. The goal is for the patient to pace the test rather than vice versa; slow patients are given needed extra time, and quick patients are allowed to proceed faster. In general, the test time is reduced but, perhaps as important, the pacing is more comfortably in tune with the patient's behavior and capabilities.

Postprocessing. During testing, the SITA visual field model makes real-time threshold estimates based on the information thus far available. After testing has been completed, a more precise recomputation of all thresholds is made. It includes a reevaluation of the time interval (window) in which to accept responses, and thereby determines which responses were likely false answers and which are to be used to determine the final threshold estimate from the Bayesian posterior probability function.

Fewer catch trials. Postprocessing also produces inferential calculation of the rate of false responses. Not only does this method produce better estimates of both false-negative and false-positive response rates, as explained later, but it saves time by eliminating the need for any false-positive catch trials and greatly reducing the number of false-negative catch trials.

The SITA strategies use an information index for each point that determines when to stop.

DETERMINING TEST RELIABILITY

To judge the reliability of the test, it is traditional to evaluate the steadiness of fixation, a tendency for false-positive responses, and a tendency for false-negative responses. These indicators of patient performance originally were determined primarily from "catch trials," but currently are supplemented increasingly or replaced by use of a gaze tracker and computational inferences.

Fixation monitoring and gaze tracking

The accuracy of perimetry strongly depends upon patient gaze stability.

The accuracy of perimetric testing results is strongly affected by the stability of the patient's gaze during testing. An ideal perimeter would determine patient gaze direction with each stimulus presentation and adjust for any gaze errors, moving the stimulus presentation site so that the desired part of the retina could be stimulated regardless of where the patient was looking,[25] or reporting the result according to the retinal location actually stimulated. Because no such ideal perimeter yet exists, current gaze tracking methods involve recording the patient's gaze behavior so that a general estimate of the usefulness of the test result may be made. Three methods are available: observation by the perimetrist, the Heijl-Krakau blind spot technique for fixation monitoring, and the recently developed gaze monitor.

Perimetrist observation. To avoid trial lens artifacts, most perimeters provide some method of observing the patient's eye position—with either a telescope, a periscope, or a video camera. This same viewing arrangement also can be used to observe the patient's gaze stability so that summary notes may be recorded in the comments section of the printout. This was the method used in the Goldmann perimeter. It still is useful for the perimetrist to observe the patient's eye movements, not only to notice wandering gaze, but also to intervene and encourage steadier fixation.

The Heijl-Krakau blind spot method. Heijl and Krakau[26] described a method of fixation monitoring in which moderately bright stimuli are presented periodically at the expected location of the physiologic blind spot. The basic assumption of this blind spot technique is that if the patient presses the response button, there must have been a gaze error large enough to have moved a bit of seeing retina into the location of the stimulus. The magnitude of such an error would be at least half the diameter of the blind spot, or about 3 degrees. Overall, approximately 5% of stimulus presentations are used to test fixation, but fixation tests are more concentrated in the early part of the session so the perimetrist can monitor the record of fixation loss and take any necessary corrective action early in the test. Such action may include coaching the patient or pausing the test to run the subroutine that locates the blind spot again.

The blind spot technique depends on the accuracy of the presumption of the blind spot's location. The perimeter begins testing by assuming the normal location, but it stops early in the test and locates the blind spot if this initial assumption seems to be in error. Specifically, if the patient does not respond to either of the first two fixation catch trials, the standard location is accepted for the rest of the test—unless the perimetrist otherwise intervenes. If the patient responds to either of the first two trials, that response is not recorded as a fixation loss; instead, a subroutine of successive stimulus presentations is undertaken to locate the top, bottom, and sides of the blind spot. On the screen (and on the subsequent printout), a triangle indicates the location used for testing.

A common source of error in the blind spot method is associated with patient head tilt, especially that which occurs if the head drifts slowly from a perfectly vertical position as the test proceeds. A tilt of only a few degrees can rotate the blind spot sufficiently to bring normal retina to bear under the stimulus. Thus, it is useful for the perimetrist to check for head tilt from time to time, especially if a large number of fixation errors are being recorded. Measurement errors also may result if, early in the test, the patient failed to respond after actually seeing the initial presentation in the presumed blind spot location (see Chapter 11 for a discussion of observing the patient during blind spot localization). Patients who frequently make false-positive responses (described later) erroneously respond to stimuli presented in the blind spot; such responses are recorded as fixation losses rather than false-positive responses. Such erroneous reports of fixation loss may be combined under the term "pseudoloss of fixation."[27]

One frequently raised question is whether changing the size of the stimulus used for blind spot checks affects the reported rate of fixation loss. Usually, size is not the issue. The standard size-III stimulus subtends 0.43 degree, compared with the blind spot's diameter of about 5 degrees by 7 degrees. Thus the size-III stimulus is small compared with the blind spot (Fig. 5-4). This is why changing the blind spot stimulus (e.g., from size III to size II or size I, which also alters the intensity to maintain equal stimulus visibility) does not appreciably change the performance of the blind spot method. Improper localization causes false reports of fixation loss, and the best way to deal with blind spot problems usually is to reinstruct the patient, straighten the head, or replot the location of the blind spot.

> A common source of error in the Heijl-Krakau method is associated with patient head tilt.

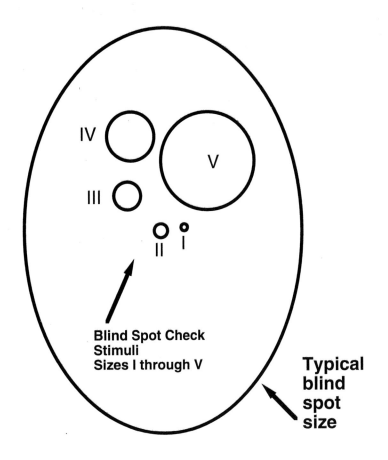

Normal Blind Spot: 5 degrees wide by 7 degrees tall

FIG. 5-4. Size of the Test Stimuli in Relation to the Size of the Physiologic Blind Spot. The normal blind spot is 5 degrees wide by 7 degrees tall. About two hundred size-3 stimuli or twelve size-V stimuli fit inside the area of the blind spot. (Courtesy of Humphrey Instruments, Inc., with permission)

The gaze monitor. Some recent models (700 series, HFA-II)[6] of the Humphrey perimeter are equipped with a full-time two-variable gaze monitor. This monitor uses image analysis methods to locate the center of the pupil and the location of the corneal reflection image of an infrared source (Fig. 5-5). The position of the corneal reflex relative to the pupil center depends strongly on gaze direction, but is much less affected by horizontal or vertical changes in head position. Gaze direction is noted only during stimulus presentation so that gaze errors in the intervals between stimulus presentations do not confuse the analysis.

The position of the light reflex also is used to calculate changes in horizontal and vertical head position. This information is used to make minuscule computer-controlled adjustments in patient head position to help keep the eye centered in the trial lens.

At the beginning of each test, a gaze monitor initialization procedure calibrates and adjusts the system to the individual patient. Mistakes in this procedure are the most common source of gaze monitor malfunction. Little is required of patients, except to look straight at the fixation point without blinking for approximately 20 seconds. The perimetrist must be careful to explain where the patient should look and how long he or she should stare without blinking.

During the test, gaze direction at the time of each stimulus presentation is charted cumulatively on the screen so that the perimetrist can intervene when necessary. Errors are indicated as upward deflections from baseline on the graph, with full scale being equal to 10 or more degrees of fixation error (Fig. 5-6). Downward deflections indicate absent pupil images or corneal reflexes, usually from a blink at the time of stimulus presentation.

One advantage of a full-time gaze monitor is that fixation is checked during 100% of the stimulus presentations, rather than 5%, as with the blind spot method. A second advantage is that no testing time is devoted to fixation check presentations, thus saving the 5% of testing time otherwise devoted to blind spot checks. This method also allows for quantification of the magnitude and direction of gaze errors and offers the possibility of future refinements (e.g., refinements in which responses associated with large fixation errors might be removed or reassigned to the proper retinal locus).

How the Two-Variable Gaze Tracker Works

Measures distance between pupil center and corneal reflex

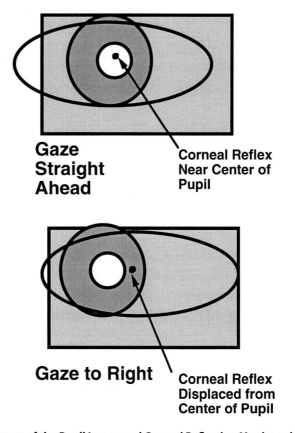

Gaze Straight Ahead

Corneal Reflex Near Center of Pupil

Gaze to Right

Corneal Reflex Displaced from Center of Pupil

FIG. 5-5. Diagram of the Pupil Image and Corneal Reflection Monitored by the Gaze Tracker. *Above,* the corneal reflex is in the position recorded when the gaze tracker is initialized (calibrated) before the test starts. *Below,* during gaze to the right, the reflex is displaced from its initial position in the pupil. If the head moves to the right without a shift in gaze angle, the pupil is no longer centered in the view, but the corneal reflex remains in nearly the same position in the pupil. (Courtesy Humphrey Instruments, Inc., with permission)

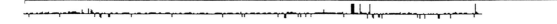

FIG. 5-6. Chart of Gaze Tracker Record. Most individuals show occasional deviations of gaze during the test, indicated by upward deflections in the tracing. Occasionally the pupil and corneal reflex are not visible to the instrument—for example, during a blink during the stimulus presentation; these are represented by downward deflections.

False-positive error rates

As catch trials detect false-positive (FP) responses, the Full Threshold and Fastpac strategies occasionally poise the hardware for presenting a stimulus but then do not actually do so. If the patient responds anyway, a false-positive response is recorded. The FP rate is the ratio of such responses to the total number of false-positive catch trial nonpresentations. In standard threshold tests these FP catch trials occur randomly once within each set of 33 successive test presentations; in suprathreshold tests they occur at a rate that gives about 10 FP catch trials in the course of the test. A running FP rate is displayed for the perimetrist to monitor the occurrence of false-positive responses.

The Sita strategy does not make explicit FP catch trials, but "listens" for false responses made before or more than a certain time after the response acceptance time windows.[18] The acceptance time window is based on the range of the patient's own response times for true responses (calculated during postprocessing taking into account that the patient's response time is affected by the stimulus intensity and may change during the test). For example, a response made 50 msec after a stimulus is too soon to be a response to a stimulus; it must be a random response or one made in anticipation of the stimulus. As another example, a response 2 seconds after a stimulus probably is too long after the stimulus; it is outside the acceptance window. Not all responses outside the acceptance interval are counted as false-positive responses. During postprocessing, some responses are "agnostic"—that is, they could be delayed true responses and thus are not counted as either true or false responses.[28]

With this method, the total "listen time" for false responses is much longer than the total time spent waiting for responses after false-positive catch trials in the non-Sita strategies, so the FP rate is determined far more precisely. During postprocessing, responses in the staircase sequence that in retrospect must have been false responses also are considered.[12] They are combined with the "listen time" data to create a maximum likelihood estimate of the false-positive rate; however, in practice these staircase false responses often do not have much effect on the FP rate that would have been calculated from the "listen time" data alone. The final result is reported as the probability of a false response during the patient's own average response interval length. The FP rate means the same as the FP ratio to catch trials, which is the number of responses per deliberate interval of waiting.

Careful patient instruction before the test and encouragement during the test can help reduce false-positive errors (see Chapter 11). High false-positive rates often occur if patients believe that they should report whenever they believe the light is on by any means of perception (seeing the light, hearing the shutter, or guessing that it is time for another stimulus) instead of simply reporting when the light is visible. False-positive responses also may occur if the patient is anxious or "trigger happy," as the result of a false impression that he must act with haste and respond while the light is still on. Patients should be told that the machine waits for a time to receive a response after the brief stimulus, and moreover, that most subjects see fewer than half of the stimuli presented. Patients who tend to make false-positive errors should be urged to make slower, more deliberate, and more certain responses. The perimetrist should pay special attention early in the test so that patients can be reinstructed and the test restarted if two or more FP responses occur early in the test.

False-negative error rates

In principle, the false-negative (FN) rate is the proportion of visible stimuli to which the patient fails to respond because of inattention. In the Full Threshold and Fastpac strategies, the FN rate is estimated at locations at which measurements of threshold sensitivity have been completed. Stimuli are presented that are 9 dB brighter than the threshold sensitivity already measured at that location. The patient is expected to see this stimulus easily, and if he fails to respond, the failure is recorded as an FN error. The intent is that the FN errors represent periods of inattention by the patient, but if the stimulus is presented in diseased locations with a broadened frequency-of-seeing curve, there are times when the stimulus is in fact not visible even to an attentive patient. The false-negative catch trials are performed randomly within each block of 33 presentations but may be skipped in the early blocks of 33 presentations if a threshold value has not yet been determined. Such FN catch trial stimuli represent about 3% of the stimulus presentations.

In the SITA strategies, the FN response rate comes from a maximum likelihood function combining two data sets.[12,14,16] One is the failure to respond in the up-and-down staircase to stimuli that should be visible. The second is a small number of explicit FN catch trials performed with stimuli intense enough to be seen with near certainty based on the slope of the frequency-of-seeing curve at that location, which in turn is assumed from the current threshold estimate at that point. A catch trial is included in the final calculation only if during postprocessing the final threshold value at that location and its corresponding frequency-of-seeing curve make it very likely that the stimulus was indeed visible.

Patient inconsistency produces a high false-negative rate. This may occur if the patient is fundamentally inconsistent in responses, changes criterion about whether a stimulus is too dim to report seeing it, has a changing state of alertness, or slows down and sometimes does not respond to a stimulus he sees, believing that it is too late to respond if the light has gone off.

High false-negative rates also are produced by patients who are reliable perimetry subjects but who have abnormal fields because visibility of near-threshold stimuli is highly variable at abnormal locations. At such locations, even an alert patient legitimately may not be able to see a stimulus much more intense than the one seen just minutes before; thus a high false-negative rate is recorded as a result of disease rather than of inattentiveness by the patient. To minimize this contribution of disease to the FN rate, SITA FN catch trials are performed only in relatively normal parts of the visual field, the intensity of the stimulus is adjusted according to the current threshold estimate, and failure to respond is counted as an FN error only if the slope of the frequency-of-seeing curve estimated after postprocessing makes it highly likely that the stimulus was indeed visible. In this way, the reported FN rate in the SITA strategy more strongly relates to patient inattention and practically is unaffected by locations with abnormal threshold sensitivity and broadened frequency-of-seeing curves from disease.

In the Full Threshold and Fastpac strategies false-negative rates are affected both by patient attentiveness and by visual field loss itself.

CURRENT THRESHOLDING ALGORITHMS: SUMMARY

Most Humphrey perimeters have two basic algorithms for determining threshold sensitivity at each test point location: the Full Threshold method and Fastpac, which is briefer but somewhat less precise. In addition, the newer Humphrey perimeters have two more efficient strategies, called SITA Standard and SITA Fast. SITA Standard gives a level of precision that is very similar to that of Full Threshold but takes about half the testing time; similarly, SITA Fast was designed to give the same precision as Fastpac in about half its testing time. Any of the strategies can be used with a 30-degree pattern of test locations, or with other patterns, such as the one that covers only the central 24 degrees of the visual field. Both the strategy chosen and the number of points tested affect the test time (Fig. 5-7).

The Full Threshold and Fastpac strategies have stood the test of time. The two SITA strategies are becoming popular, give the practitioner additional useful options, and may soon replace the older strategies for many clinicians. SITA Standard has been shown more clearly to be highly reliable, but for elderly or easily fatigued patients, the shorter SITA Fast algorithm sometimes provides a clearer diagnostic picture. Taking into account all previous experience, we believe that the 30-2 and 24-2 patterns, a white size-III test stimulus, and either the Full Threshold or the SITA Standard strategy are the appropriate choices for the majority of common clinical circumstances. When a short test is needed, 24-2 testing with Fastpac or with SITA Fast may be chosen. Details of other test options and appropriate test selection, especially for less frequent clinical needs, are covered in Chapter 8.

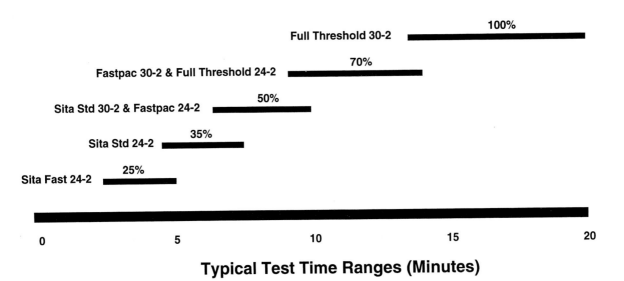

Typical Test Time Ranges (Minutes)

FIG. 5-7. Comparative Test Times for Four Mainstream Test Algorithms. Percentages are relative to typical test time for Full Threshold 30-2 testing. (Courtesy Humphrey Systems, with permission)

SUPRATHRESHOLD TESTS

Threshold tests are designed to estimate or measure the threshold sensitivity. Suprathreshold tests determine whether the visual sensitivity at a particular location is better than some chosen criterion. Such a test may detect an abnormality and outline its location and extent but does not quantify its depth. The obvious advantage of the test is that the test time is short if there is only one stimulus presentation at each test location. Its main uses are to detect an abnormality (screening), to characterize the topographical nature of an abnormality (diagnosis), and to quantify the boundary of the visual field (e.g., to calculate disability or document the effect of ptosis).

As with threshold testing, a pattern of points is chosen that blankets the area of diagnostic interest, and often this may be the same 76 locations represented in the 30-2 threshold test. In some strategies, if the stimulus is not visible, the depth of the defect may be further categorized.

One of the three methods described next is commonly used for setting the level of stimulus intensity for suprathreshold testing, and any of these three strategies may be used to categorize the level of any loss that may be found.

Three methods for level setting

For screening and diagnostic purposes, the stimulus intensity may be set based on age,[29] on individual threshold sensitivity—measured at a few points at the beginning of the test (threshold-related screening), or on a useful standard. *Age-related screenings* are performed in the Humphrey perimeter with stimuli 8 dB (0.8 log unit) more intense than the mean age-corrected normal sensitivity at each test point. *Threshold-related screenings* are based on the second most sensitive of actual threshold measurements made at the four standard locations at the beginning of the test, after which suprathreshold testing is performed at all test locations, with stimuli 6 dB more intense than the expected threshold sensitivity at each location (adjusting for sector and eccentricity). *Single intensity screenings* are conducted with the same stimulus intensity at all locations. The intensity is selected to represent some standard for quantifying disability, determining the extent of field needed for driving, and for similar purposes (most often a 10-dB stimulus, equivalent to Goldmann's III-4e stimulus, is selected).

In general, for detection and diagnosis, we lean toward the use of age-related instead of threshold-related suprathreshold tests. Age-related testing takes less time than threshold-related procedures because it eliminates preliminary thresholding of points, and it usually is sufficiently sensitive to detect signs of disease. Age-related testing also may be more consistent because it is not dependent on the patient's ability early in the test to respond to near-threshold stimuli. However, localized scotomas may not be isolated by age-related testing in patients who have significant media opacities. In such cases, sensitivity is reduced at all locations, and the relatively greater loss at a few locations is masked. Moreover, threshold-related testing may detect shallow relative scotomas in a person with supranormal visual sensation. Theoretically, in such cases, threshold-related testing has the advantage of tailoring the testing protocol to each patient's overall hill of vision. However, age-related testing seems more practical when shallow relative scotomas are infrequent or inconsequential and there is also an opportunity to retest patients with broad depression of visual sensation that might mask localized defects.

Three strategies to categorize loss

In the standard suprathreshold procedure of the Humphrey perimeter, missed stimuli automatically are repeated before the location is recorded as not seeing the stimulus. Before the test, the perimetrist chooses whether such locations are further characterized. There are three choices:

1. With the Two-Zone mode, there is no further testing, and points missed twice are marked on the printout with a black symbol indicating abnormal sensitivity at that location (Fig. 5-8).

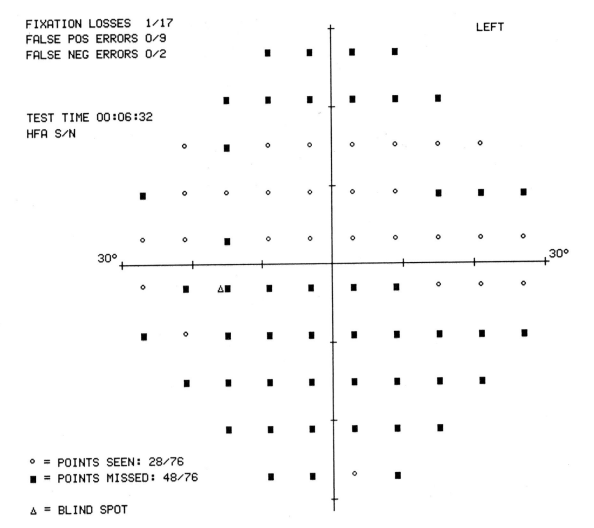

FIXATION LOSSES   1/17
FALSE POS ERRORS 0/9
FALSE NEG ERRORS 0/2

LEFT

TEST TIME 00:06:32
HFA S/N

30°   30°

o = POINTS SEEN: 28/76
■ = POINTS MISSED: 48/76

△ = BLIND SPOT

FIG. 5-8. Central 76-Point Suprathreshold Screening Test; Two-Zone Strategy. The test points are in the same locations as the central 30-2 pattern used for threshold testing. Black squares indicate where the test stimulus was not seen, given two opportunities.

2. The Three-Zone mode takes the further step of exposing twice-missed locations to a maximal luminance 10,000-asb (0-dB) stimulus. If the maximal stimulus is not seen, the location is categorized as having an "absolute" defect, but if the maximal stimulus is seen, the location is categorized as having a relative defect (Fig. 5-9).

3. The Quantify Defects mode actually intensifies the stimulus level in 4-dB steps until it is finally seen, and then dims it again in 2-dB steps until again it is not seen. Thus, the Quantify Defects mode is a screening procedure in which missed points are thresholded, and threshold sensitivity loss is displayed relative to the expected hill of vision for that patient. If very many locations are thresholded, the test becomes lengthy—longer than the standard threshold tests, which save time by determining the most efficient starting intensity for the thresholding sequence.

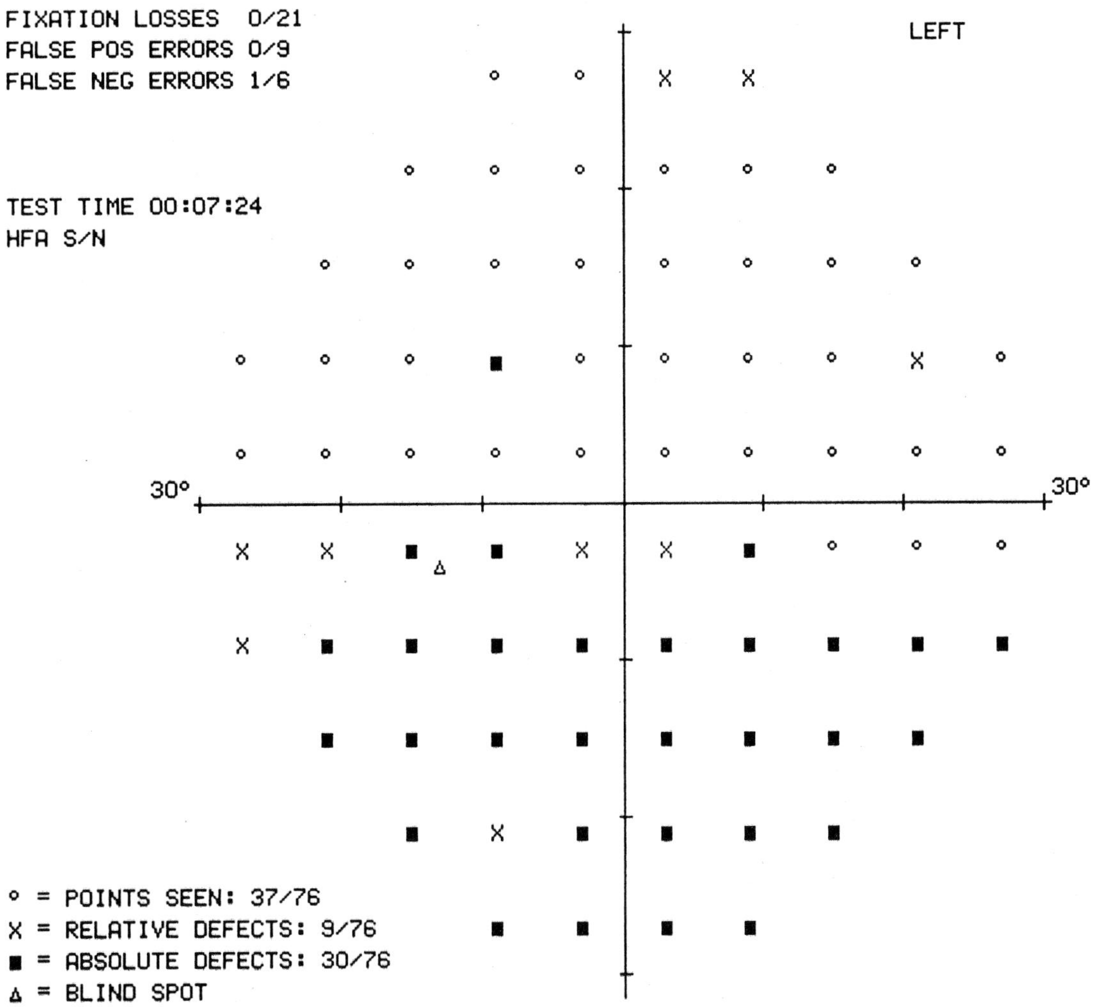

FIXATION LOSSES 0/21
FALSE POS ERRORS 0/9
FALSE NEG ERRORS 1/6

LEFT

TEST TIME 00:07:24
HFA S/N

30°   30°

○ = POINTS SEEN: 37/76
X = RELATIVE DEFECTS: 9/76
■ = ABSOLUTE DEFECTS: 30/76
Δ = BLIND SPOT

FIG. 5-9. Three-Zone Strategy. Again, a central 76-point screening pattern was tested. Defective locations are classified as relative or absolute.

Suprathreshold testing vs. thresholding

For glaucoma management, threshold testing is preferable to suprathreshold screening.

The balance between the time needed for testing and the amount of information obtained affects the choice of whether to use a thresholding method or the briefer and simpler suprathreshold strategy. At least for glaucoma, it generally has become accepted that the more detailed information provided by threshold testing is useful for detecting early cases in an office setting, and it is certainly the standard method for following the course of the disease.[11] However, there are times when suprathreshold tests are practical for detecting and characterizing visual deficits (see Chapter 8). Population screening,[30] or even uncovering and diagnosing suspected neurologic disease,[29] may be well addressed by suprathreshold tests, although the familiar 30-2 threshold testing remains the more frequently used and generally accepted standard for definitive diagnosis and for detection of subtle abnormality.

STRUCTURING THE TEST CONDITIONS

Patient instruction

Threshold perimetric testing is a demanding and unfamiliar task for patients. Moreover, threshold perimetry is performed only when signs, symptoms, or history suggests the presence of disease, and patients often are justifiably anxious as a result. Most test stimuli are presented at or below the threshold of vision—a procedure guaranteed to cause further anxiety in patients already alerted to the possibility of vision loss. The test is administered by a computerized instrument in a dark room—hardly a reassuring experience, especially if the patient has no idea how long the test will last. The test is perceptually complex, with some stimuli being easily seen, others only faintly seen, and still others not seen at all; the test spots also may show up anywhere in the visual field at any time. The bowl is for the most part featureless and sometimes becomes disorienting. If the patient's non-dominant eye is being tested, retinal rivalry may produce a visual perception alternating between that of the bright bowl and that of the darkly occluded dominant eye; the background illumination of the bowl will seem to be alternately dim and bright. Refractive correction is accomplished using a lens held stationary relative to the instrument—and not necessarily stationary relative to the patient; thus, the patient must take care to remain aligned relative to the lens, or artifactual field loss may be recorded. Staying motionless for the duration may be tiring.

The perimetrist affects the test quality.

All of these considerations highlight the importance of the interaction between perimetrist and patient. Careful attention from the perimetrist can make all the difference; it can make the patient's experience far more pleasant and acceptable, and it can help yield test results that make the interpretation task far simpler for the doctor. To relieve anxiety and improve performance, the patient should be told that the machine will seek the dimmest stimulus that the patient can see, and therefore many of the stimuli will be very dim or even invisible. It is very helpful if the technician recognizes that he is performing the test with the use of the perimeter, and not that the perimeter is performing the test with the perimetrist simply monitoring or supervising.

The perimetrist's tasks include patient instruction and monitoring, as well as the technical details of using the proper lens and pausing and interacting with the machine when needed (these technical skills are covered in Chapter 11). The perimetrist should, at the beginning of the test, tell patients carefully and sympathetically the importance of the test, what to expect, and what to do. If the technician watches the patient with particular care for the first minute or so of testing, errors can be caught early, and lengthy and disconcerting retests may be avoided. If, during the test, the technician offers a word or two of encouragement, anxiety is reduced, test reliability is increased, and future compliance is improved. An investment of attentive instruction during the first field test will pay dividends on future tests.

Mydriatics and pupil size

The visibility of a stimulus depends heavily on the contrast between the stimulus and the background; fortunately, when the pupil size changes, the light intensity of both the stimulus and the background change in proportion, and contrast is unaffected. However, visibility also depends somewhat on retinal adaptation, determined by the total amount of light reaching the retina, and thus is not completely independent of pupil size. Pupil size also determines which part and how much of the crystalline lens is used to focus the retinal image; and the optical properties of the center and periphery of the lens may not be the same. Optical properties change from one person to another and when disease (e.g., nuclear sclerosis) is present. Moreover, light scatter (e.g., from cortical spokes, posterior subcapsular lens opacities, or capsular opacity in pseudophakic patients) has considerable effect on the retinal image contrast.

Thus, the clinician must decide whether to dilate patients undergoing perimetry. The decision may affect the clinician's ability to judge abnormality and his patient's ability to judge change (progression) of the field. In general, testing with the spontaneous pupil size is best, and patients should not be dilated unless there is a clear reason. Diagnostic tests performed after a full eye examination with pupil dilation may prove difficult to interpret. A subcapsular cataract that seriously impedes vision in the undilated state may be an example of an exception. A patient also may be dilated if necessary to facilitate other aspects of the office visit, (e.g., optic disk evaluation), as long as the pupil size is consistent with what was present at baseline; this approach adds an element of unpredictability because the amount of dilation may vary from visit to visit, but the procedure may be necessary to improve clinic flow.

All Humphrey normal data were collected from subjects with natural, undilated pupils. When the objective is to decide whether the field is normal, the data analysis aids provided with the instrument are best applied to patients having natural pupils. When the objective is to judge the progression of disease, consistency of pupil size is more important than the size per se. Even with statistical aids like the Glaucoma Change Probability analysis, it must be realized that the test-retest variability empirically found in glaucoma patients, which is the basis of the

> All Humphrey normals data were collected from subjects having natural, undiluted pupils.

analysis, was obtained from patients in whom no change in pharmaceutical regimen was made.

> Carefully recording pupil size at each visit helps to identify inconsistencies caused by variations in pupil size.

Carefully recording pupil size at each visit helps to identify inconsistencies caused by variations in pupil size. Automatic measurement of pupil size is now an available option on one model of the Humphrey perimeter. This method offers higher precision than generally can be achieved by conventional observation and may end up providing greater availability of pupil size data because the perimetrist no longer will have to remember to make the measurement at the time of each perimetric examination.

Refractive correction

The use of trial lenses should be avoided when the refractive state of the eye permits. Although more than 1 D of blur can affect the result, it is also true that the trial lens holder frequently causes artifactual field defects that can seriously complicate interpretation and statistical data analysis (see Chapters 2 and 7). Therefore, when a standard size-III stimulus is used, refractive corrections of less than 1 D probably are best ignored in the interest of keeping the trial lens holder out of the way. Additionally, it is best to use the weakest lens that will permit the patient to focus clearly on the fixation light; for example, 3-D myopes of any age will not need a lens, and others who have not undergone lens extraction or been given cycloplegic agents may be young enough to use part of their accommodation comfortably for the test duration. The Humphrey perimeter is programmed to suggest a trial lens that is consistent with this philosophy. In any case, the patient always should be asked to confirm that the fixation light is reasonably clear before testing (see Chapter 11) in the event that, for example, a -3.00-D lens is inadvertently placed in the lens holder instead of the intended $+3.00$-D lens. The effect of a 6-D error in a lens used for perimetry is illustrated in Figures 2-6 and 2-7. Anyone is capable of such a mistake.

The testing environment

For standard white-on-white Humphrey perimetry, room lighting should be low, but it need not be completely dark. The perimeter will alert the operator if the room is too bright. To some degree, the instrument is capable of correcting for the effects of localized shadows in the bowl caused by uneven room lighting, although it is best to avoid routine reliance on this corrective function. If SWAP testing is being performed, lighting conditions must more carefully be kept low, and the bowl must be kept free of shadows because of the specific wavelengths used in illuminating the bowl (see Chapters 2 and 8).

Tests require the patient to concentrate and should be performed in a quiet room, away from the bustle of the clinic and the noise of the waiting room. It is possible to have more than one perimeter operating in a room at the same time, although some difficulties may be encountered if one patient overhears and acts on instructions intended for another. Some patients may require more isolation from distraction than others.

The patient should be seated in an upright position in a low, comfortable office chair. Use of clinic stools can be both dangerous and uncomfortable because of a lack of stability and body support. The newer, smaller perimeters make it easier to provide comfortable access even for large and obese patients. More details on patient comfort are given in Chapter 11.

REFERENCES

1. Heijl A: Perimetric point density and detection of glaucomatous visual field loss, *Acta Ophthalmol* [Copenh] 71:445-50, 1993.
2. Heijl A: Humphrey Field Analyzer. In Drance SM, Anderson DR: *Automatic perimetry in glaucoma: A practical guide,* p 129, Orlando, Fla, 1985, Grune & Stratton.
3. Heijl A: The Humphrey Field Analyzer: Construction and concepts, *Doc Ophthalmol Proc Ser* 42:77-84, 1985.
4. Heijl A: The Humphrey Field Analyzer: Concepts and clinical results, *Doc Ophthalmol Proc Ser* 43:55-64, 1985.
5. Haley MJ (editor): *The Field Analyzer primer,* ed 2, San Leandro, Calif, 1987, Allergan Humphrey.
6. Johnson CA, Cioffi GA, Drance SM et al: A multicenter comparison study of the Humphrey Field Analyzer I and the Humphrey Field Analyzer II, *Ophthalmology* 104:1910-1917, 1997.
7. Iwase A, Kitazawa Y, Kato Y: Clinical value of Fastpac: A comparative study with the Standard Full Threshold method. In Mills RP, Wall M, editors: *Perimetry update 1992/93: Proceedings of the Xth International Perimetric Society Meeting, Kyoto, 1992,* p 365, Amsterdam, 1993, Kugler.
8. O'Brien C, Poinoosawmy S, Wu J, Hitchings R: Statpac-Fastpac comparison in glaucoma. In Mills RP, Wall M, editors: *Perimetry update 1992/93: Proceedings of the Xth International Perimetric Society Meeting, Kyoto, 1992,* p 369, Amsterdam, 1993, Kugler.
9. Hatch W, Flanagan JG, Trope GE: Evaluation of repeatability of Fastpac in glaucoma. In Mills RP, Wall M, editors: *Perimetry update 1994/95: Proceedings of the XIth International Perimetric Society Meeting, Kyoto, 1994,* p 239, Amsterdam, 1995, Kugler.
10. O'Donnel NP, Birch MK, Wishart PK: Fastpac error is within the long-term fluctuation of Standard Humphrey threshold visual field testing. In Mills RP, Wall M, editors: *Perimetry update 1994/95: Proceedings of the XIth International Perimetric Society Meeting, Washington, DC, 1994,* p 231, Amsterdam, 1995, Kugler.
11. Mills RP, Barnebey HS, Migliazzo CV, Li-Y: Does saving time using FASTPAC or suprathreshold testing reduce utility of visual fields? *Ophthalmology* 101:1596-603, 1994.
12. Olsson J, Rootzén H, Heijl A: Maximum likelihood estimation of the frequency of false positive and false negative answers from the up-and-down staircases of computerized threshold perimetry. In Heijl A, editor: *Perimetry update 1988-89: Proceedings of the VIIIth International Perimetric Society Meeting, Vancouver, 1988,* p 245, Amsterdam, 1989, Kugler.
13. Olsson J, Åsman P, Rootzén H, Heijl A: Improved threshold estimates using full staircase data. In Mills RP, Heijl A, editors: *Perimetry update 1990-91, Proceedings of the IXth International Perimetric Society Meeting, Malmö, 1990,* p 245, Amsterdam, 1991, Kugler.
14. Olsson J, Heijl A, Bengtsson B, Rootzén H: Frequency-of-seeing in computerized perimetry. In Mills RP, editor: *Perimetry update 1992/1993, Proceedings of the Xth International Perimetric Society Meeting, Kyoto, 1992,* p 551, Amsterdam, 1993, Kugler.
15. Olsson J, Bengtsson B, Heijl A, Rootzén H: New threshold algorithms for automated static perimetry. In Mills RP, Wall M, editors: *Perimetry update 1994/95, Proceedings of the XIth International Perimetric Society Meeting, Washington, DC, 1994,* p 265, Amsterdam, 1995, Kugler.
16. Olsson J, Bengtsson B, Heijl A, Rootzén H: Improving estimation of false-positive and false-negative responses in computerized perimetry. In Mills RP, Wall M, editors: *Perimetry update 1994/95, Proceedings of the XIth International Perimetric Society Meeting, Washington, DC, 1994,* p 219, Amsterdam, 1995, Kugler.
17. Bengtsson B, Olsson J, Heijl A, Rootzen H: A new generation of algorithms for computerized threshold perimetry, SITA, *Acta Ophthlamol Scand* 75:368-375, 1997.

18. Olsson J, Bengtsson B, Heijl A, Rootzen H: An improved method to estimate frequency of false positive answers in computerized perimetry, *Acta Ophthalmol Scand* 75:181-183, 1997.

19. Bengtsson B, Heijl A, Olsson J: Evaluation of a new threshold visual field strategy, SITA, in normal subjects, *Acta Ophthalmol Scand* 76:165-169, 1998.

20. Bengtsson Boel, Heijl Anders: Evaluation of a new threshold visual field strategy, SITA, in patients with suspect and manifest glaucoma. *Acta Ophthalmol Scand* (in press), 1998.

21. Bengtsson Boel, Heijl Anders: SITA Fast, a new rapid perimetric threshold test. Description of methods and evaluation in patients with manifest and suspect glaucoma, *Acta Ophthalmol Scand* (in press), 1998.

22. Olsson J, Rootzén H: An image model for quantal response analysis in perimetry, *Scand J Statistics* 21(4):375-387, 1994.

23. Olsson J, Heijl A, Rootzén H: US patent number 5,461,435, issued Oct 24, 1995.

24. Olsson J, Heijl A, Rootzén H: US patent number 5,381,195, issued Jan 10, 1995.

25. Tate GW, Lynn JR: *Principles of quantitative perimetry: Testing and interpreting the visual field,* p. 279, New York, 1977, Grune Stratton.

26. Heijl A, Krakau CET: An automatic static perimeter: Design and pilot study, *Acta Ophthalmol* [Copenh] 53:293-310, 1975.

27. Sanabria O, Feuer WJ, Anderson DR: Pseudo-loss of fixation in automated perimetry, *Ophthalmology* 98:76-78, 1991.

28. Olsson J, Heijl A, Rootzén H: US patent number 5,598,235,issued Jan 28, 1997.

29. Siatkowski RM, Lam B, Anderson DR et al: Automated suprathreshold static perimetry screening in neuro-ophthalmology, *Ophthalmology* 103:907-917, 1996.

30. Sponsel WE, Ritch R, Stamper R et al for the Prevent Blindness America Glaucoma Advisory Committee: Prevent Blindness America visual field screening study, *Am J Ophthalmol* 120:699-708, 1995.

CHAPTER 6

The single field printout

The standard single field Statpac printout presents the raw test results of a single 30-2, 24-2, or 10-2 threshold test along with a statistical analysis of the results relative to age-corrected normal data. There are several different packets of information presented on the printout, including:

1. Basic identification of patient and test;
2. Indicators of test reliability;
3. Raw unprocessed threshold sensitivity measurements;
4. Deviations of measured sensitivities from age normal (total deviation);
5. Deviations from normal after adjustment for the patient's overall sensitivity (pattern deviation);
6. Overall indices of normality (global indices); and
7. Plain-language analysis (the Glaucoma Hemifield Test).

BASIC IDENTIFICATION

> Puzzling diagnostic problems may be resolved by confirming basic data: birth date, eye tested, stimulus size, test used.

The section at the top of the printout identifies the patient by name and date of birth and indicates which eye was tested. It also lists which test was used and how and when the test was administered. All too often seemingly difficult diagnostic problems can be resolved simply by confirming these basic data. Erroneously entered birth dates or incorrectly sized stimuli can wrongly suggest that the visual field is abnormal or has changed. Testing a normal right eye when the instrument expects a left eye can produce results that look quite pathological. Mistaking a 10-2 test for a 30-2 test can result in misinterpretation, as can mistaking a test performed in 1985 for one performed in 1995. All these mistakes have been made and will happen again to anyone who is not careful enough to routinely verify the basics before interpreting test results.

RELIABILITY PARAMETERS

During a perimetric test, three types of reliability parameters are generated: those to estimate the stability of patient gaze (fixation); those intended to estimate the patient's tendency to make false-positive response errors; and those intended to estimate the rate of false-negative response errors.

Gaze stability

Perimetric testing depends on knowing where the patient is looking so stimuli may be presented at known locations in the visual field. The accuracy of the test results can be strongly affected by the strength or weakness of the patient's ability to stay focused on the fixation target during the test. The Heijl-Krakau blind spot method described in Chapter 5 can be used to monitor and record a patient's fixation loss (FL) rate during the test. Field analyzers of the 700 series (HFA-II) are equipped with a gaze monitor, which can be used in addition to or in place of the blind spot checking technique.

When the blind spot checking method is used, the FL rate is recorded on the printout as the ratio of the number of times the patient responded to the blind spot stimulus divided by the total number of such presentations. The letter X is printed twice next to the FL rate whenever the ratio exceeds 20% (Fig. 6-1).

Perimeters equipped with a gaze monitor show fixation errors on the screen during the test so that the perimetrist can make adjustments or instruct the patient when necessary. A tracing appears at the bottom of the printout (see Fig. 5-6), and its interpretation is covered in Chapter 7.

False-positive error rates

The perimetric false-positive (FP) error rate in the non-SITA strategies is the frequency with which the patient presses the button during FP catch trials, which are pauses during which no stimulus is presented. The number of erroneous

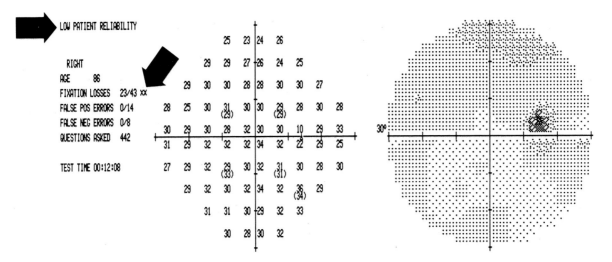

FIG. 6-1. Example of Field Test Indicated as Unreliable. See Figures 7-1 through 7-10 for other examples.

responses per catch trial is given as a ratio. The letter X is printed twice next to the FP ratio when it exceeds 33%.

The SITA strategies do not make explicit FP catch trials but calculate FP rates from responses at unexpected times during the test. The SITA false positive rates are expressed as percentages and represent the probability that the patient would make an FP response during the acceptance interval after a stimulus presentation (the duration of which is determined separately according to the individual's response times). The details of this calculation are given in Chapter 5.

False-negative error rates

The perimetric false-negative (FN) error rate is the frequency with which the patient fails to press the response button when a visible stimulus is presented. A high FN rate represents an inconsistent responsiveness of the patient or loss of attentiveness to the task at hand. For tests run using the Full Threshold and Fastpac strategies, the false negative rate (FN) is expressed on the printout as the ratio of the number of times the patient failed to respond to a stimulus 9 dB more intense than the previously determined threshold estimate divided by the total number of such FN catch trials. As with false-positive responses, an XX appears next to the FN rate on the printout when it exceeds 33%.

For tests using the SITA strategies, the result is displayed as a percentage instead of a ratio. The recorded parameter more closely represents the percentage of time the patient fails to respond to visible stimuli because of inconsistency or inattentiveness because the strategy does not consider any failure to respond during the test that might be caused by disease (see Chapter 5).

Tests labeled as having low reliability

Tests become increasingly unreliable with FP rates over 10 to 15%.

When the Humphrey perimeter was first developed and a database of normal values was collected as a basis for statistical evaluation of the results of the Full Threshold strategy, fields in the database were not included if they had suspect reliability indices. The purpose was to exclude unreliable test takers from the normative database. Thus, fields were excluded if the fixation loss rate was greater than 20%, or if either the false-positive rate or the false-negative rate exceeded 33%. For the Statpac statistical calculations based on the normal values to be strictly valid, the patient must have met these same criteria. Therefore, XX is printed next to the tabulation of each reliability parameter ratio that exceeds these limits, and a caution message, "low patient reliability," appears on the printout. The same criteria are used for the Fastpac strategy.

Accumulated experience currently suggests that the caution message might better read, "broader limits of normal values may apply than the ones used by the Statpac analysis" (see Chapter 7). The caution message therefore should be considered only a warning that the statistical analysis from the normative database is not completely valid because patients with these reliability parameters were excluded from the database. The test marked "low patient reliability" does not necessarily lack useful information. One first must make an effort to discern the cause for the inappropriate responses in this particular test. *High FL rates* often are "pseudolosses" of fixation from undetected patient misalignment; frequently the patient's gaze was perfectly stable throughout testing, and the test result is perfectly valid. *High FP rates* almost always indicate an unreliable test; in fact FP rates of only 10% to 15% may produce unreliable test results. When FP catch trials are used to determine the FP rate, the small number of catch trials (1 per 33 stimulus presentations) may fail to detect moderately trigger-happy patients (see Figs. 7-1 through 7-3). When using the Full Threshold and Fastpac strategies, *high FN rates* in abnormal visual fields are common in perfectly attentive patients who consistently respond to visible stimuli (the SITA strategies reduce the link of field abnormality and elevated FN rates). In normal visual fields, high FN rates usually mean that the patient is inconsistent or became inattentive late in the test; usually in such instances there are areas falsely labeled with subnormal visual sensation, and the test result appears abnormal. When FN rates are high, separating truly abnormal fields from those that falsely appear to be abnormal can be a problem in the non-SITA strategies. The details of interpretation are covered later (Chapter 7).

> High FL rates often are due to patient misalignment rather than to unsteady fixation.

QUESTIONS AND TEST TIME

The "Questions asked" report on the printout is perplexing until it is understood that the question, "Do you see this?" represents each stimulus presentation. The number of stimulus presentations (questions asked) is tabulated and is closely correlated to the recorded test time. Fields characterized by irregular threshold values or inconsistent responses (e.g., high pattern standard deviation, short-term fluctuation [SF], FP, FL) require the longest time, whereas tests of severely abnormal fields often are very short. These parameters help the clinician select efficient test strategies to reduce the time the patient must spend in concentrated effort. The numbers represent the time spent presenting stimuli and do not include time spent on set-up and explanations to the patient.

RAW TEST RESULTS

Threshold sensitivity values

Decibel threshold sensitivity values are displayed as a map (sensitivity value table), except that the sensitivity value at the fovea is listed over to the side along with the reliability parameters. In classical (Full Threshold and Fastpac) strategies, repeat determinations of threshold at a location are given in parentheses underneath the values initially determined (Fig. 6-2). With the SITA strategies, only one value is given because the nature of the test is to probe all locations with additional stimuli until a single best estimate of threshold sensitivity comes within a predefined confidence limit or is as reliable as can be obtained practically.

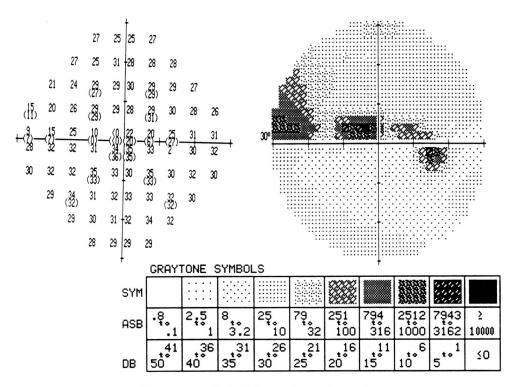

FIG. 6-2. Threshold Value Table and Greyscale.

Interpolated greyscale

To develop a greyscale printout, interpolated threshold sensitivity values are assigned to locations between the test points and threshold sensitivities are combined into groups 5 dB in width, so that the range from 1 to 40 dB is assigned to eight levels of grey. Thus, the greyscale is another way of displaying raw threshold data and is not a statistical or normative analysis.

The greyscale (see Fig. 6-2) is helpful in identifying general patterns of field loss and in calling attention to locations that may be abnormal. However, this analysis can be misleading, and the clinician must examine thoughtfully the actual sensitivity values in areas called to his attention by the greyscale appearance. For example, two locations with different degrees of grey may be only 1 dB apart (e.g., 21 dB vs. 20 dB), or they actually may differ in sensitivity by as much as 9 dB (e.g., 16 dB vs. 25 dB). On printouts with only two levels of grey, all values are within 10 dB of each other; three or more levels of grey mean that some locations are at least 10 dB different from others. Some parts of the visual field may appear dark and yet not be associated with disease (e.g., dark areas caused by eyelid artifacts or the normal reduction in sensitivity that occurs with age). Thus the clinician also must look to other analyses, such as the probability maps described later, to confirm any impressions gleaned from the greyscale. The darkness or greyness of a given region also is affected by the freshness of the ribbon in dot matrix printers

> The greyscale may not highlight mild, but definite visual field loss.

and differences in the spacing and size of the dots with other printers. The clinician must take this into account when comparing a series of visual fields produced on different printers. Finally, black areas with less than 0 dB of sensitivity represent regions at which the maximal stimulus available was not seen, but they may not represent a total loss of visual function at that location; a larger stimulus might be seen, as might objects in the environment during daily activities.

Reliability parameters, sensitivity values, and the greyscale represent the raw data obtained during a test session. The remainder of the printout contains analyses in which the raw data are compared with a normal database.

TOTAL DEVIATION (FROM NORMAL VALUES FOR AGE)

> The TOTAL deviation probability map highlights test points that are significantly less sensitive than normal.

Total Deviation is the difference at each test point between the patient's measured threshold sensitivity and the median normal value for the patient's age. The total deviation display has two parts: a table of numeric values, which represents the actual decibel deviation from age-normal, and below that, a probability plot showing symbols that indicate the statistical significance of each measured deviation.[1-5]

A past rule of thumb, based on initial observations with automated static threshold perimetry, was that a sensitivity value was considered abnormal if it was more than 5 dB worse than the mean normal value for age, and the suggested use of probabilities was based on Gaussian statistics.[1] Subsequent empirical studies of normal subjects with the Humphrey perimeter showed that deviations of less than 5 dB may be noteworthy near the center of the field and that even 10-dB deviations near the edge of the visual field may well be within the normal range.[6] The perimeter's computer is programmed with this empirical information in the form of significance limits for the differing normal variability at each location, thus relieving the practitioner of the burden of memorizing a mass of information.

A key to the probability symbols is shown near the bottom of the printout. The symbols increase in darkness as the deviation becomes more significant. The significance limits used were empirically derived by direct non-Gaussian statistics as one-tailed percentiles within a database of normal field examinations.[2] Thus, for example, marking a test location with the symbol for $p < 1\%$ means that fewer than 1% of reliable normal fields in the age-corrected database have a sensitivity value that low.

In both the numeric and probability displays of total deviation, the two points nearest the typical location of the physiologic blind spot are not represented because little diagnostic information is contained in points that are physiologically expected to be blind or at least highly variable from one person to another.

The deviation from the normal probability display can call attention to subtle abnormalities (deviations from normal) in diagnostically typical locations, even when the greyscale fails to highlight the defective region (Fig. 6-3). Conversely, it may sometimes indicate that a dark region on the greyscale is not outside normal limits.

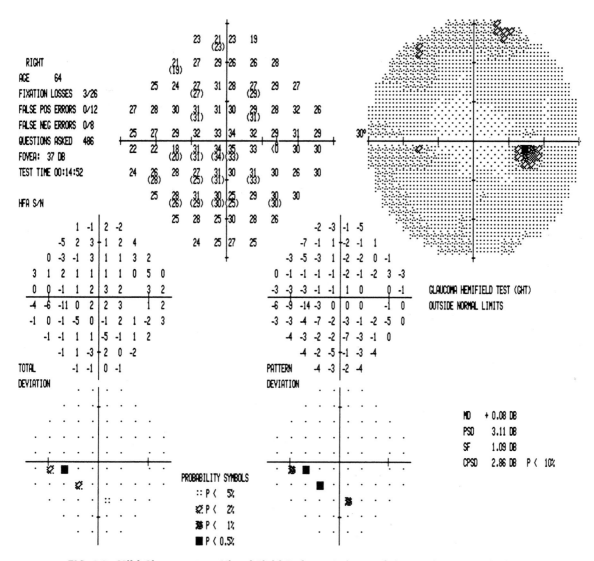

FIG. 6-3. Mild Glaucomatous Visual Field Defect. A cluster of abnormal points in the lower nasal quadrant, evident in the total and pattern deviation probability maps, may be overlooked or of uncertain significance in the other displays.

PATTERN DEVIATION (LOCALIZED LOSS)

The PATTERN deviation probability map highlights significant localized loss, and ignores generalized field changes.

The function of the Pattern Deviation plot is to expose localized defects that may be masked by either a generalized depression or an elevation of the hill of vision. This is accomplished by making an adjustment of the threshold values according to the "General Height" (GH) of the visual field.

If, for example, a cataract depresses the visual field (see Chapter 9), almost all test points may be abnormal enough to be represented by very dark probability symbols in the total deviation plot. In this case, the total deviation plot will be of no help in differentiating moderately deep overall loss from moderate loss with even deeper localized defects; all points are outside the statistical range of normal. By removing the effects of any generalized depression, the Pattern Deviation plot may allow localized defects to be unmasked.

In the opposite direction, if the sensitivity of a field is unusually *high* at normal locations, test points forming a shallow relative arcuate defect may have values in the statistically normal range, although the values are lower than would be expected from the high-normal values elsewhere in the visual field of this eye. This is rare in standard white perimetry, but it is not uncommon in blue-yellow testing (SWAP).

The concept behind making an adjustment for the General Height of the hill of vision is important to understand, although the details need not be remembered. The adjustment is made based on the threshold determined at a representative point in the least diseased portion of the visual field and its deviation from the age-normal threshold value for that point. For the 24-2 and 30-2 patterns, only the points of the 24-2 pattern (a subset of those of the 30-2 pattern) are considered, and thus the same set of points is used for both patterns. The three points nearest the normal location of the physiologic blind spot are ignored. (These are the points 15 degrees temporal that lie 3 degrees above the horizontal, 3 degrees below, and 9 degrees below, respectively.)

Of the remaining 51 locations, the six points with the highest sensitivity compared with normal are not considered because a certain number of points may have had a falsely high estimate of sensitivity as a statistical accident. Thus, of the 51 points that are finally considered, the seventh-highest sensitivity value relative to age-normal is taken to represent the overall General Height of the hill of vision. This is the 85th percentile best point. In forming the pattern deviation plot, the deviation of this point from its normal value is subtracted from the deviations from normal of all tested points. The pattern deviation of the seventh best point thus becomes zero (Fig. 6-4), and the deviations of all other test locations are adjusted by the same amount. The calculations are made to the nearest 10th of a decibel but are reported on the plot rounded to the nearest integer. In the case of the 10-2 pattern, all 68 points are considered, and the 85th percentile best point is used to determine General Height.

In the same manner used for the Total Deviation plot, probability symbols highlight test points where the decibel Pattern Deviation values approach the end of the normal range by non-Gaussian statistics. All these determinations and

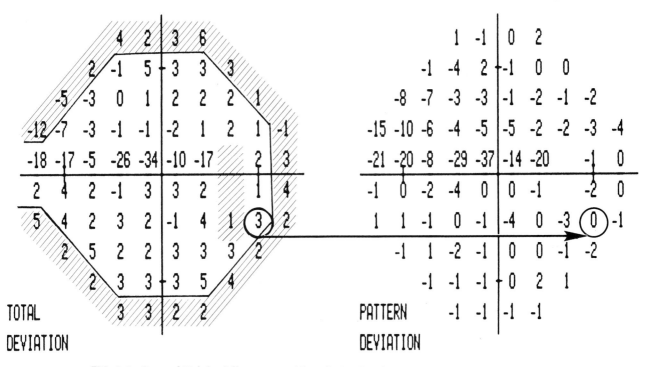

FIG. 6-4. General Height Adjustment. After eliminating the points shaded, the seventh most sensitive (compared with normal) point of the remaining 51 points is adjusted to zero deviation.

adjustments are made before rounding, but the numeric values displayed in the printout are rounded to the nearest integer.

Because many points are analyzed in the Total and Pattern Deviation plots, it is expected that a normal field may randomly contain a few scattered points outside the statistical normal range. Thus, the finding of a few marginally abnormal points is not sufficient to conclude that a field is abnormal. Abnormality of the field must be judged on the basis of finding a sufficient degree of abnormality in points clustered in a typical location or pattern that is in accordance with the clinical circumstance, as will be discussed in Chapter 7.

GLOBAL INDICES

As many as four global indices are provided by the Statpac analysis (Fig. 6-5), including Mean Deviation (MD), Pattern Standard Deviation (PSD), Short-term Fluctuation (SF), and Corrected Pattern Standard Deviation (CPSD). In contrast to the point-by-point total and pattern deviation analyses, each global index summarizes and characterizes one aspect of the complete test as a single index value. Significance limits are provided for each index so that abnormal findings (values infrequent among normal subjects) can be identified in an easy and consistent manner. Global indices conveniently reduce the test result to a few simple values but simultaneously conceal important information about the location and pattern of field loss. Thus, global indices are best used in combination with pattern-oriented information such as that supplied in greyscales and probability plots.

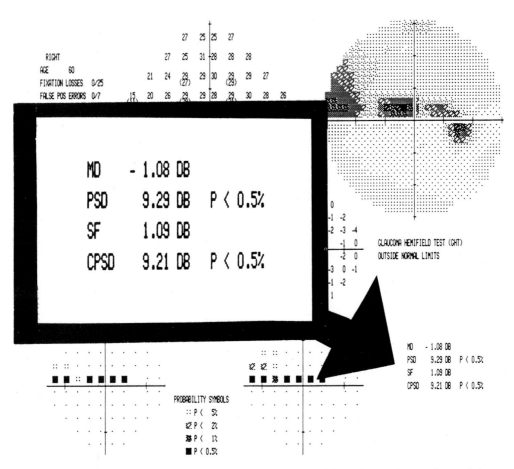

FIG. 6-5. Global Indices. The MD and PSD indices are derived from the numbers in the total deviation plot. The SF index is derived from the preselected 10 locations that have duplicate threshold determinations. The CPSD index is calculated from the PSD and SF indices.

Mean Deviation

The MD index signifies average overall severity of field loss. In principle, it is the average of all the numbers shown in the Total Deviation plot. In detail, it is calculated from a weighted mean of all the age-corrected deviations from normal displayed in the Total Deviation plot. All tested locations are included in the calculation except for the two nearest the typical location of the physiologic blind spot. The deviation from normal at each point is weighted according to the variance of the normal values at that location. Thus points with low variance—that is, closer to fixation—affect the MD value more than do the more eccentric points, which have a higher variance. The formula for calculation of the mean deviation is:

$$\frac{\dfrac{1}{n}\sum_{i=1}^{n}\dfrac{X_i - N_i}{S_{1i}^2}}{\dfrac{1}{n}\sum_{i=1}^{n}\dfrac{1}{S_{1i}^2}}$$

where X_i is the measured threshold, N_i is the normal reference threshold at point i, and S^2_{1i} is the variance of normal field measurements at point i. The number of test points (excluding the blind spot) is denoted by n.

Because MD is an index of average severity of field loss, it is affected both by the degree of loss and by the number of affected locations. Thus an MD of -4.00 dB may indicate a 4-dB depression of sensitivity everywhere in the field, an 8-dB depression of sensitivity over one half of the field, or a 16-dB depression over one fourth of the field. A positive number indicates that the average sensitivity is above-average normal for age, whereas a negative number indicates that the average sensitivity is below the average normal value. If the MD is lower than that found in 10% of the normal subjects in the perimeter's database, a significance level is printed ($p < 10\%$, $p < 5\%$, $p < 2\%$, $p < 1\%$, or $p < 0.5\%$), making it unnecessary to memorize the corresponding limits of normality. No probability statement is given for supernormal findings.

Pattern Standard Deviation

Pattern Standard Deviation (PSD) is an index of the roughness of the hill of vision and indicates the degree to which the numbers in the total deviation plot are not similar to each other. Specifically, the PSD index is the standard deviation around the mean that constitutes the MD index. If all values in the field are equally abnormal, the expected value at each location would be the normal value adjusted by the Mean Deviation, but the variance around the mean value would not be affected. In making the calculation of PSD, the difference of each sensitivity value from this expected value is weighted according to the variance of the normal values at that location in the visual field. The formula is:

$$\sqrt{\left\{\frac{1}{n}\sum_{i=1}^{n} S^2_{1i}\right\} \cdot \left[\frac{1}{n-1}\sum_{i=1}^{n}\frac{(X_i - N_i - MD)^2}{S^2_{1i}}\right]}$$

where X_i is the measured threshold, N_i is the normal reference threshold at point i, S^2_{1i} is the variance of normal field measurements at point i, MD is the mean deviation index, and n is the number of test points (excluding the blind spot).

PSD is small in a normal field or in a field in which all points are equally abnormal (e.g., the PSD would be 0 if all points were depressed by exactly 7 dB). PSD becomes large as some points become more affected than others do; thus the PSD is an index of unequalness in the amount of field loss. A single moderately deep scotoma can produce a PSD value that is clearly abnormal; if the scotoma enlarges, or if new scotomas develop, the PSD becomes increasingly abnormal. In very advanced or end-stage loss, PSD starts decreasing again as many points have threshold values close to 0 dB, the deviations from normal cluster around maximal values, and few or none of the points remain normal. Significance limits are displayed if the PSD exceeds that found in 90% of normal reliable fields.

PSD quantifies localized loss as a single value and is most useful in identifying early defects.

Short-term fluctuation

The Short-term Fluctuation (SF) is in principle the standard deviation of multiple measurements of threshold within a test session. It is an index of intratest measurement variability. It is estimated from duplicate measurements made at 10 standard locations, weighted according to the normal population variance at those locations. This estimate of SF is available as a frequently used option with the standard Full Threshold and Fastpac strategies, but not with the SITA strategies, which do not make duplicate threshold determinations.

Except for the weighting and a different selection of points used, the SF value calculated by the Humphrey perimeter is the same as the SF of the Octopus perimeter, which is calculated as the root mean square (RMS) of the standard deviations estimated at the locations that underwent duplicate testing (see Chapter 2). In making the SF calculation, locations with thresholds of 0 dB or less are not considered. The formula for SF used by the Octopus perimeter was given in Chapter 2. The formula for SF with the Humphrey perimeter is:

$$\sqrt{\left\{\frac{1}{10}\sum_{i=1}^{10} S_{2j}^2\right\} \cdot \left\{\frac{1}{10}\sum_{i=1}^{10} \frac{(X_{j1} - X_{j1} - X_{j2})^2}{2 \cdot S_{2j}^2}\right\}}$$

where X_{j1} is the first and Xj_2 the second threshold value. The normal intratest variance in point i is denoted by $S^2{}_{2j}$.

SF usually is between 1 and 2.5 dB in reliable normal fields. SF becomes high to the degree that duplicate determinations at the 10 preselected locations tend to be different. Such variable responses are typical of abnormal locations in the visual field with a broad frequency-of-seeing curve (see Chapter 2) and thus are at least in part an abnormality index. Variable threshold values also may result in part from patient testing inconsistencies, and thus SF also is in part a reliability index. As a global index, it is used to correct the PSD index to produce CPSD, as explained in the next section.

Corrected Pattern Standard Deviation (CPSD)

The Corrected Pattern Standard Deviation (CPSD) index is calculated as an adjustment to the PSD. The adjustment is made because part of the variability above or below expected values (represented in the PSD) is a result of the imperfect reproducibility of threshold determination (represented by SF). In an effort to create an index that more purely represents actual unevenness in the amount of field loss, the testing variability, as represented by the SF, is removed from the PSD to produce the CPSD.

Much of the theoretical superiority of CPSD over PSD is lost in practice. One reason is that an SF value estimated from only 10 duplicate measurements tends to be less reliable than the basic PSD measurement itself; thus, the use of SF to make a correction introduces its own errors. Moreover, the "corrected" PSD is calculated to remove the influence of patient unreliability as represented in the SF index. However, the SF index may be high by virtue of variable responses inherent in diseased areas of the visual field. The use of SF to correct the PSD inadvertently removes not only the impact of patient errors but also some of the impact of the presence of disease, thus diminishing the diagnostic content of the CPSD index. In balance, the CPSD is not always a better representation of localized field loss than the uncorrected PSD.

To calculate CPSD, variances rather than standard deviations are subtracted, and a correction factor, k, is applied (1.28 for the 30-degree field and 1.14 for the 24-degree field) because the spatial distribution of the 10 points involved in the SF calculation is narrower than the distribution of the points included in the PSD calculation. Thus the formula is:

$$(CPSD)^2 = (PSD)^2 + k(SF)^2.$$

If $k(SF)^2$ happens to be larger than $(PSD)^2$, the CPSD is assigned a value of 0 dB. Again, percentile values are given on the printout if fewer than 10% of the normal population have the calculated CPSD or one that is higher. The CPSD is not calculated if SF was not estimated during the test.

Octopus indices

The Octopus program G1 provides four equivalent global indices,[7-10] including the MD, loss variance (LV) (corresponding to PSD), Short-term Fluctuation (SF), and corrected loss variance (CLV) (corresponding to CPSD). They differ in that the calculations are not weighted, the positive values of MD represent loss of sensitivity, and the indices of localized loss are given as the variance (dB^2) instead of the standard deviation (dB). Conceptually they have the same diagnostic implications as the Humphrey indices.

PLAIN LANGUAGE ANALYSIS

> The Glaucoma Hemifield Test gives a plain language interpretation, assuming glaucoma is the diagnosis being considered.

The Humphrey Glaucoma Hemifield Test (GHT)[11-15] gives a plain language analysis of the visual field test result. The analysis takes into account groups of points along the paths of nerve fiber bundles and thus is more finely tuned to detecting a patch of early glaucomatous visual field loss than are the global indices. As implemented in the Humphrey GHT, the analysis takes into account the non-Gaussian distribution of normal values and weights the values according to the population variance at that location. The GHT is provided for 30-2 and 24-2 tests performed using standard Full Threshold or either of the SITA strategies. No GHT analysis is available for the Fastpac strategy.

In the GHT, five zones in the upper field (Fig. 6-6) are compared with five zones in mirror-image locations in the lower field. The zones are constructed in the approximate patterns of retinal nerve fibers, and thus the GHT is directed primarily at the diagnosis of glaucomatous visual field loss, and not other diseases, such as vertical hemianopia. A score is assigned to each zone based on the percentile deviations in the pattern deviation plot of the points in the zone. A comparison of each upper zone is made with the corresponding lower zone, and the difference in scores between the upper and lower zones is compared with significance limits

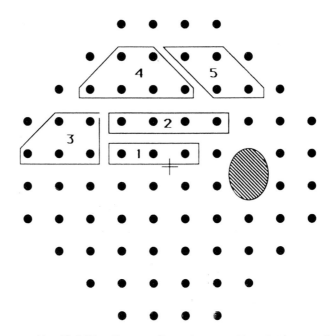

FIG. 6-6. Glaucoma Hemifield Test Zones. (From *Statpac 2 Users Guide;* reproduced with permission from Humphrey Systems.)

taken from a database of normal subjects. The General Height of the field is determined in the manner described earlier in this chapter to detect both overall depression and overall elevations of sensitivity.

Five possible messages may appear as the summary result of the GHT. The only two that can appear simultaneously are "borderline" and "general reduction of sensitivity" (Fig. 6-7). The five messages are:

1. **Outside normal limits.** This message means that one of two conditions has been met: (1) when the scores in the upper zones are compared with those of the lower zones, at least one sector pair's score difference must exceed that found in 99% of the normal population; or (2) the individual zone scores in both members of any zone pair exceed that found in 99.5% of normal individuals.

2. **Borderline.** In comparing the upper zones with the lower zones, at least one zone pair difference exceeds that found in 97% of normal individuals.

3. **General reduction of sensitivity.** This message appears only if neither of the conditions for the "outside normal limits" message is met, but the General Height calculation shows the best part of the field to be depressed to a degree that occurs in fewer than 0.5% of the normal population.

4. **Abnormally high sensitivity.** The General Height calculation shows the overall sensitivity in the best part of the field to be higher than that found in 99.5% of the population. This message supersedes and suppresses all others. In the face of abnormally high sensitivity, the comparison of upper zones with lower zones is not made.

5. **Within normal limits.** This message appears if none of the preceding four conditions is met.

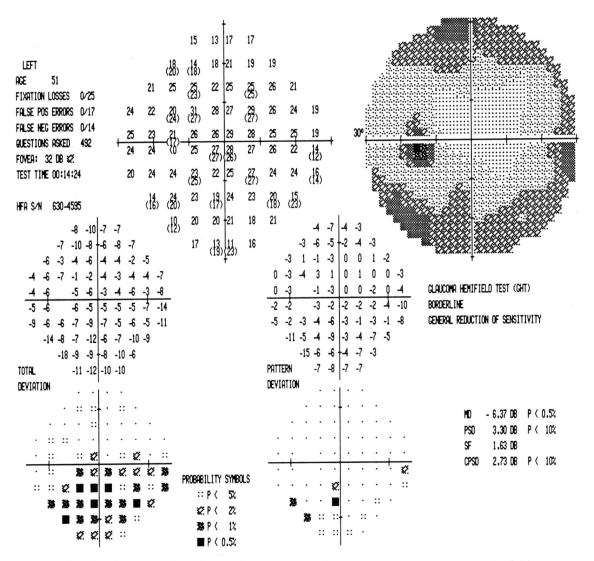

FIG. 6-7. Glaucoma Hemifield Test. In this example, two messages appear because the field generally is depressed and has equivocal asymmetry in the depression of the upper and lower halves of the field.

The GHT was designed to have an expected specificity of approximately 94% (1% false-positives from each of 5 zone pairs, plus 0.5% for general reduction and 0.5% for abnormally high sensitivity). Expected sensitivity depends heavily on the mix of mild, moderate, and severe cases of glaucoma in the clinical sample. Empirically reported sensitivity and specificity findings have varied but generally have been quite good.[16] Experienced interpreters of visual field tests may override the analysis in making diagnostic judgments after recognizing an artifact or an atypical field pattern (Fig. 6-8). However, if for clinical or research purposes a single objective statistical criterion for glaucoma is sought that does not depend on subjective clinical judgment, none has proved better than the mirrored hemifield comparison of nerve fiber zones made with the GHT.

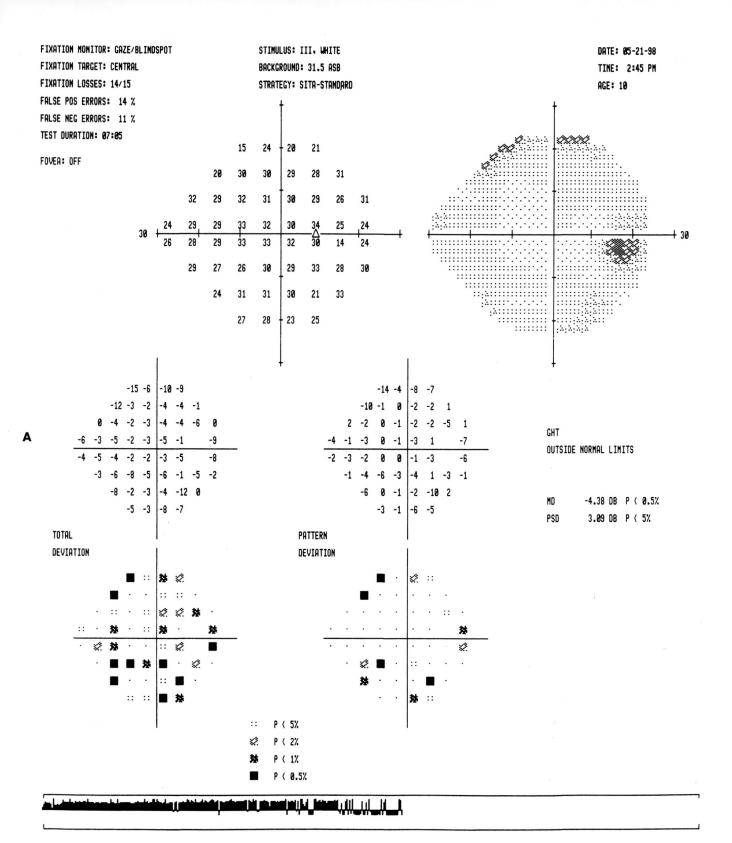

FIXATION MONITOR: GAZE/BLINDSPOT   STIMULUS: III. WHITE   DATE: 05-21-98

FIXATION TARGET: CENTRAL   BACKGROUND: 31.5 ASB   TIME: 2:45 PM

FIXATION LOSSES: 14/15   STRATEGY: SITA-STANDARD   AGE: 10

FALSE POS ERRORS: 14 %

FALSE NEG ERRORS: 11 %

TEST DURATION: 07:05

FOVEA: OFF

A

```
        15  24   20  21
      20  30   30   29  28  31
    32  29  32   31   30  29  26  31
  24  29  29  33   32   30  34  25  24
30
  26  28  29  33   33   32  30  14  24
    29  27  26  30   29   33  28  30
      24  31  31   30   21  33
        27  28   23  25
```

```
    -15 -6  -10 -9
  -12 -3 -2  -4 -4 -1
 0 -4 -2 -3  -4 -4 -6  0
-6 -3 -5 -2 -3  -5 -1      -9
-4 -5 -4 -2 -2  -3 -5     -8
 -3 -6 -8 -5  -6 -1 -5 -2
  -8 -2 -3  -4 -12  0
   -5 -3  -8 -7
```

```
    -14 -4  -8 -7
  -10 -1  0  -2 -2  1
 2 -2  0 -1  -2 -2 -5  1
-4 -1 -3  0 -1  -3  1     -7
-2 -3 -2  0  0  -1 -3    -6
 -1 -4 -6 -3  -4  1 -3 -1
  -6  0 -1  -2 -10  2
   -3 -1  -6 -5
```

GHT

OUTSIDE NORMAL LIMITS

MD   -4.38 DB   P < 0.5%

PSD   3.09 DB   P < 5%

TOTAL DEVIATION

PATTERN DEVIATION

```
::  P < 5%
⧄  P < 2%
❋  P < 1%
■  P < 0.5%
```

FIG. 6-8. Normal Field Despite GHT Message. The gaze tracker record and fixation loss (FL) index suggests that this 10-year-old patient searched for the stimuli throughout the test especially in the right eye (**A,** this page), but also in the left eye (**B,** facing page). Poor fixation, along with elevated rates of false-negative (FN) and false-positive (FP) responses, produced abnormal Mean Deviation (MD) and Pattern Standard Deviation (PSD) indices; and the irregular threshold values were sufficient to cause the Glaucoma Hemifield Test (GHT) to be "outside normal limits." However, the clinician overrides the statistically based diagnostic statement, recognizing the scattered, irregularly abnormal points in the probability plots to represent an artifact.

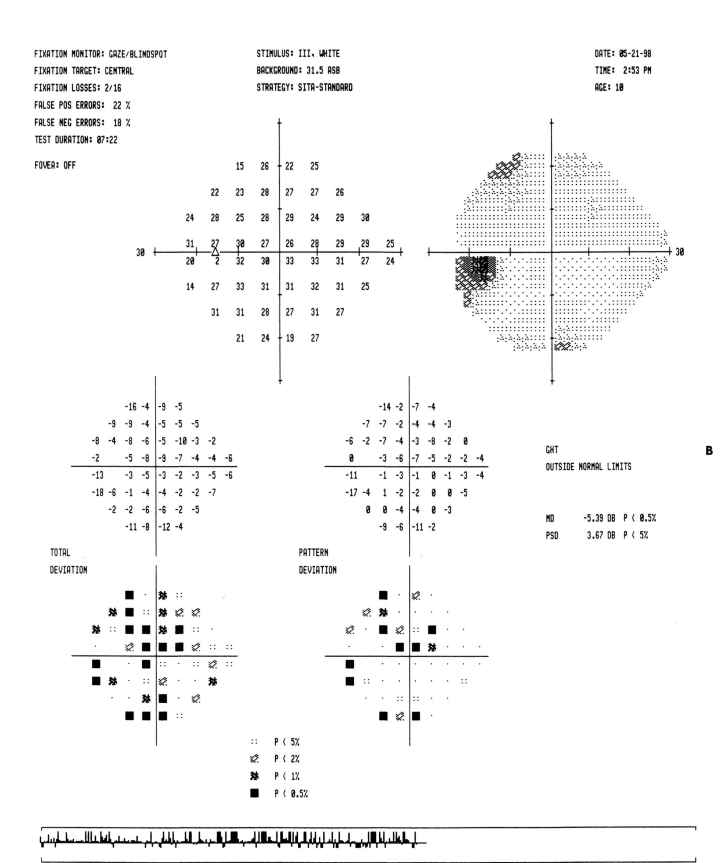

FIXATION MONITOR: GAZE/BLINDSPOT
FIXATION TARGET: CENTRAL
FIXATION LOSSES: 2/16
FALSE POS ERRORS: 22 %
FALSE NEG ERRORS: 18 %
TEST DURATION: 07:22

FOVEA: OFF

STIMULUS: III, WHITE
BACKGROUND: 31.5 ASB
STRATEGY: SITA-STANDARD

DATE: 05-21-98
TIME: 2:53 PM
AGE: 10

```
            15  26   22  25
        22  23  28   27  27  26
    24  28  25  28   29  24  29  30
    31  27  30  27   26  28  29  29  25
    20   2  32  30   33  33  31  27  24
    14  27  33  31   31  32  31  25
        31  31  28   27  31  27
            21  24   19  27
```

```
        -16 -4  -9  -5
     -9  -9 -4  -5  -5  -5
  -8 -4 -8 -6  -5 -10 -3 -2
  -2    -5 -8  -9  -7 -4 -4 -6
 -13    -3 -5  -3  -2 -3 -5 -6
 -18 -6 -1 -4  -4 -2 -2 -7
     -2 -2 -6  -6 -2 -5
        -11 -8 -12 -4
```

TOTAL
DEVIATION

```
        -14 -2  -7  -4
     -7  -7 -2  -4  -4 -3
  -6 -2 -7 -4  -3 -8 -2  0
   0    -3 -6  -7 -5 -2 -2 -4
 -11    -1 -3  -1  0 -1 -3 -4
 -17 -4  1 -2  -2  0  0 -5
      0  0 -4  -4  0 -3
        -9 -6 -11 -2
```

PATTERN
DEVIATION

GHT   B
OUTSIDE NORMAL LIMITS

MD   -5.39 DB P < 0.5%
PSD   3.67 DB P < 5%

::   P < 5%
⊠   P < 2%
▨   P < 1%
■   P < 0.5%

FIG. 6-8, cont'd.

119

REFERENCES

1. Schwartz P, Nagin P: Probability maps for evaluating automated visual fields. In Greve E, Heijl A, editors: *Sixth International Visual Field Symposium, Santa Margarita, Liqure, 1984,* Dordrecht, 1985, Dr. W. Junk Publishers. Documenta Ophthalmologica Proceedings Series 1984;42:39-48.

2. Heijl A, Lindgren G, Olsson J: A package for the statistical analysis of computerized fields. In *Seventh International Visual Field Symposium,* Amsterdam, 1986, Dordrecht, Martinus Nijhoff/Dr. W. Junk Publishers. Documenta Ophthalmologica Proceedings Series 1987;49:153-168.

3. Heijl A, Åsman P: A clinical study of perimetric probability maps, *Arch Ophthalmol* 107:199-203, 1989.

4. Heijl A, Lindgren G, Olsson J, Åsman P: Visual field interpretation with empirical probability maps, *Arch Ophthalmol* 107:204-208, 1989.

5. Heijl A, Lindgren G, Lindgren A et al: Extended empirical statistical package for evaluation of single and multiple field in glaucoma: Statpac 2. In Mills RP, Heijl A, editors: *Perimetry Update 1990/91,* p 303, Amsterdam, 1991, Kugler.

6. Heijl A, Lindgren G, Olsson J: Normal variability of static perimetric threshold values across the central visual field, *Arch Ophthalmol* 105:1544-1549, 1987.

7. Bebie H: Computerized techniques of visual field analysis. In Drance SM, Anderson DR, editors: *Automatic perimetry in glaucoma: A practical guide,* p 147, Orlando, FL, 1985, Grune Stratton.

8. Flammer J, Jenni F, Bebie H, Keller B: The Octopus G1 program, *Glaucoma* 9:67-72, 1987.

9. Flammer J, Drance SM, Augustiny L, Funkhouser A: Quantification of glaucomatous visual field defects with automated perimetry, *Invest Ophthalmol Vis Sci* 26:176-181, 1985.

10. Flammer J: The concept of visual field defects, *Graefes Arch Klin Exp Ophthalmol* 224:389-392, 1986.

11. Åsman P, Heijl A: Glaucoma Hemifield Test: Automated visual field evaluation, *Arch Ophthalmol* 110:812-9, 1992.

12. Åsman P: Computer-assisted interpretation of visual fields in glaucoma, *Acta Ophthalmol* 70[Suppl 206]:1-47, 1992.

13. Åsman P, Heijl A: Evaluation of methods for automated hemifield analysis in perimetry, *Arch Ophthalmol* 110:820-6, 1992.

14. Åsman P, Heijl A: Weighting according to location in computer-assisted glaucoma visual field analysis, *Acta Ophthalmol* [Copenh] 70:671-678, 1992.

15. Åsman P, Heijl A, Olsson J, Rootzen H: Spatial analyses of glaucomatous visual fields: A comparison with traditional visual field indices, *Acta Ophthalmol* [Copenh] 70:679-686, 1992.

16. Katz J, Sommer A, Gaasterland DE, Anderson DR: Comparison of analytic algorithms for detecting glaucomatous visual field loss, *Arch Ophthalmol* 109:1684-1689, 1991.

ADDITIONAL READING

Haley MJ, editor: *The Field Analyzer Primer,* p 130, ed 2, San Leandro, CA, 1987, Allergan Humphrey.

Introducing Statpac 2, San Leandro, CA, 1989, Allergan Humphrey.

Statpac Users Guide, San Leandro, CA, 1986, Allergan Humphrey.

CHAPTER 7

Interpretation of a single field

Most visual field examinations are performed with a specific diagnostic goal in mind. Before approaching this diagnostic decision, one must look for artifacts and confounding features of the examination. For example, if the field seems normal, but the examination was unreliable, might a defect have been missed? If the field seems abnormal, but the examination was unreliable, is the defect real or an artifact produced by an imprecise examination?

RELIABILITY

The database used in Statpac for the Full Threshold and Fastpac strategies was constructed from data of normal subjects, after elimination of those results which were most unreliable, based on a 33% limit for false-positive (FP) and false-negative (FN) rates and a 20% limit for fixation loss (FL). Should any of these limits be exceeded in a standard visual field test undergoing Statpac analysis, the aberrant value is highlighted with a double X (XX), and a warning message ("low patient reliability") is given (see Fig. 6-1). This message should not be construed to mean that the field is necessarily lacking in any useful diagnostic interpretation or that it is not useful as a baseline for following the progress of glaucoma. A more focused interpretation of the message is that caution is needed when interpreting the Statpac statistical analysis that compares the visual field test results with the normal database, which did not include subjects with high FP, FN, or FL parameters. Patients without disease but with a tendency for high FP, FN, or FL parameters may have a broader range of "normal" values; however, patients with disease may have defects that are hidden by FP responses.

The normative database for the SITA strategy does not exclude normal subjects with high FN or FP rates; it requires that patients be free of ocular disease and that their FL be less than 20%.

When interpreting visual field data or its statistical analysis with any testing algorithm, the type and degree of any bad information or invalid analyses that may appear on the printout should be considered. This explains our initial attention to indicators of test reliability.

> The "low patient reliability" warning suggests caution, but does not necessarily prevent interpretation of results.

False-positive responses

The FP rate represents the tendency for patients to push the button, not in response to seeing a stimulus, but at random, in expectation of a stimulus, or in response to a nonvisual cue. False-positive responses begin to have an effect on the test results well before reaching the 33% rate that was used to exclude data from the initial Statpac database and that indicates frankly unreliable field tests.

Among these effects is that some points will have unusually high sensitivity values. Just as the patient responds when there is no stimulus at all, he or she also may respond when there is a real but unperceived stimulus, perhaps because the time seems right or because there is an audible clue. This response is recorded as meaning that the patient saw the stimulus, and a high sensitivity value is reported. On the greyscale printout there may be scattered, very light areas or "white

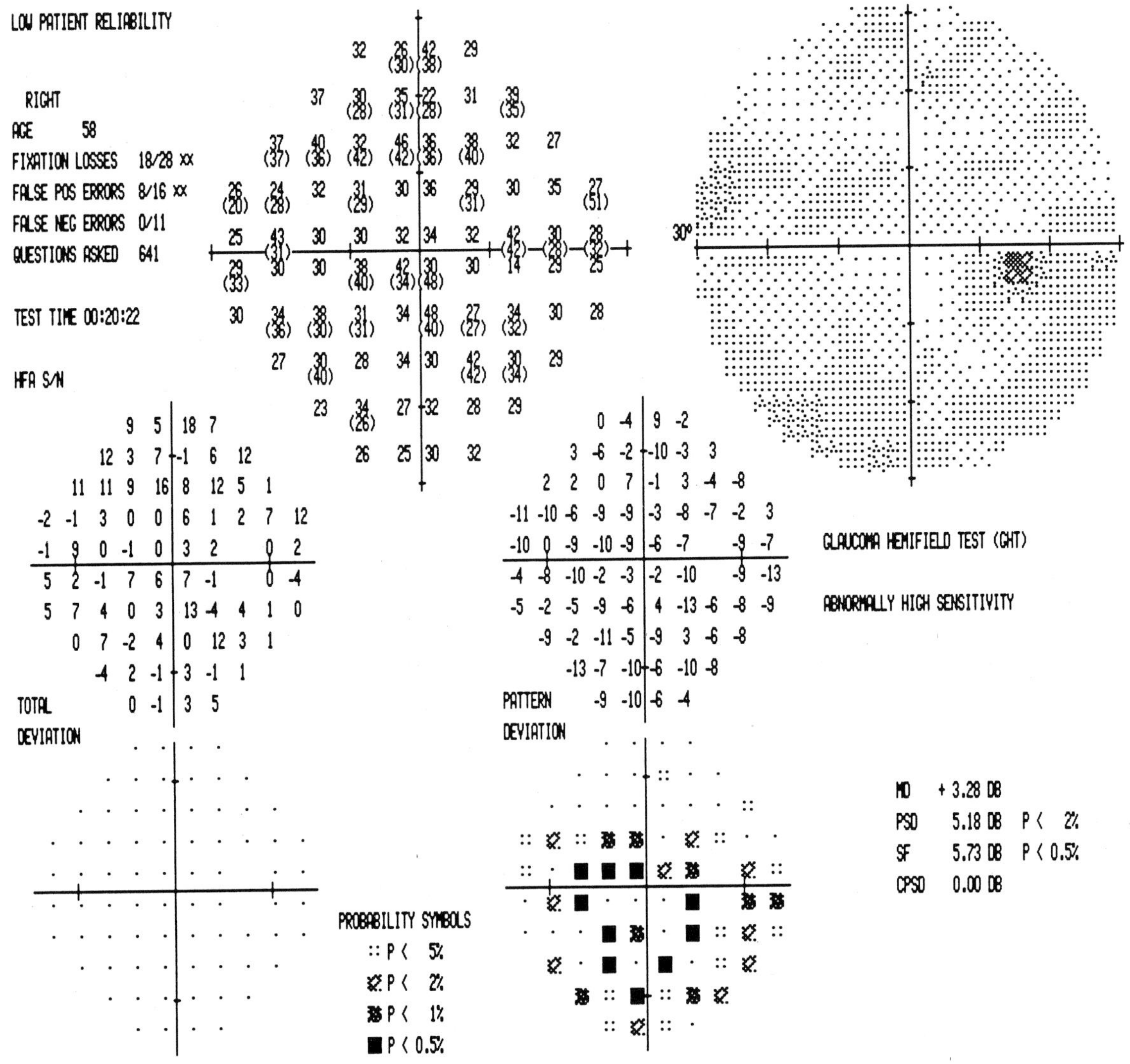

FIG. 7-1. High False-Positive Rate. Most of the features mentioned in the text are present, except that the CPSD is spared. (Courtesy of Alfred Sommer, MD)

scotomas" representing peaks of high sensitivity. In the numeric printout, threshold values of 37 or 40 dB (or even higher) may be recorded, which represent stimuli not visible to most people.

If one of the four primary points has been determined (falsely) to have a very high sensitivity value, the entire quadrant is influenced because the sensitivity at the primary point is used to determine the initial stimulus intensity at adjacent points. For these surrounding points, any inconsistency in the patient's responses may cause the end point for threshold determination to be reached prematurely by accident, and the reported sensitivity value tends to be closer to the starting stimulus intensity.

If the test result shows meaningfully high sensitivity values at more than 15% of the points, there are two additional consequences. First, the GHT indicates

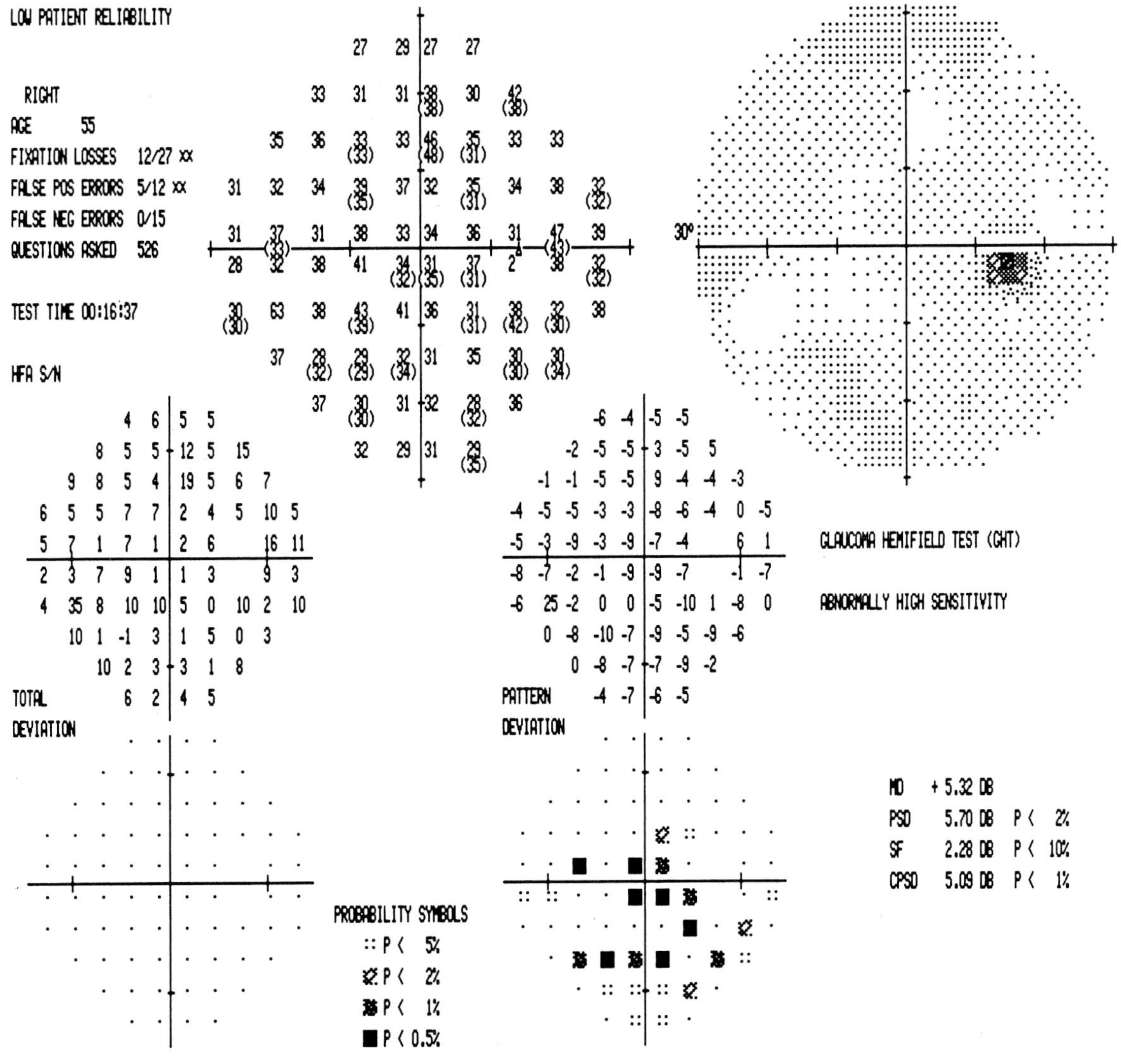

LOW PATIENT RELIABILITY

RIGHT
AGE   55
FIXATION LOSSES   12/27 xx
FALSE POS ERRORS   5/12 xx
FALSE NEG ERRORS   0/15
QUESTIONS ASKED   526

TEST TIME 00:16:37

HFA S/N

TOTAL DEVIATION

PATTERN DEVIATION

GLAUCOMA HEMIFIELD TEST (GHT)

ABNORMALLY HIGH SENSITIVITY

MD   + 5.32 DB
PSD   5.70 DB   P < 2%
SF   2.28 DB   P < 10%
CPSD   5.09 DB   P < 1%

PROBABILITY SYMBOLS
:: P < 5%
⊗ P < 2%
▨ P < 1%
■ P < 0.5%

FIG. 7-2. High False-Positive Rate with Abnormal CPSD. On repeat examinations this patient always tends to have a high FP rate, sometimes with a normal CPSD.

"abnormally high sensitivity." Second, the pattern deviation probability plot erroneously shows points with statistically significant loss compared with values expected by virtue of the General Height correction.[1]

In addition, the mean deviation (MD) index may have a strikingly positive value. Because of irreproducible and inconsistent threshold determinations, both pattern standard deviation (PSD) and short-term fluctuation (SF) usually are high. Corrected pattern standard deviation (CPSD) may or may not be affected. With many points seeming to have sensitivity unlike their neighbors, many points are doubly determined, and the examination may have been a lengthy one, with many questions asked.

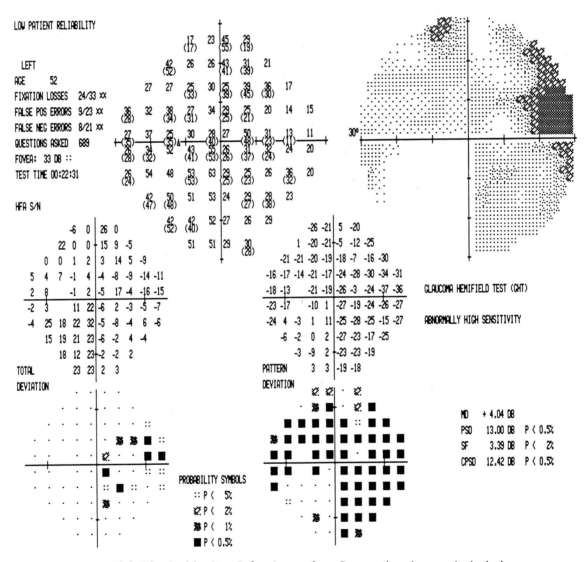

FIG. 7-3. High False-Positive Rate Before Instruction. Because the primary point in the lower temporal quadrant had an initial threshold determination of 53 dB, the entire quadrant has high measurements and is white on the greyscale printout. The patient was coached and the follow up is shown in Figure 7-4.

When a patient responds even when the stimulus is not seen, the recorded FL rate is high, not because fixation is poor, but because the patient responds to stimuli correctly presented in the blind spot that he or she cannot see. If it happens that a point with an excessively high threshold value is selected for a subsequent FN catch trial, the stimulus may not be seen, and a high FN rate results. True scotomas, including the physiologic blind spot, may not be discovered because the patient responded even though the stimulus was unseen.

Because of all these effects, a high FP rate is particularly devastating to the accuracy of the visual field examination. In fact, a serious impact on the field result occurs at a much lower level than the 33% rate that triggers the "low patient

> False-positive responses affect the result, even when the FP rate is well under 33%.

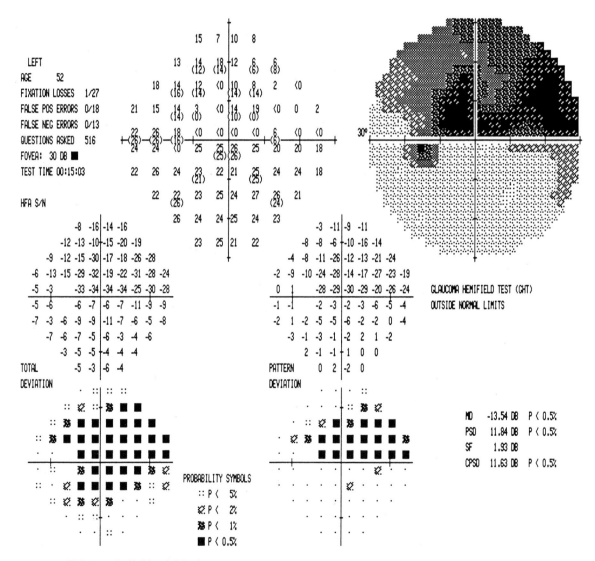

FIG. 7-4. Reliable Field After Instruction. Three weeks after the examination shown in Figure 7-3, the patient performed reliably and the field abnormality was accurately quantified. Note the change in MD from Figure 7-3.

reliability" message. Moreover, FP catch trials represent a small percentage of the presentations during the test, and therefore may not fully reveal that the patient tends to push the button at some times when he or she does not see a stimulus.

Not many patients give false-positive responses, but the clinician studying a field test diagram must be alert to note any sign of such behavior, particularly when a few locations have unusually high threshold values. Even if the reported FP rate is not high in such cases, irregularities in the field sensitivity values should not be attributed automatically to a disease state, and it should be recognized that abnormally reduced sensitivities might not have been fully revealed. Although infrequent, this is an important and correctable problem, so when FP responses occur, the patient should be coached gently, as detailed in Chapters 6 and 11. The majority of patients with this problem respond to suitable instruction (see Figs. 7-3 and 7-4), although there are a few who can never be tested reliably. When such a patient is encountered, the perimetrist should help the clinician understand the patient's limitations and how to interpret the field printout by writing on the diagram that an unacceptably high FP rate persisted despite reinstruction of the patient. The clinician will know that the technician and the patient both did their best.

False-negative responses

Another form of inconsistency is the failure of the patient to respond when a visible stimulus is presented. If the patient fails to respond to visible stimuli because he is unable to concentrate but has in fact a normal visual field, the measured threshold values may seem abnormally low, because some visible stimuli did not produce a patient response. These failures to respond produce falsely low estimates of sensitivity at various locations and a negative MD index. Most likely, some points are randomly more affected than others are, so the PSD and SF indices become abnormal. Because the falsely low sensitivity values determine the starting stimulus intensity for testing of adjacent points, and points, and false-negative responses lower the sensitivity estimate even more, there is some clustering of points with reduced sensitivity (resembling scotomas), but perhaps not in diagnostically typical locations. If inattention becomes worse toward the end of the test, sensitivity may tend to be progressively worse away from the primary points so that patches of depressed sensitivity occur at the edge of the field, which is tested last (Fig. 7-5).

One characteristic type of false field defect that accompanies a high FN is the result of either fatigue or hysteria (in the medical sense). If the patient becomes progressively less responsive as the examination proceeds, the primary points may show normal sensitivity, but points tested later seem to have depressed sensitivity. In such cases, the higher sensitivity values at the four primary points produce a distinctive cloverleaf pattern in the greyscale printout (Figs. 7-6 and 7-7). The FN rate is high, because later in the test the patient fails to respond to stimuli 9 dB more intense than stimuli he saw previously. An increasing tendency not to respond exaggerates the tendency noted in Figure 7-5 for the sensitivity to be artificially lower at more peripheral points.

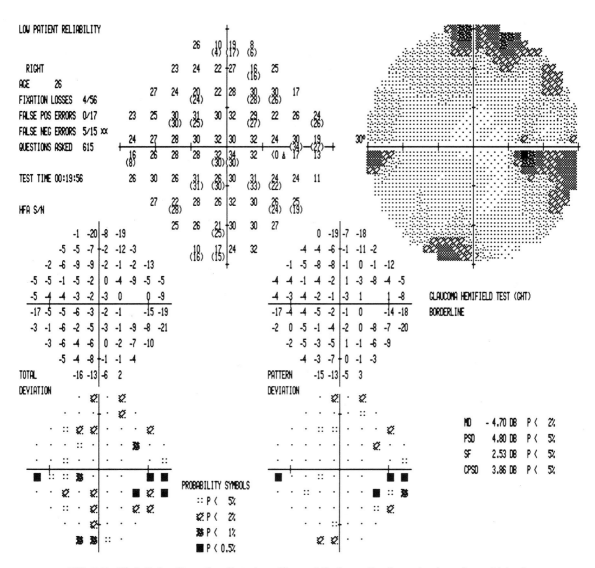

LOW PATIENT RELIABILITY

RIGHT

AGE   26
FIXATION LOSSES   4/56
FALSE POS ERRORS 0/17
FALSE NEG ERRORS 5/15 xx
QUESTIONS ASKED   615

TEST TIME 00:19:56

HFA S/N

TOTAL
DEVIATION

PATTERN
DEVIATION

GLAUCOMA HEMIFIELD TEST (GHT)
BORDERLINE

PROBABILITY SYMBOLS
    :: P < 5%
    ▨ P < 2%
    ▩ P < 1%
    ■ P < 0.5%

MD   - 4.70 DB   P < 2%
PSD   4.80 DB   P < 5%
SF   2.53 DB   P < 5%
CPSD   3.86 DB   P < 5%

FIG. 7-5. High False-Negative Rate In a Normal Patient. Patchy reduction of sensitivity in clusters toward the edge is typical. (Courtesy of Alfred Sommer, MD)

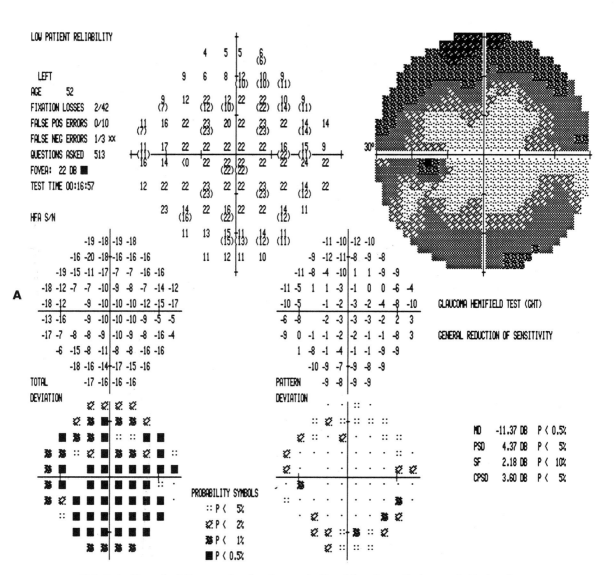

LOW PATIENT RELIABILITY

LEFT

AGE 52
FIXATION LOSSES 2/42
FALSE POS ERRORS 0/10
FALSE NEG ERRORS 1/3 xx
QUESTIONS ASKED 513
FOVEA: 22 DB ■
TEST TIME 00:16:57

HFA S/N

TOTAL
DEVIATION

PATTERN
DEVIATION

GLAUCOMA HEMIFIELD TEST (GHT)

GENERAL REDUCTION OF SENSITIVITY

PROBABILITY SYMBOLS

:: P < 5%
⧄ P < 2%
▨ P < 1%
■ P < 0.5%

MD	-11.37 DB	P <	0.5%
PSD	4.37 DB	P <	5%
SF	2.18 DB	P <	10%
CPSD	3.60 DB	P <	5%

A

FIG. 7-6. Cloverleaf Pattern On the Greyscale Resulting From Fatigue. A, Notice the test time of 16:57 after a similarly long test on the right eye. This patient was already tired when the fovea and primary points were tested, giving depressed threshold values of 22 to 23 dB, and later became even less responsive as more peripheral locations were tested.

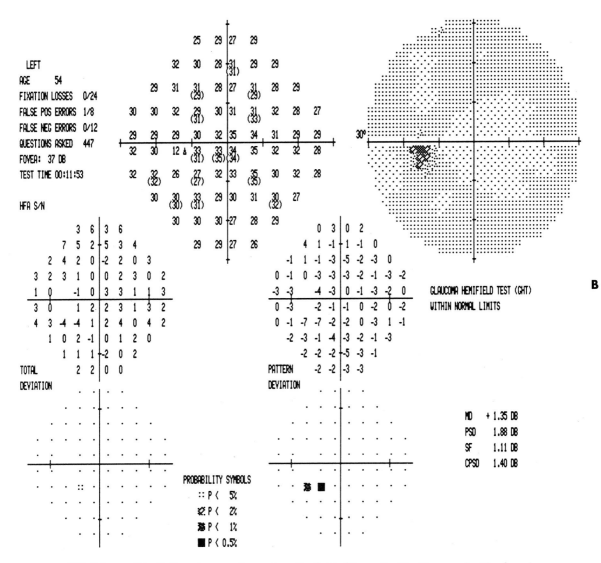

LEFT

AGE   54
FIXATION LOSSES   0/24
FALSE POS ERRORS   1/8
FALSE NEG ERRORS   0/12
QUESTIONS ASKED   447
FOVEA: 37 DB
TEST TIME 00:11:53

HFA S/N

                25   29 27   29

        32 30 28 31   29   29
                   (31)
    29 31 31   28 27   31   28   29
            (29)   (29)
30 30 32 29   30 31   31   32   28   27
            (31)   (33)
29 29 29 30   32 35   34   31   29   29
32 30 12 ▲ 33   33 34   35   32   32   28
            (31) (35)(34)
    32 32 26 27   32 33   35   32   28
        (32)   (27)   (35)
        30 30   33 29 30   31   30   27
            (30) (31)   (32)
            30   30 30 27   28   29

            29   29 27 26

         3   6 3   6
      7 5 2 5   3   4
   2 4 2 0 -2   2   0   3
3 2 3 1 0 0   2   3   0   2
1 0   -1 0 3   3   1   1   3
3 0   1 2 2   3   1   3   2
4 3 -4 -4 1 2   4   0   4   2
   1 0 2 -1 0   1   2   0
      1 1 1 -2   0   2
TOTAL   2 2 0   0
DEVIATION

                      0   3 0   2
                   4 1 -1 1 -1   0
               -1 1 -1 -3 -5 -2 -3   0
            0 -1 0 -3 -3 -3 -2 -1 -3 -2
           -3 -3   -4 -3 0 -1 -3 -2   0
            0 -3   -2 -1 -1 0 -2   0 -2
            0 -1 -7 -7 -2 -2 0 -3   1 -1
              -2 -3 -1 -4 -3 -2 -1 -3
                 -2 -2 -2 -5 -3 -1
PATTERN   -2 -2 -3 -3
DEVIATION

GLAUCOMA HEMIFIELD TEST (GHT)
WITHIN NORMAL LIMITS

MD   + 1.35 DB
PSD   1.88 DB
SF   1.11 DB
CPSD   1.40 DB

PROBABILITY SYMBOLS

    :: P < 5%
    ▨ P < 2%
    ▩ P < 1%
    ■ P < 0.5%

B

FIG. 7-6, cont'd.   B, On subsequent occasions, the field of the patient in *A* is normal, with a foveal threshold of 37 dB.

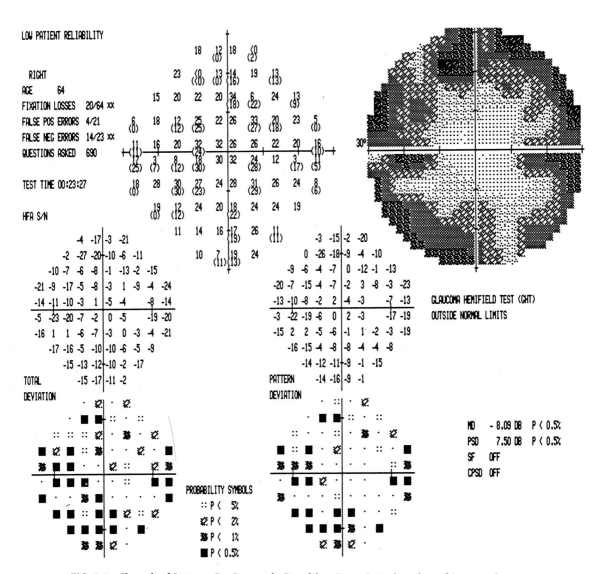

FIG. 7-7. Cloverleaf Pattern On Greyscale Resulting From Deterioration of Responsiveness as the Test Proceeds. High FN rate with the best sensitivity at the four primary points is typical. (Courtesy of Alfred Sommer, MD)

The interpretative problem is this: a high FN, combined with a high SF and high PSD, is also an expected feature of a reliable test of a truly abnormal field with true defects,[2-4] at least with the traditional FN catch trials of the non-SITA strategies (Fig. 7-8). Two pathologic psychophysical elements seem to account for this phenomenon.[5-11]

First, a region of the field affected by disease not only has a reduced sensitivity but also characteristically shows considerable inconsistency in whether a given stimulus is visible (represented in a broadened frequency-of-seeing curve with a more shallow slope). Thus a moderate reduction of sensitivity might have been determined by the staircase strategy at a particular point. Later, when a stimulus 9 dB more intense is presented as a catch trial at that location, the stimulus truly may not be seen because of pathologic variability in visibility at this abnormal location.

Second, psychophysical fatigue (not of the person but of the visual sensitivity apparatus) may occur preferentially at abnormal points. Thus a point in the field becomes less sensitive with repeated testing. As a result of either psychophysical cause, the traditional catch trial stimulus is not seen, and a lack of response is recorded as an FN response.

A distinct and important modification in the SITA strategies is an effort to remove these two disease-induced effects on the reported FN rate. Therefore a high FN rate more reliably indicates inattention rather than disease.

Thus, at least with the traditional non-SITA testing, the clinician must look for certain clues to distinguish between a normal field made to look abnormal by FN responses and an abnormal field with numerous FN responses as one of its features. True defects may be in an arcuate distribution, whereas pseudodefects (Figs. 7-9 and 7-10) may be randomly patchy, most typically at the edge (the last points to be tested). Either true defects or pseudodefects may appear as a dense concentric loss that leaves only a central island of vision, although careful inspection of glaucomatous contraction of the field often shows a recognizable nasal step (see Fig. 7-10). Knowledge of the clinical setting helps. Is the intraocular pressure elevated? Is there excavation of the optic disc? True defects may be unequal in the two eyes and are particularly recognizable if the visual field asymmetry is accompanied by asymmetric intraocular pressure or disc excavation. An inconsistent patient may tend to be equally unreliable in both eyes.

Thus, a field may be judged reliable despite a high FN rate determined by traditional catch trials, if there is a reproducible field defect that is characteristic of the disease in question, especially if there are no other signs of unreliability in the visual field. However, a reported high FN rate is cause for considering the field test unreliable if a cloverleaf pattern is seen in the greyscale, if there is a nondiagnostic pattern of patchy irregularity in the sensitivity values (especially causing edge points, tested last, to appear irregularly abnormal), or if a visual field abnormality simply is not expected, given the rest of the clinical findings. In any case, the required action is often the same. Newly diagnosed field abnormalities require confirmation through a repeat field examination or through the presence of other clinical signs. Likewise, seemingly unreliable field tests may require a repeat test.

False-negative responses reflect patient inattention. In non-SITA strategies, the presence of disease also raises the FN rate.

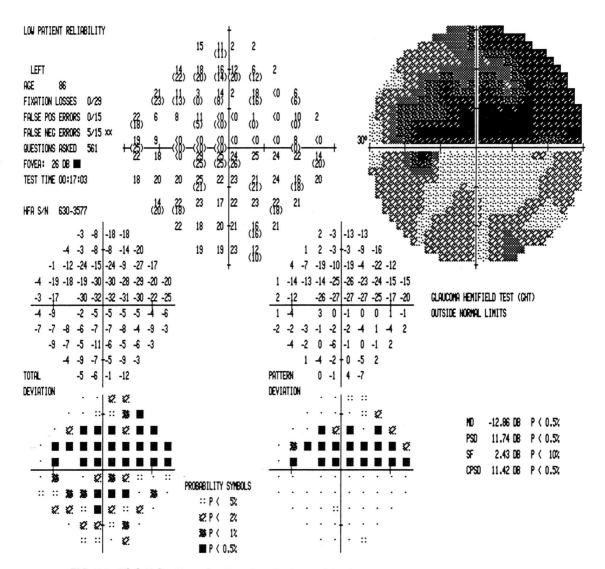

LOW PATIENT RELIABILITY

LEFT

AGE 86

FIXATION LOSSES 0/29

FALSE POS ERRORS 0/15

FALSE NEG ERRORS 5/15 xx

QUESTIONS ASKED 561

FOVEA: 26 DB ■

TEST TIME 00:17:03

HFA S/N 630-3577

```
                15  (11) 2   2
         14  18  16 (12) 6   2
        (22)(20)(14)(20)(12)
      21  11   3  14  2  18  (0)  6
     (23)(13) (0) (8)    (16)    (6)
  22   6   8  11  (0) (0)  1  (0) 10   2
 (18)           (5)(8)        (0)
  19   9  (0) (0) (0) (0  (0  (0   8  (0
 (25)    (0) (0) (0)
  22  18  (0)  24  25  24  22  14
        (0)(25)(25)(26)        (20)
  18  20  20  25  22  23  21  24  16  20
        (21)       (21)       (18)
     14 (0) 23  17  22  23  22  21
    (20)(18)              (18)
        22  18  20 21  16  21
                  (16)
```

```
   -3  -8  -18 -18
 -4  -3  -8 -8 -14 -20
-1 -12 -24 -15 -24 -9 -27 -17
-4 -19 -18 -19 -30 -30 -28 -29 -20 -20
-3 -17   -30 -32 -32 -31 -30 -22 -25
-4 -9  -2 -5 -5 -5 -5 -4 -6
-7 -7 -8 -6 -7 -7 -8 -4 -9 -3
  -9 -7 -5 -11 -6 -5 -6 -3
    -4 -9 -7 -5 -9 -3
```

TOTAL   -5 -6 -1 -12

DEVIATION

```
              19  19 23  12
                      (10)
        1   2  -3 -3 -9 -16
     4  -7 -19 -10 -19 -4 -22 -12
  1 -14 -13 -14 -25 -26 -23 -24 -15 -15
  2 -12   -26 -27 -27 -27 -25 -17 -20
  1 -4   3  0 -1  0  0  1 -1
 -2 -2 -3 -1 -2 -2 -4  1 -4  2
    -4 -2  0 -6 -1  0 -1  2
      1 -4 -2  0 -5  2
```

PATTERN   0 -1 4 -7

DEVIATION

```
              2  -3 -13 -13
```

PROBABILITY SYMBOLS

:: P < 5%

✛ P < 2%

▩ P < 1%

■ P < 0.5%

GLAUCOMA HEMIFIELD TEST (GHT)

OUTSIDE NORMAL LIMITS

MD   -12.86 DB   P < 0.5%

PSD   11.74 DB   P < 0.5%

SF   2.43 DB   P < 10%

CPSD   11.42 DB   P < 0.5%

FIG. 7-8. High False-Negative Rate In a Patient With Glaucoma. The field seems otherwise reliable, and the high FN rate apparently results from inconsistent responses in the region of the field with relative sensitivity reduction.

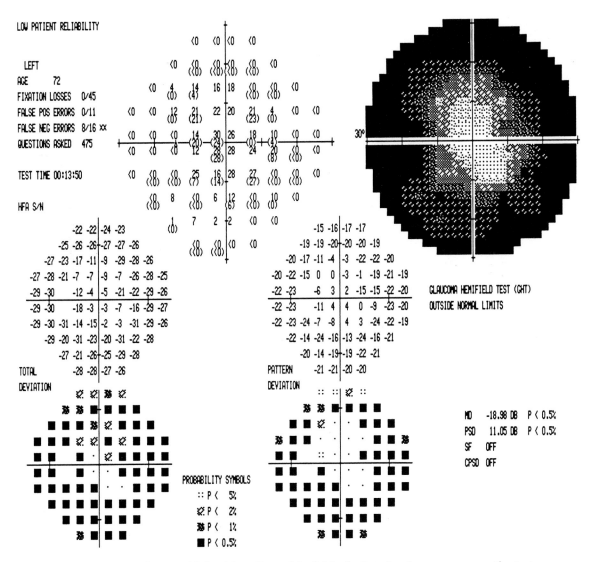

FIG. 7-9. Pseudocentral Island In a Normal Individual. Deteriorating responses as the test proceeds explain both the high FN rate and the contracted appearance of the field. The patient simply stopped responding as the test proceeded, so it seemed that he could see only in the central regions.

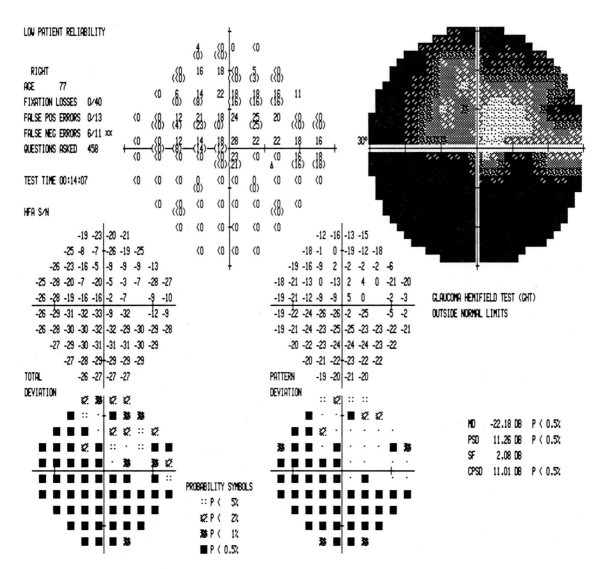

FIG. 7-10. Central Island From Glaucoma With a High False-Negative Response Rate. The asymmetry between the upper and lower hemifields suggests that this is a true defect that encroaches the point of fixation from the lower nasal quadrant; note also the small region of preserved vision temporal to the blind spot. It is, however, the presence of elevated pressure and extensive cupping that makes this diagnostic impression certain, in contrast to Figure 7-9. (Courtesy of Alfred Sommer, MD)

Fixation losses

The third official reliability index, when the Heijl-Krakau blind spot method is used, is the fixation loss (FL) rate. If the patient is not maintaining fixation, the patient sees a stimulus presented at the location where the blind spot would be during properly positioned gaze. If the FL rate is low, one can feel confident that good fixation was maintained, provided that by other indications the patient was suitably responsive (there are areas of detected visual sensation in the field and the FN rate is low).

A high FL rate (> 20%) is a common reason for a field examination to be labeled "unreliable,"[12-15] although often it is in fact reliable. A high FL rate is difficult to interpret because loss of fixation is not the only reason that the patient might respond to the FL catch trial. As previously noted, a patient with a high FP rate will respond even when he does not see the FL catch trial stimulus presented in the blind spot of a well-fixated eye. A stimulus in the blind spot also might be potentially visible when the nasal field of the other eye is not occluded.

Most often, however, a falsely high FL rate (pseudoloss of fixation) occurs because the physiologic blind spot of the well-fixated eye is not in the expected position. This may be caused by slight changes in the head tilt, which rotate the physiologic blind spot in and out of the selected test position as the examination proceeds.

> The FL index may falsely suggest poor fixation.

Pseudoloss of fixation presents a dilemma of interpretation. A field examination certainly is less reliable if there is true loss of fixation (Fig. 7-11), but in many clinical settings a recorded high FL rate occurs as pseudoloss of fixation in a perfectly reliable visual field examination. It is a reasonably safe assumption that the field test was reliable if the blind spot method yields a high FL rate, if all other indications are that the field is reliable (i.e., the FN, FP, and SF values are small, and the visual field defects are nicely delineated, in keeping with the clinical expectation, and perhaps reproducible on other examinations). It is reassuring if the test location 15 degrees temporal to fixation at 3 degrees below the horizontal has the expected poor sensitivity of a point in the blind spot position.

An attentive perimetrist can help greatly with this problem.[16-18] If a high FL rate is accumulating from blind spot catch trials in the early stages of the examination, and if it appears on the monitor that fixation is indeed unsteady, the patient needs encouragement. Conversely, if fixation appears steady, the test should be paused and the blind spot relocated, so that the clinician is not misled while interpreting the test results. Perhaps after the patient is repositioned comfortably, he will be able to maintain a steady head position for the rest of the examination. (At times the blind spot simply cannot be localized because, for example, it is connected with a large, dense arcuate field defect; in such cases the fixation monitor can be turned off.) If, throughout the remainder of the test, the patient's fixation is steady on the monitor, it is very helpful for the perimetrist to record on the printout that fixation was observed to be steady.

In some clinics it is standard procedure to turn off the fixation monitor routinely (or selectively, in lieu of relocating the blind spot to overcome falsely reported fixation loss). However, when interpreting such a field, one loses the reassurance one has in many field tests with a low FL rate. Therefore, unless a gaze tracker is being used, we prefer that the perimetrist recognize early in the

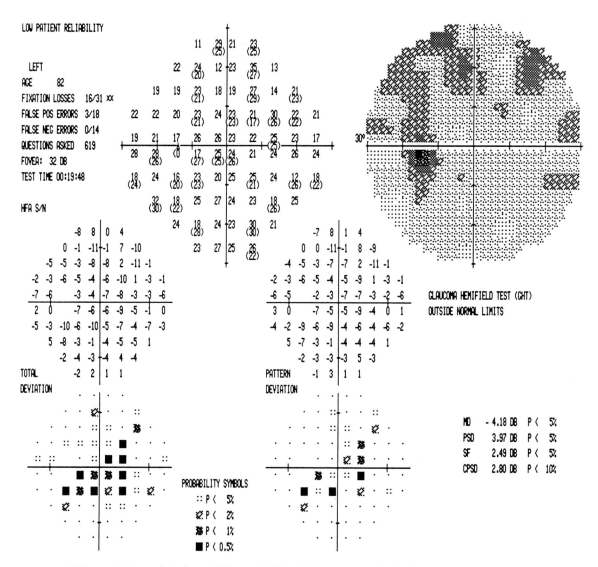

FIG. 7-11. Normal Patient With Unreliable Field Because of Fixation Loss. The acuity is 20/25. Foveal sensitivity is high (32 dB) when the patient is looking at the stimulus and knows where it will be presented. The reduced sensitivity surrounding the center may result from his not keeping the eye directed straight ahead when stimuli in the central 10 degrees were presented; thus, he did not see stimuli he might have seen if he had been centrally fixated. However, this same field appearance could result from a cataract combined with pseudoloss of fixation in a reliable examination. (Courtesy of Alfred Sommer, MD)

examination any false reports of fixation loss and correct the problem by having the blind spot relocated. Only if this fails should the fixation monitor be turned off.

When a tracing is available from the gaze tracker of the HFA-II, the blind spot technique need not be used or its results need to be interpreted in light of the gaze-tracker record. The gaze tracker gives the additional information of the gaze position at each stimulus presentation. The history of gaze stability during the test may help the clinician interpret certain findings. For example, if fixation deteriorated toward the end of testing of the second eye, the test results are less reliable for points tested last—namely, those near the edge (Fig. 7-12).

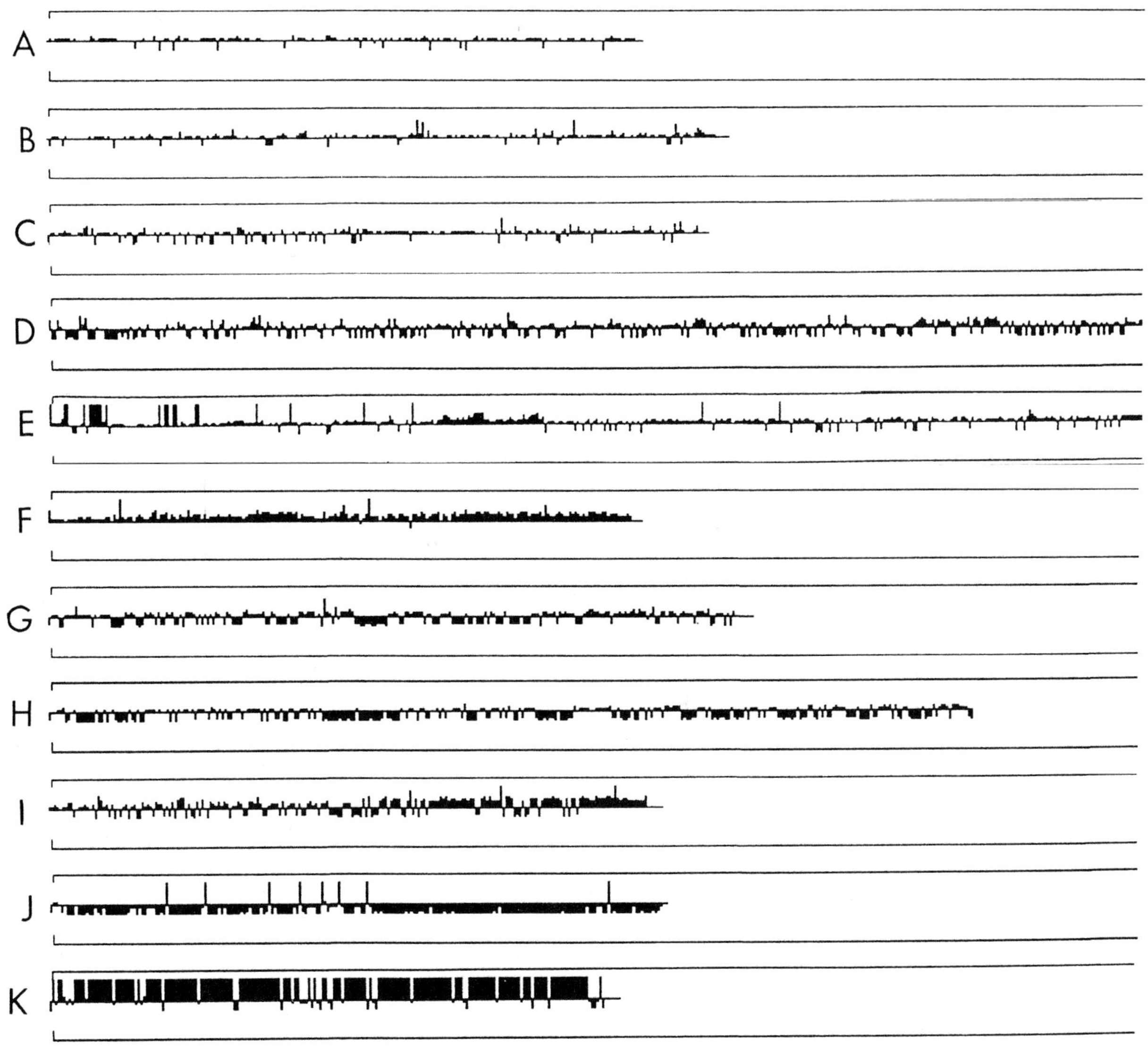

FIG. 7-12. Composite of Tracings From the Gaze Tracker. The position of the eye is recorded during each stimulus presentation (but not between presentations), with a vertical bar or a blank space for each stimulus. Downward deflections indicate that either the corneal reflection or the pupil image was not adequate to calculate gaze direction at that moment. Upward deflections indicate the magnitude of the gaze misalignment (up to 10 degrees maximum) in any direction. **A,** During this test, there were scattered instances when gaze alignment was indeterminate (downward deflections), and the rest of the time gaze was perfectly aligned within the precision of the measurement (about 1 to 2 degrees). An occasional downward deflection usually occurs because the stimulus happens to be presented during a blink. **B,** A few large deviations (upward deflections) occur, but the steadiness of fixation is rarely better than that shown on this record. The frequency of gaze errors is certainly less than the 20% generally accepted with the blind spot method. **C,** Again, both the performance of the gaze tracker and the fixation of the patient are exceptionally good. **D,** Although the gaze tracker image was not always adequate to provide a measurement, for the majority of presentations the tracker was able to show excellent alignment throughout this lengthy test. **E,** Early in the test gaze was errant, but as the patient settled into the test with encouragement from the perimetrist, fixation became remarkably steady. **F,** It is exceptional for the gaze tracker to have a readable image on every presentation (no downward de-flections), and the patient's fixation also is very acceptable. **G,** During nearly every presentation in which the tracker could provide information, the gaze was in good alignment. **H,** Again, although the tracker often had an inadequate image (downward deflections), fixation was steady at all other times, and the number of times fixation was successfully checked is greater than that provided by the blind spot technique. **I,** In this case, fixation became less steady late in the test, which is helpful information when determining confidence in the threshold values reported for the peripheral points, which are tested toward the end of the test session. The blind spot method also was used in this test; it checked fixation more frequently in the earlier parts of the test and hence reported an FL rate of only 2/17. If downward deflections had become more frequent late in the test, it might have suggested eyelid lag from fatigue. **J,** The gaze tracker rarely had an adequate image; when it did, gaze seemed highly deviant. This record indicates that the initialization (calibration) of the gaze tracker failed. If the perimetrist had been attentive, he would have tried to reinitialize the gaze tracker as soon as the problem was evident. However, eyelid ptosis or miotic pupils may make it difficult or impossible to obtain the required images in some cases. **K,** The gaze tracker had an acceptable image but incorrectly reported large deviation errors in this well-fixing patient (1/17 FL by the blind spot method during this same test). Again, the perimetrist could have tried to reinitialize the gaze tracker early in the test because, for example, the patient may not have been gazing straight ahead during the original initialization. Other field tests on this patient showed tracings of high quality.

Short-term fluctuation

The short-term fluctuation (SF) index is calculated in hopes that it will call attention to inconsistencies in repeat threshold measurements. The clinician must interpret whether the inconsistencies result from disease with reduced threshold and broadened frequency-of-seeing curves, from unreliable patient responses, or from both. Not only is the SF index affected by both disease and unreliability, but it also suffers because it is not measured accurately, and in any event, it is different in every location, so that diagnostic information is lost when SF is represented by a single number meant to represent the field globally.

A high SF index is an expected result of patient inconsistency and accompanies abnormal FP, FN, and FL reliability parameters. Figures 7-1, 7-3 (but not 7-4), 7-5, and 7-13 show that SF reflects the inaccuracy of measurement in unreliable fields. The SF index also reflects the presence of abnormality, if some or all of the 10 points used to determine the index happen to fall within the visual field defect (Figs. 7-14 through 7-16). It was already noted that disease-related variability might produce a high FN rate in addition to a high SF index.

To judge whether a high SF index (and FN rate) is a sign of patient inattention or a sign of disease, the clinician should examine the 10 points that constitute the basis for the SF calculation. If the two threshold determinations agree at normal points, but there is a marked discrepancy at moderately abnormal locations, the abnormal SF can be interpreted as reflecting that the field is abnormal without suggesting inattentiveness or inconsistency on the part of the patient (see Fig. 7-15). This may be confirmed if in fact the test-retest reproducibility is good at all the normal locations, and the reliability indices may further show that the patient is by nature consistent. However, if the test-retest difference is high even at normal locations, the patient may by nature be inconsistent, and this may be confirmed if the FP and FL rates are also high.

With the Sita strategies, no global estimate of test-retest variation (i.e., SF) is made. Compared with the older strategies, patient reliability is better determined from the improved FP and FN reliability parameters, and abnormality of the field is better determined by the threshold estimates, the probability deviation plots, and the GHT.

Text continued on p. 143

There are better indicators of reliability and of disease than the estimated average SF.

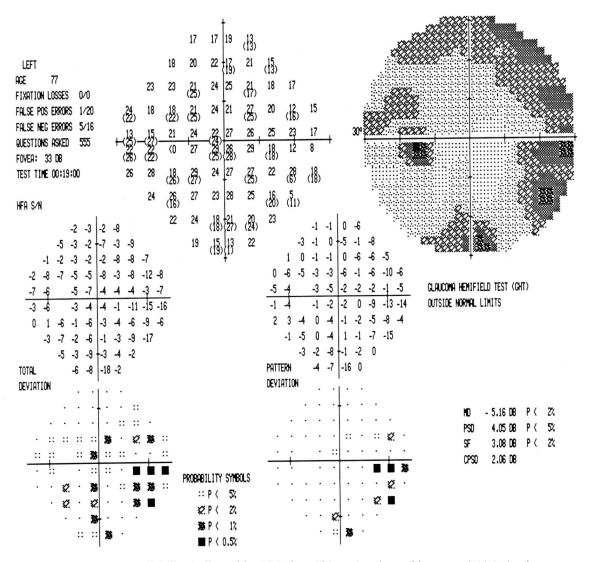

FIG. 7-13. Unreliability Indicated by SF Index. This patient has mild cataract (20/40 visual acuity), accounting for mild general depression. She has a tendency not to respond to visible stimuli because of inattention but the false-negative response rate is just within the 33% limit of "reliability" (5/16). However, because of failure to respond, scattered points have underestimated thresholds of varying degree, affecting the PSD index. The SF index is abnormal because of inconsistent duplicate threshold determinations. The CPSD index is normal because most of the variation in the PSD index is accounted for by short-term fluctuation. The total and pattern deviation plots show patchy deviation from normal values. Apart from mild cataract, the patient has no ocular abnormalities. The visual field examination was performed in both eyes because of uniocular secondary glaucoma in the other eye. The clue to the unreliability of the examination resides in the SF index, a borderline false-negative error rate, and the lack of any cause for visual deficit on ophthalmoscopic examination.

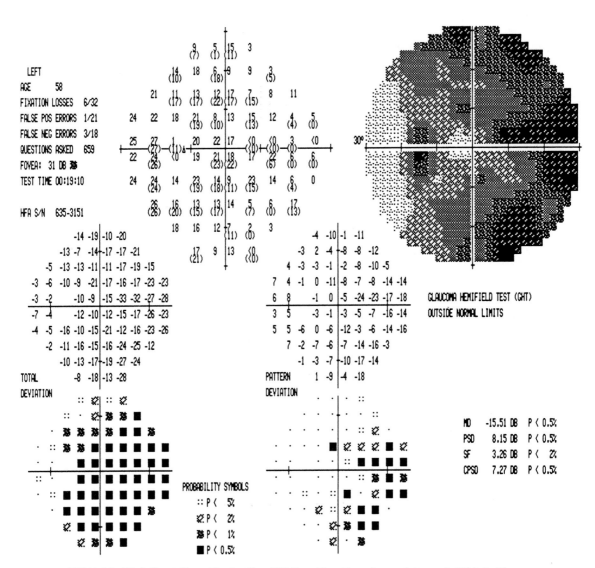

FIG. 7-14. High Short-Term Fluctuation (SF) Resulting From Inconsistency In Widely Abnormal Field Caused By Glaucoma. The false-negative responses are only slightly elevated (3/18). This patient's other eye is normal and the SF of the field of the other eye is 1.37, so the patient is reliable.

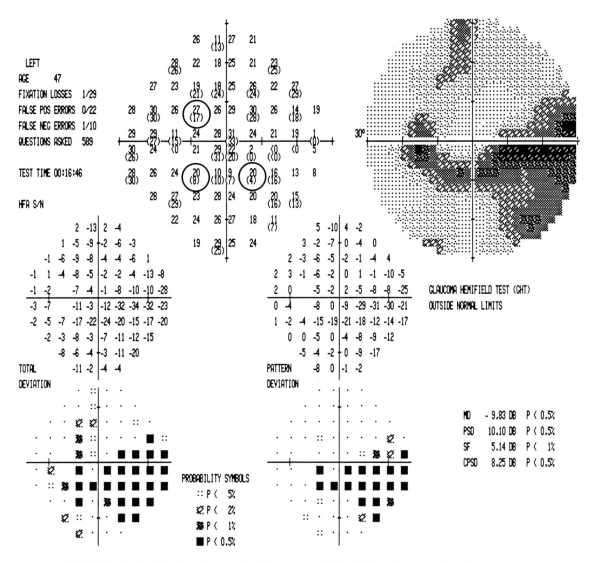

FIG. 7-15. High SF Index Caused By Glaucoma. Of the 10 locations used for SF calculation, only the three in the abnormal zone are inconsistent. The seven locations with normal threshold are reproducible.

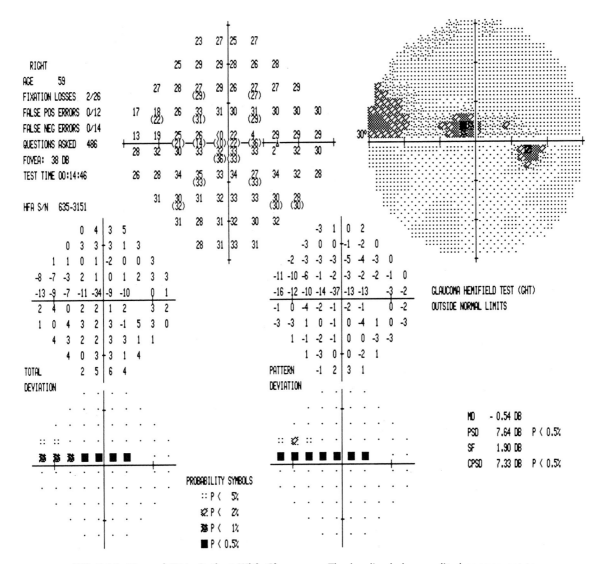

FIG. 7-16. Normal SF In Patient With Glaucoma. The localized abnormality happens not to involve any of the 10 points used to estimate SF.

IS THE FIELD ABNORMAL?

By now, halfway through the book and well into this chapter, readers may wonder if we ever will consider how to determine whether the field is normal, and if it is abnormal, which disease it represents. Such interpretation is best made after thoroughly understanding the basis of the perimetric test and for individual fields cannot be undertaken without an awareness of what transpired while the examination was being conducted, as reflected in the indicators of test reliability.

Most clinicians, after studying the reliability parameters, glance at the interpolated greyscale. The more experienced then quickly turn to the probability plots of total and pattern deviations, scan the global indices, and note the GHT message. These all are helpful distillates of the raw data. It is also sensible to look selectively at the actual sensitivity values in the relevant affected regions, based on the statistical distillates.

Two types of abnormalities are identified: generalized and localized.

Generalized depression

The term "generalized depression" sometimes is used to imply that all regions of the field are abnormal to an equivalent degree. Some use the term less strictly to mean that all parts of the field are affected to some degree early in the disease, even if unequally so. As suggested by Heijl, and to be clear in communication among ourselves (the purpose of language, after all), the term "widespread loss" might be used to mean that most or all locations are abnormal, but not necessarily to the same degree. For now, it is important to realize that not everyone attaches the same meaning to the term "generalized depression."

Identifying pure, generalized depression of sensitivity (widespread depression of equal degree) requires first that there be no evidence of localized abnormality. The PSD and CPSD indices must be normal, the Glaucoma Hemifield Test (GHT) must be neither borderline nor abnormal, and the pattern deviation plot must not reveal that some regions are more abnormal than others are.

Second, the field as a whole must be recognizably abnormal. The depression of sensitivity is recognized by comparison of the obtained threshold values with normal values, with the values in the other eye, or with previously recorded values in this individual patient.

Comparison with normal. Comparison with the average normal value is given point by point in the Total Deviation plot, and the weighted average is summarized in the MD index. Figures 7-17 through 7-19 show the typical features of the printout. In the Total Deviation plot, minus values of approximately equal magnitude may be recognized. The probability plot may show abnormality in the total deviation plot that is eliminated in the Pattern Deviation plot. The MD index averages the measurement errors at the 74 points and, in the absence of localized loss, quantifies the degree of overall generalized depression.

Unfortunately, the normal range is reasonably wide, so several decibels of depression must occur before the MD index falls outside the normal range, even at the 5% level. It also must be remembered that when the one-tailed percentile

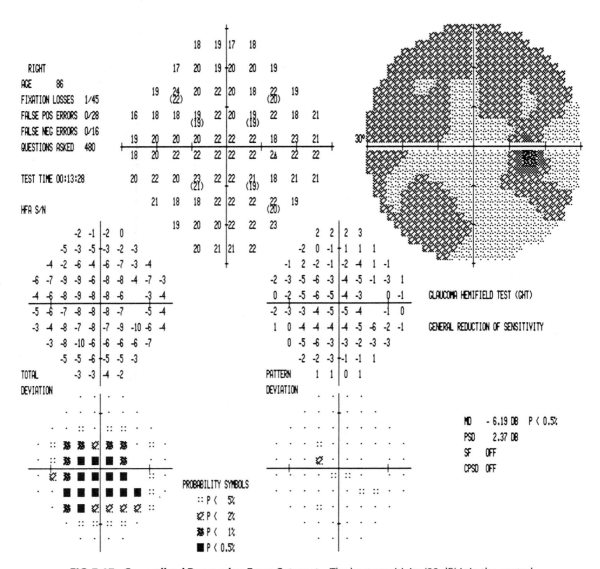

FIG. 7-17. Generalized Depression From Cataract. The best sensitivity (22 dB) is in the central 10 degrees. The depression from normal values (Total Deviation plot) is more marked centrally than toward the edge. Because of this and because the range of normal is smaller near the center, the statistical significance in the Total Deviation probability plot tends to be greater at the center.

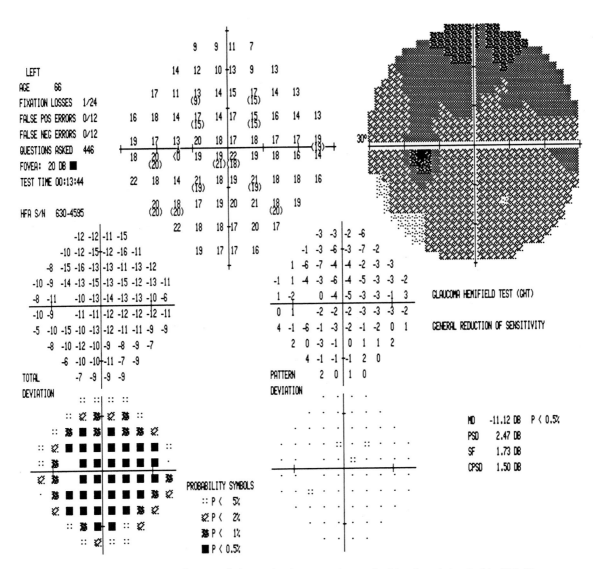

LEFT
AGE 66
FIXATION LOSSES 1/24
FALSE POS ERRORS 0/12
FALSE NEG ERRORS 0/12
QUESTIONS ASKED 446
FOVEA: 20 DB ■
TEST TIME 00:13:44

HFA S/N 630-4595

```
                    9    9  |11   7
               14  12   10 +13   9   13
          17  11   13   14  15   17   14  13
                   (9)          (15)
     16  18  14   17   14 |17   15   16  14  13
                  (15)         (15)
     19  17  13   20   18 |17   18   17  17   19
                                              (18)
     18   20   <0   19   19 +22   18   19  18  16   14
          (20)           (21) (18)
     22  18  14   21   18 |19   21   18  18  16
                  (19)         (19)
          20   18   17  19 |20   21   18   19
          (20) (20)              (20)
               22  18   18 +17   20   17
                         19  17 |17  16
```

```
-3  -3 |-2  -6
                                     -1  -3  -6 +-3  -7  -2
                                   1  -6  -7  -4 |-4  -2  -3  -3
                               -1   1  -4  -3  -6 |-4  -5  -3  -3  -2
                                1  -2    0  -4 |-5  -3  -3  -1    3
                                0   1    -2  -2 |-2  -3  -3  -3  -2
                                4  -1  -6  -1  -3 |-2  -1  -2   0   1
                                   2   0  -3  -1 | 0   1   1   2
                                        4  -1  -1 +-1   2   0
PATTERN                             2   0   1   0
DEVIATION
```

```
           -12  -12 |-11  -15
      -10  -12  -15 +-12  -16  -11
  -8  -15  -16  -13 |-13  -11  -13  -12
-10  -9  -14  -13  -15 |-13  -15  -12  -13  -11
-8  -11     -10  -13 |-14  -13  -13  -10  -6
-10  -9     -11  -11 |-12  -12  -12  -12  -11
-5  -10  -15  -10  -13 |-12  -11  -11  -9  -9
  -8  -10  -12  -10 |-9  -8  -9  -7
      -6  -10  -10 +-11  -7  -9
TOTAL        -7  -9 |-9  -9
DEVIATION
```

GLAUCOMA HEMIFIELD TEST (GHT)

GENERAL REDUCTION OF SENSITIVITY

PROBABILITY SYMBOLS
:: P < 5%
✘ P < 2%
▨ P < 1%
■ P < 0.5%

MD   -11.12 DB   P < 0.5%
PSD   2.47 DB
SF   1.73 DB
CPSD   1.50 DB

FIG. 7-18. Cataract. The overall depression is more advanced, with a foveal threshold of 20 dB and MD index of −11.12 dB. Note that the upper hemifield is normally less sensitive than the lower hemifield, and attention is called to this by the darkened greyscale of a depressed field. Because of a wide range of normal in the upper field, its greater depression does not yield greater significance in the Pattern Deviation probability plot. The hemifield analysis did not yield significant or even borderline asymmetry of the upper and lower regions but only a general reduction of sensitivity.

145

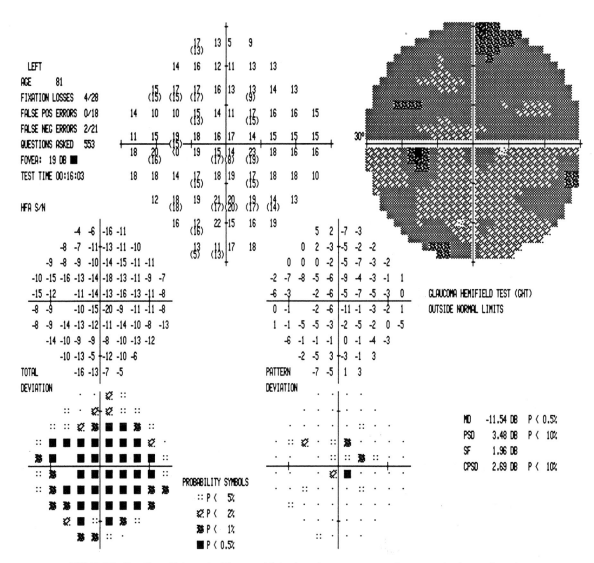

FIG. 7-19. Another Cataract. The sensitivity is quite even except for several edge points that produce a borderline CPSD index. Because the range of normal is narrower near the center, the depression at the center is marked as statistically significant in the pattern deviation plot. This pattern should not be taken to indicate a central scotoma (for example, from macular disease) unless the actual central sensitivity level is less than its surround. See Figure 3-2, in which several points have actual sensitivities less than their surround.

ranking is $p < 5\%$, 1 of 20 reliable field examinations of normal eyes shows mean sensitivity levels this low. Thus, if visual field examinations were performed on 20 eyes without disease, an MD depressed to this level would be expected approximately once, just by chance or as a normal variant.

The GHT also may indicate generalized depression with the message "general reduction of sensitivity." For this message to appear, the General Height calculation (see Chapter 6) must have shown the best part of the field to be depressed to a degree that occurs in fewer than 0.5% of the normal population, while at the same time the mirror-image comparison of the upper and lower hemifields must have been within normal limits or borderline.

A distinct, pure generalized depression is most typical of preretinal optical abnormality. Rarely would the MD index fall outside the normal range by virtue of glaucoma without first producing one of the diagnostic signs of a localized defect (to be enumerated in the next section). The example in Figure 7-20 may be about the only one in existence. Even in that example, careful inspection suggests an upper arcuate defect. If the MD index has fallen outside the normal range without accompanying signs of a localized field defect, the cause is almost surely nonglaucomatous; more likely it is another disease (such as cataract) or an artifact (such as a small pupil or improper refractive correction).

There are two additional ways to recognize generalized depression. They may be more sensitive than comparing the field with the normal range for the purpose of recognizing the infrequent cases of mild depression due to glaucoma: comparison with the other eye and comparison with a previous baseline in that individual.

Comparison with the other eye. Even if both values are within the normal range, a 2-dB difference of the MD index between the two eyes probably is not accidental, although confirmation by a second test is prudent. An average 1.5-dB difference must be maintained on two consecutive tests to yield confidence at the 5% level that true asymmetry exists. An average difference as small as 1 dB on four consecutive tests is statistically significant and potentially meaningful.

These criteria identify that one eye has, overall, a depressed sensitivity compared with the other. Localized perturbations in the visual field (real or artifactual) cause an MD difference between the two eyes. In the absence of such a localized element to the loss, glaucoma can be considered the cause of mild generalized depression only if there are other signs of glaucoma, and there is no evidence of nonglaucomatous causes of asymmetric visual sensitivity (e.g., asymmetric pupil size, mild asymmetric cataract, anisometropia, amblyopia). The diagnosis of glaucoma is most firm when the asymmetry of the MD index is reproducible on other occasions and corresponds to an asymmetry of intraocular pressure or of disc cupping.[19,20]

Comparison of the Mean Deviation (MD) index with an established baseline. The MD index can be compared with an established baseline. The principle is the same as when judging a pair or series of visual field test results for progression of disease (see Chapter 9). In one approach, a plot and regression analysis of the MD over time (Change Analysis printout or Glaucoma Change Probability printout) is analyzed to look for a statistically significant decline in the MD index. A

Text continued on p. 152

Glaucoma rarely affects MD appreciably without first producing a localized defect.

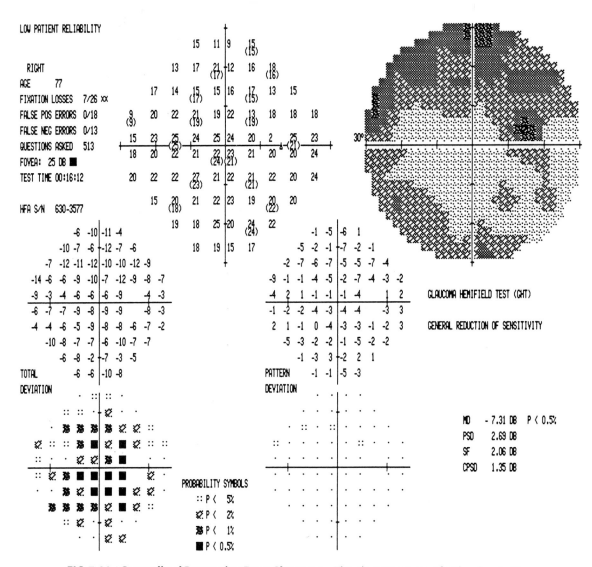

FIG. 7-20. Generalized Depression From Glaucoma. The glaucoma is manifest by elevated intraocular pressure and extensive cupping (0.95 cup/disc ratio), with a very thin but even rim of tissue around the disc circumference. A diffuse loss from glaucoma of this degree without more evidence of localized loss is very rare. As with the cataract example, the best sensitivity is in the central 10 degrees, with a foveal threshold of 25 dB (visual acuity of 20/60). The greatest deviation from normal is in the upper hemifield, but given normal variation in the upper field and possible eyelid artifacts, the Pattern Deviation probability gives only a hint of localized abnormality. The CPSD index is normal and the GHT failed to find statistically significant hemifield asymmetry, even at the borderline (third percentile) level. No cataract accompanied the glaucoma. This eye is not more myopic than the other eye (Fig. 7-21) and the media are of equal clarity in the two eyes on slit lamp and fundus examination.

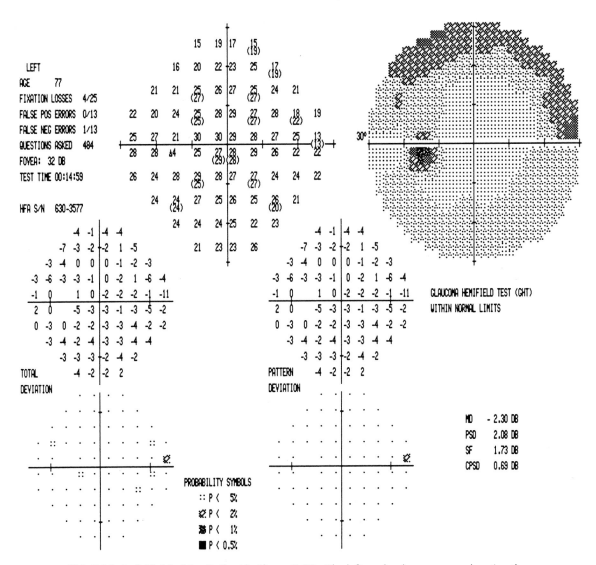

FIG. 7-21. Left Field of the Patient in Figure 7-20. The left eye has less pressure elevation than the right eye and a moderate sized (0.7 cup/disc ratio) round cup. The only clinically evident difference between the two eyes is reduced acuity, higher pressure, and a much larger excavation of the disc in the right eye.

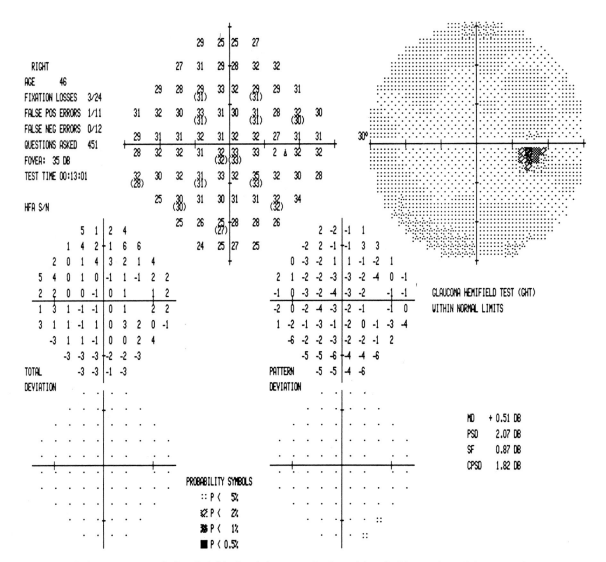

FIG. 7-22. Normal Visual Field of a Right Eye. The foveal threshold is 35 dB and the MD index is +0.51.

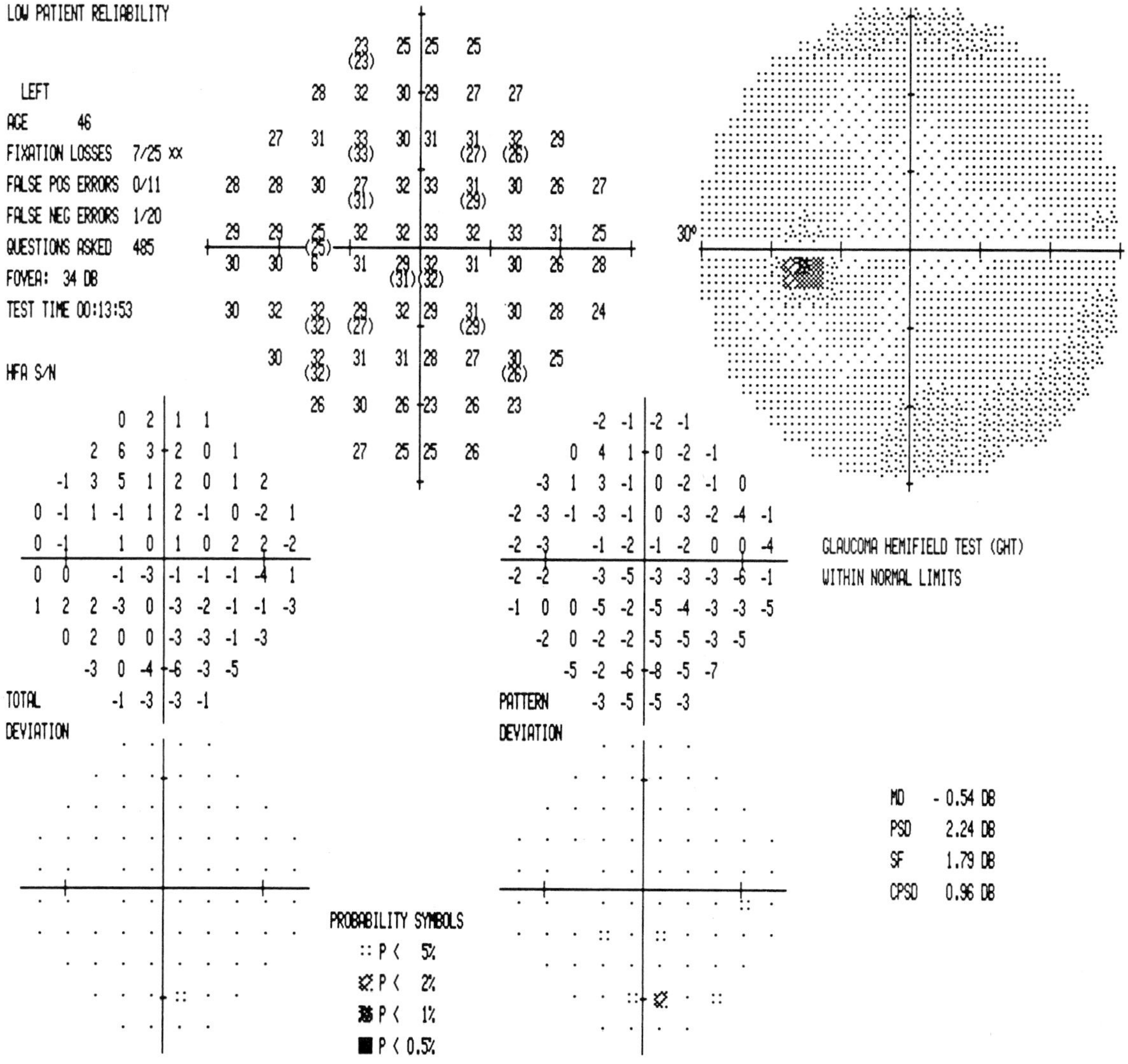

LOW PATIENT RELIABILITY

```
                              23
                             (23)  25  25   25

    LEFT                 28   32  30 |29  27  27
AGE      46
FIXATION LOSSES  7/25 xx    27  31  33   30  31  31   32  29
                                   (33)            (27) (26)
FALSE POS ERRORS  0/11  28  28  30  27   32  33  31   30  26  27
                                   (31)          (29)
FALSE NEG ERRORS  1/20  29  29  25  32  32 |33  32   33  31  25
                               (25)
QUESTIONS ASKED  485    30  30   6   31  29 (31)(32) 31   30  26  28
FOVEA:  34 DB
TEST TIME 00:13:53      30  32  32  29   32 |29  31   30  28  24
                               (32)(27)          (29)

HFA S/N                     30  32  31  31 |28  27  30  25
                               (32)                  (26)
                              26  30  26 |23  26  23
```

```
             0   2   1   1                                -2  -1 |-2  -1
         2   6   3 |2   0   1                27  25 |25  26     0   4   1 |0  -2  -1
    -1   3   5   1 | 2   0   1   2                        -3   1   3  -1 |0  -2  -1   0
 0  -1   1  -1   1 | 2  -1   0  -2   1                 -2  -3  -1  -3  -1 |0  -3  -2  -4  -1
 0  -1       1   0 | 1   0   2   2  -2                 -2  -3      -1  -2 |-1  -2   0   0  -4
 0   0      -1  -3 |-1  -1  -1  -4   1                 -2  -2      -3  -5 |-3  -3  -3  -6  -1
 1   2   2  -3   0 |-3  -2  -1  -1  -3              -1   0   0  -5  -2 |-5  -4  -3  -3  -5
     0   2   0   0 |-3  -3  -1  -3                      -2   0  -2  -2 |-5  -5  -3  -5
        -3   0  -4 |-6  -3  -5                             -5  -2  -6 |-8  -5  -7
TOTAL      -1  -3 |-3  -1                     PATTERN       -3  -5 |-5  -3
DEVIATION                                     DEVIATION
```

GLAUCOMA HEMIFIELD TEST (GHT)
WITHIN NORMAL LIMITS

MD   - 0.54 DB
PSD   2.24 DB
SF   1.79 DB
CPSD   0.96 DB

PROBABILITY SYMBOLS
:: P < 5%
⊠ P < 2%
▩ P < 1%
■ P < 0.5%

FIG. 7-23. Subtle Depression of the Left Field of the Patient in Figure 7-22. Although the visual acuity is 20/15 in each eye, the foveal threshold of the left eye is 34 dB. The MD is −0.54 dB, 1.05 dB less than the other eye. The pressure in this eye usually is higher, and its disc has a noticeably larger excavation. Only by comparison with the other eye would either the disc or the field be suspected of being abnormal. Such subtle visual field depression needs confirmation on a second and third occasion (which was done in this patient) to be accepted as real. In any event, it represents very mild disease that may never amount to much, and therapeutic decisions cannot be based on the visual field findings alone. This example simply illustrates that very mild glaucomatous damage can be recognized with careful attention to a quantified field examination.

Glaucoma rarely affects MD appreciably without first producing a localized defect.

second approach is to compare the MD to that of a baseline field or a baseline pair and note if the difference is statistically significant (Glaucoma Change Probability printout). With either approach, if the decline is statistically significant, one must be cautious regarding changes caused by long-term fluctuation. If there seems to be a genuine generalized decline in the MD index without a localized defect appearing, it usually is nonglaucomatous. To diagnose glaucoma, other causes must be ruled out and the clinician must have other, confirming evidence, such as an enlarging excavation or an uncontrolled intraocular pressure.

Localized defects

It usually is more rewarding diagnostically to look for localized defects than to identify generalized depression. The Statpac Single Field Printout gives a number of useful statistics. It calls attention to the points that are at the lower end of the normal threshold sensitivity range, provides global indices and their normal prevalence percentiles, and provides the results of the GHT. Several criteria seem to be useful as guidelines for recognizing the presence of localized defects. These criteria refer only to the visual field element of diagnosis and therapeutic decision making. As always, the clinical setting and other clinical signs also must be considered.

For topographical diagnosis, the clinician may try to distinguish one pattern of localized defect from another. When trying to diagnose the presence or absence of a specific disease, such as glaucoma or chloroquine retinopathy, one already has the expected pattern in mind, and the question is whether the abnormality exists. At this point we consider only the second diagnostic problem—how to determine whether the visual field has evidence of a particular disease, and more specifically, whether there is a glaucomatous nerve fiber bundle defect.

Three criteria for minimal abnormality. Well-established defects, such as those shown in Chapter 4, can be recognized without difficulty. The question at hand is how to recognize accurately the mildest defect without falsely labeling normal fields as glaucomatous. In the correct clinical context, reliable fields can be considered to have a localized glaucomatous defect if the pattern deviation probability plot shows a cluster of three or more nonedge points that have sensitivities occurring in fewer than 5% of the normal population ($p < 5\%$), and one of the points has a sensitivity that occurs in fewer than 1% of the population ($p < 1\%$). The points must be in a cluster in an expected location. By chance, several of the 76 tested points may exceed the percentile criterion in a normal field, and there is even a tendency for such points to be grouped in a normal field,[21,22] but a cluster in a nerve fiber bundle pattern indicates glaucoma if there is already reason to suspect that particular disease. Edge points are not included because of frequent artifacts at these locations, but confidence in a group of three abnormal nonedge points is greater if the adjacent edge points also are abnormal.

A second sensitive and specific criterion is that the PSD (or CPSD) has a value that occurs in less than 5% of normal reliable fields ($p < 5\%$).

A third criterion is that the GHT indicates that the field is abnormal. The hemifield analysis probably is the most accurate overall; some other criteria may be indistinguishably equal to the GHT, but none is clearly better.[23]

Sensitivity in recognizing subtle nerve damage is greatest if it is accepted that meeting any one of these three criteria is sufficient to make the test result abnormal. However, specificity falls if the clinician decides to accept any one of them in isolation. He should reserve diagnostic judgment on isolated findings but seek confirmation by meeting other criteria, by consistent findings on repeat testing, or perhaps more reliably by finding an independent clinical sign, like glaucomatous cupping or a disc hemorrhage.

These three criteria seemingly are the easiest and the most accurate of any currently proposed for use in an office practice. Even with widespread loss, these criteria typically are met (see Fig. 4-20). Application of these criteria also is demonstrated in Figure 6-3 and Figures 7-22 through 7-31. There must be some flexibility in the criteria according to the clinical setting, as discussed theoretically in the next section.

Other criteria. The aforementioned criteria derive an element of their usefulness from the use of mean normal values and also from the probability rankings of the obtained thresholds and indices in healthy eyes. Other criteria have been used in clinical and research settings when full normative data are not available.

One such criterion is that three nonedge points must be deepened by 5 dB, and one must be deepened by 10 dB; the 5- and 10-dB criteria both must be met in comparison with the point-wise mean normal value and also with a normal or a less-affected region of the field (to ensure that there is a localized defect in addition to any general involvement that may be present). Although the mean normal value still must be known, an advantage of this kind of criterion is that it does not require knowledge of the *range* of normal values point by point. The concurrent disadvantage is that the criterion may falsely label edge points as abnormal and fail to discern slight abnormality near the center.

Another criterion that has been used in scientific study is complex, requiring 5 to 9 dB (depending on location) of depressed sensitivity in the total deviation plot. A cluster of three points so depressed (or two points depressed to that degree in the company of one point depressed by 12 dB) constitutes abnormality. Only points in the central 24-2 pattern are considered.[23,24]

Another approach is a mirror-image analysis, similar to the Statpac hemifield analysis, performed on threshold data transferred into a personal computer.[25-28] This method is advantageous in a research setting when working with raw threshold data independent of a normative database.

These various criteria have been shown to be suitably sensitive and specific[23] for some office diagnoses and research purposes in the past decade, but currently they may be replaced by the more refined criteria, described in the previous section.

The unreliable field. When an examination is not perfectly reliable, some signs of localized defects may be produced falsely. If the patient has an unusually high rate of false-positive or false-negative responses, the visual sensitivity values are less accurate. The field is likely to show considerable unevenness in threshold values because one point may have an overestimated visual sensitivity and its neighbor an underestimated visual sensitivity. Consequently, the PSD index will be high. The SF may or may not be equivalently elevated, so the CPSD may or may not be abnormal. In addition, in a session with numerous false-positive and false-negative responses, the sensitivity values obtained are influenced even more than usual by the starting value used in the threshold determination, which was based on the threshold determination at the primary points (which in turn may have been faulty). Consequently, points with abnormal values may be grouped,

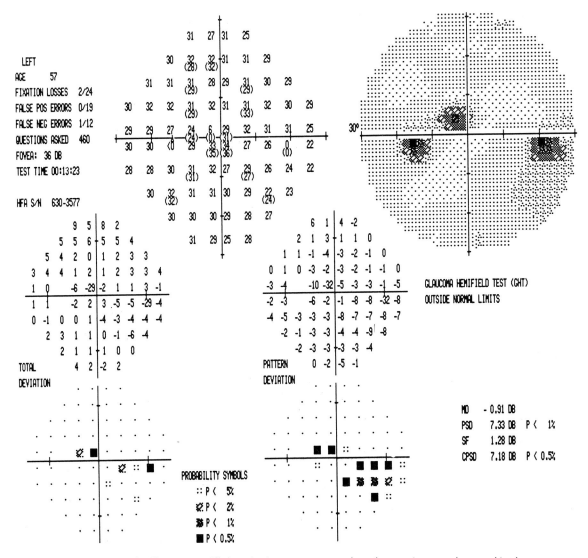

FIG. 7-24. Early Glaucoma. All the criteria are met: more than three points are abnormal in the pattern deviation probability plot; the CPSD index is very abnormal; and the GHT is outside normal limits. Although attention is called to the two deeply scotomatous regions on the greyscale, the pattern deviation plot reveals that the lower nasal quadrant is broadly involved as well.

and the criterion that three adjacent points be abnormal may be met. With the thresholds of adjacent points artificially close to one another, and perhaps different from the matching group in the opposite hemifield, the hemifield analysis also may be affected. The most significant flaw in an unreliable examination is causing a normal field to seem abnormal.[28-30] It is unusual for an abnormal field to appear normal because of unreliable performance by the patient.

To repeat an important point, the basis for statistical calculations in the printout is a normative database, which for Full Threshold and Fastpac (but not SITA) required FN and FP to be under 33%. Therefore the calculations do not completely apply to fields that fail to meet the same reliability criteria as the corresponding normative database. In cases that do not, the calculations are faulty, but the clinician still may discern important diagnostic information. *Text continued on p. 162*

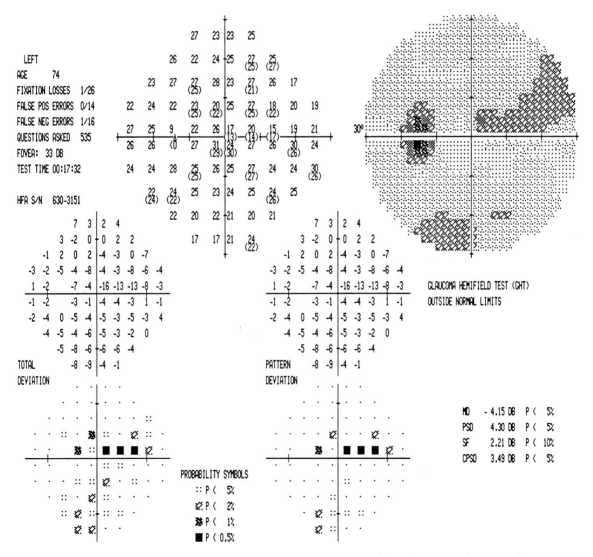

FIG. 7-25. Mild Glaucoma. The field is more diffusely involved but the pattern deviation plot calls specific attention to the points above the nasal horizontal meridian. The CPSD index and GHT are abnormal.

155

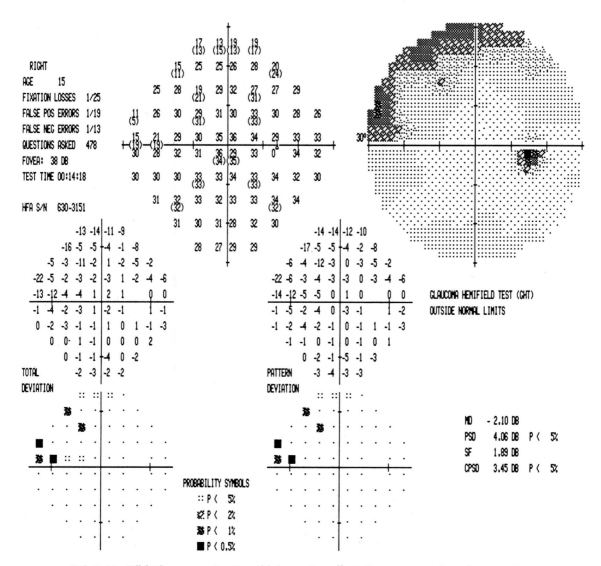

RIGHT

AGE 15

FIXATION LOSSES 1/25

FALSE POS ERRORS 1/19

FALSE NEG ERRORS 1/13

QUESTIONS ASKED 478

FOVEA: 38 DB

TEST TIME 00:14:18

HFA S/N 630-3151

GLAUCOMA HEMIFIELD TEST (GHT)
OUTSIDE NORMAL LIMITS

MD   - 2.10 DB

PSD   4.06 DB   P <   5%

SF   1.89 DB

CPSD   3.45 DB   P <   5%

PROBABILITY SYMBOLS

:: P <   5%

P <   2%

P <   1%

■ P < 0.5%

FIG. 7-26. Mild Glaucoma. Spotty mild depression affects the upper nasal quadrant, particularly near the edge. The abnormality falls short of having a cluster of three nonedge points abnormal in the pattern deviation plot but excavation toward the inferior pole of the disc in the presence of high pressures, along with the reproducibility of these findings on repeated examination, suggest that the defect is real.

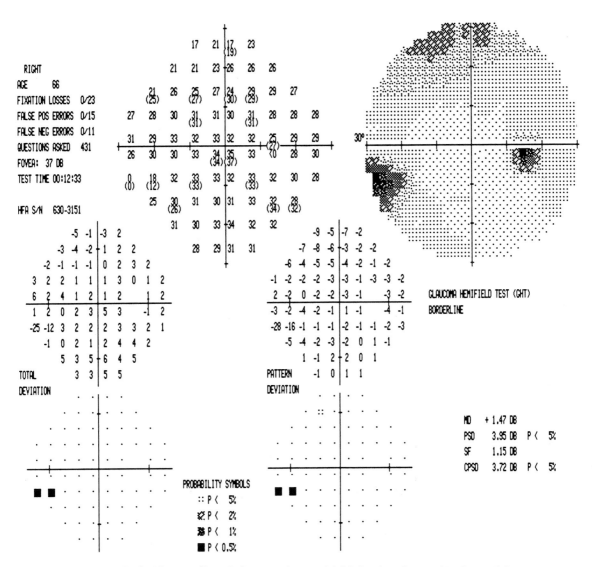

FIG. 7-27. Early Abnormality. Only two points are highlighted as abnormal in the total deviation plot, and one of these is an edge point. The CPSD abnormality is caused by the reduced sensitivity at the lower nasal edge, which could be an artifact. Because of the uncertain location of the abnormality, the GHT gives a borderline result. However, this defect is in keeping with the appearance of the optic disc and is reproducible on other occasions; thus, it undoubtedly is real.

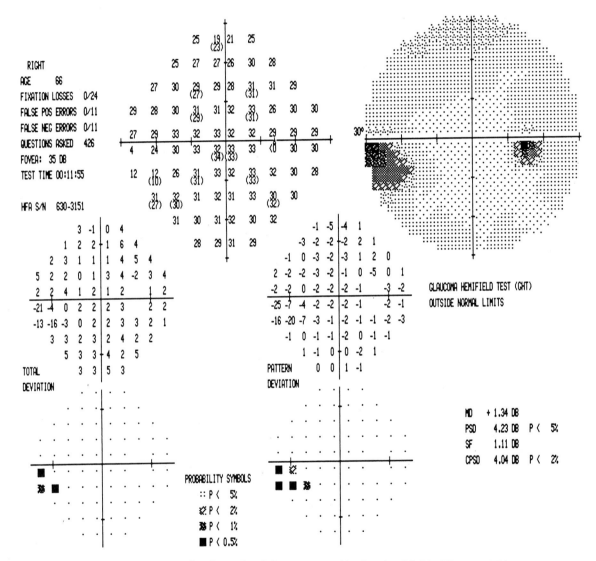

FIG. 7-28. Repeat Examination. The defect uncovered in the visual field of Figure 7-27 is not only confirmed but more clearly evident.

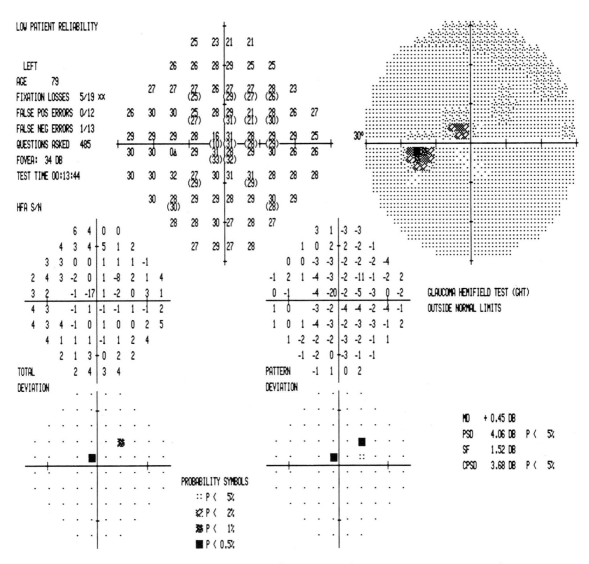

LOW PATIENT RELIABILITY

```
                              25   23  21   21

    LEFT                   26   26   28  29   25   25

AGE      79           27   27   27   26  27   27   28   23
                                  (25)    (29) (27) (26)
FIXATION LOSSES  5/19 xx

FALSE POS ERRORS  0/12    26  30   30   25   28  31   21   28   26   27
                                       (27)    (31) (21) (30)
FALSE NEG ERRORS  1/13

QUESTIONS ASKED  485   29  29  29   28   16  31   28   28   29   25
                                       (10) (31) (28) (25)
FOVEA:  34 DB          30  30   04   29   31  28   30   28   26
                                       (33) (32)
TEST TIME 00:13:44     30  30   32   27   30  31   31   28   28   28
                                       (29)    (29)

                       30   28   29   29   28   29   30   29
                             (30)                       (28)
HFA S/N
                              28   28   30  27   28   27
```

```
       6   4   0   0                              3   1  -3  -3
     4   3   4   5   1   2             27  29  27  28       1   0   2   2  -2  -1
   3   3   0   0   1   1   1  -1                        0   0  -3  -3  -2  -2  -2  -4
 2   4   3  -2   0   1  -8   2   1   4              -1   2   1  -4  -3  -2 -11  -1  -2   2
 3   2      -1 -17   1  -2   0   3   1               0  -1      -4 -20  -2  -5  -3   0  -2
   4   3      -1   1  -1  -1   1  -1   2              1   0      -3  -2  -4  -4  -2  -4  -1
 4   3   4  -1   0   1   0   0   2   5               1   0   1  -4  -3  -2  -3  -3  -1   2
   4   1   1   1  -1   1   2   4                      1  -2  -2  -2  -3  -2  -1   1
     2   1   3   0   2   2                             -1  -2   0  -3  -1  -1
TOTAL      2   4   3   4              PATTERN       -1  -1   1   0   2
DEVIATION                            DEVIATION
```

GLAUCOMA HEMIFIELD TEST (GHT)

OUTSIDE NORMAL LIMITS

```
MD      + 0.45 DB
PSD       4.06 DB   P <  5%
SF        1.52 DB
CPSD      3.68 DB   P <  5%
```

PROBABILITY SYMBOLS

:: P < 5%

P < 2%

P < 1%

■ P < 0.5%

FIG. 7-29. Another Mild Defect. Two small scotomas in the upper arcuate region, one adjacent to fixation, do not meet the criterion for abnormality in the pattern deviation plot. However, the GHT and CPSD indices in the absence of any edge artifacts are reasonably conclusive. The findings are in keeping with the appearance of the optic disc and the abnormalities were confirmed on other occasions.

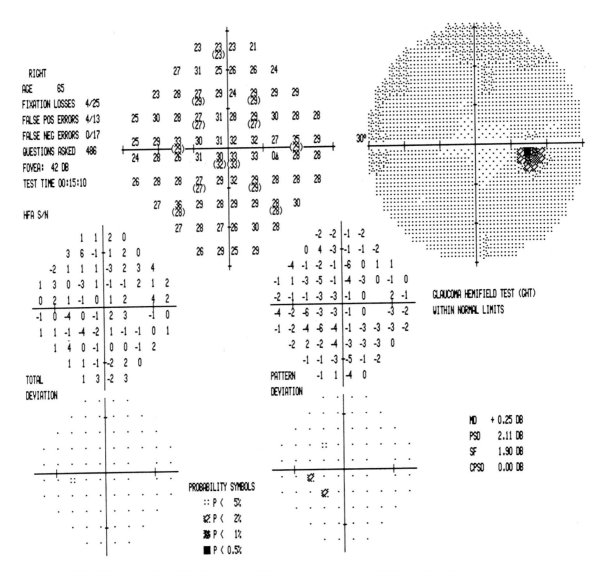

RIGHT

AGE 65
FIXATION LOSSES 4/25
FALSE POS ERRORS 4/13
FALSE NEG ERRORS 0/17
QUESTIONS ASKED 486
FOVEA: 42 DB
TEST TIME 00:15:10

HFA S/N

GLAUCOMA HEMIFIELD TEST (GHT)
WITHIN NORMAL LIMITS

TOTAL
DEVIATION

PATTERN
DEVIATION

PROBABILITY SYMBOLS
:: P < 5%
▨ P < 2%
▧ P < 1%
■ P < 0.5%

MD + 0.25 DB
PSD 2.11 DB
SF 1.90 DB
CPSD 0.00 DB

FIG. 7-30. Questionable Glaucoma. This eye has a pressure of 28 mm Hg, with a disc excavation that is slightly larger than the excavation in the disc of the other eye. The two points reduced 4 dB from normal in the lower nasal quadrant may represent a beginning abnormality, but an identical equivocal finding could occur in a normal eye. Therefore definitive identification of these points as a glaucomatous defect depends on the reproducibility, or perhaps even evolution, of the abnormality on subsequent examinations.

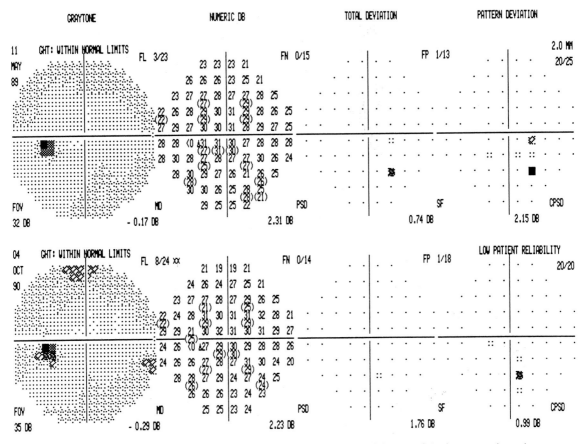

FIG. 7-31. Suspicious Glaucoma. This patient, with pseudoexfoliation of the lens capsule and variable, sometimes elevated intraocular pressure, shows four abnormal points in the lower nasal quadrant during the first examination, and this is confirmed during follow up. Note that the same region is affected but not necessarily the same points, which is consistent with the concept that beginning field loss often is represented by a region of variable responses rather than by a very localized but deep scotoma (see Heijl A: Perimetric point density and detection of glaucomatous visual field loss, *Acta Ophthalmol (Copenh)* 71:445-450, 1993). Only further follow up will prove whether this was the beginning of glaucoma. At this time the CPSD index and GHT are normal.

Diagnosis and statistics

Some important epidemiologic and statistical principles affect the interpretation of a diagnostic field examination. Separating the diseased from the healthy solely on the basis of "normal values" is faulty. If a test result found in few normal subjects (e.g., a CPSD value with a probability value < 5%) is judged as evidence of disease, then 5% of *normal* people tested have a "positive test" even if very few (perhaps 1%) of the group tested really have diseased visual function. In view of this, one might adopt more stringent criteria, demanding that the value be that found in fewer than 1% of normal individuals before accepting it as diagnostic. In that case, a new problem arises. Individuals in the early stage of disease truly may have mild optic nerve damage, but the threshold values or statistical parameters may have declined only from the midnormal range to a borderline value (e.g., the 10th percentile). Even if the value of the diagnostic parameter declines to the 2.5 percentile, the damage will be undetected if meanwhile the more stringent criterion is applied that requires decline to the 1% level for a diagnosis to be established.

The unavoidable dilemma, classic in statistical and epidemiologic circles, is that the desire for high specificity (few falsely positive tests) clashes with the desire for high sensitivity (no missed diagnoses). The escape from the dilemma is to recognize that there are no set criteria for deciding whether a field is abnormal. The prevalence or likelihood of disease independent of (or before) the visual field test result must be taken into account. The statistician's statement is that the predictability of a test result depends on prevalence in addition to sensitivity and specificity; the clinician's statement is that the test result must be interpreted in light of the other clinical findings.

There are several points to consider. First, the statistical printout of a visual field test gives only the relationship of parameter values to the distribution of these values in normal subjects. Whatever the test parameter, the range of values in the normal population and how rare the obtained value is in the absence of disease must indeed be known. However, the distribution of values among the diseased population also must be considered. A cutoff criterion for diagnosis depends on how much the distributions of diseased and healthy populations overlap; the useful cutoff point is not determined by the percentile ranking in the normal population but by the overlap of values in the groups with and without disease. Unfortunately, a range, frequency, distribution, or percentile ranking of abnormal values cannot be defined accurately. Glaucoma, like many other diseases, occurs in varying degrees of severity. Separation of severely abnormal cases from normal is easier than separation of mild cases from normal. One "range of abnormal" values might be found if tabulated from a group of individuals with glaucoma in which moderate or severe cases predominate. The range might be quite different in another group with many cases that were recognized early and included in the cohort. If it were possible, the trick would be to find some criterion that is exceedingly rare among normal individuals but quite common in those with glaucoma, even with mild glaucoma. In the real world, a clean separation is not possible. A compromise criterion that at least allows the optimum separation must be sought.

"Outside the normal range" is not the same as "Inside the disease range."

Second, the test itself and which strategy is used are not the only determinants of the diagnostic predictability of the test result. The test per se has no particular sensitivity or specificity, but simply provides threshold values and calculated parameters. The sensitivity and specificity depend on the criterion chosen as the dividing line between healthy and diseased.

Third, the practical meaning of the test result depends heavily on the clinical circumstances, which other signs are present, and which decisions are made as a result of the test. Making such judgments constitutes the art of practicing medicine. For example, if a patient has asymmetrically elevated intraocular pressure and asymmetric cupping of the optic disc, with thinning of the inferior rim in one eye, a subtle depression in the upper hemifield may reflect mild axon loss. The same visual field finding in a patient with healthy discs, perhaps with prominent eyebrows, may be interpreted as not representing glaucomatous disease.

A crisp diagnostic decision may not be needed in either case, if the major use of the field test will be to recognize any future deterioration. If the management decision is based more on severity of nerve damage than on the presence or absence of such damage, there may be little practical difference between equivocal presence or equivocal absence of a visual field defect; the decision may be governed more strongly by other clinical findings and the course of the disease. In other words, it may not be important to have crisp criteria for disease in a real clinical setting, if therapeutic decisions are based on a combination of findings and if intervention may not be indicated in the preclinical stage of disease. The moderate or severe cases usually are not diagnostic problems; it is finding a criterion to distinguish individuals with early or mild disease from healthy individuals that is most difficult and occupies considerable attention (but may not be really so important in daily practice).

Fourth, in a contrasting circumstance of population screening[31] (see Chapter 8), both the test strategy and the criterion applied to the test result may be selected intentionally to ignore equivocal findings. In the first place, equivocal findings are more likely to represent false results and, if genuine, they are likely to represent mild disease that is less important to detect. The benefit of detection is higher among those with moderately advanced disease, and the cost of sorting mild disease from nondisease is high. In other words, it may be disquieting not to have crisply accurate and universally applicable criteria for abnormality, but common sense and clinical judgment are just as important as statistical considerations in deciding whether a test result represents a clinical circumstance that requires action.

Finally, the needs in scientific studies differ from clinical needs. Flexible criteria are a source of bias if the evaluators, for example, deduce to which diagnostic or therapeutic group an individual subject belongs. Thus, he often cannot be permitted knowledge of the clinical circumstances that would help with interpretation in a clinical setting. When two groups are compared scientifically, the interest is in an average difference between them. The result is not affected by occasional false calls equally divided between the two groups. Thus, inflexible criteria fit the needs of scientific studies. In clinical practice, however, astute flexibility represents sound clinical judgment, and the individual patient is ill served by inflexibility. For

Equivocal early diagnosis is not a good guide to management. Passage of time helps separate "healthy" from "mildly diseased."

example, the fields in Figures 7-27 and 7-29 through 7-32 are by themselves too nonspecific to be diagnostic for a scientific study but are worthy of cautious attention in a clinical setting.

HOW ADVANCED IS THE DISEASE?

The severity of glaucomatous disease influences clinical decisions and in research may affect or correlate with the findings of the scientific study. The severity rating of a patient's disease may depend on other clinical findings as well; moreover, both disease scores and visual field scores are somewhat arbitrary. Yet, it may be useful to use criteria similar to those of your colleagues, so reference is made in this chapter to some published criteria currently in use.

The number of axons damaged should relate to the average defectiveness of the field, which is perhaps best represented by the MD index. Classification based simply on the MD index may be particularly appropriate when designating pathogenic severity of the disease.

> Context determines if severity ratings should relate to the quantity of damage or also take into account the location and impact of visual loss.

Symptomatic impact is affected also by the location of the defect and is especially important if near or at fixation, in particular below fixation. With these considerations in mind, one classification[32] to guide clinical decisions considers the field abnormality to be an *early defect* if there is a defect and the field meets *ALL* the following requirements:

1. The MD is better than −6 dB;
2. Fewer than 18 of the 76 points in a 30-2 pattern (25%) are defective in the total deviation probability plot at the 5% level;
3. Fewer than 10 points are defective at the 1% level; AND
4. No point in the central 5 degrees has a sensitivity less than 15 dB.

A *moderate defect* exceeds one or more of the criteria required to keep it in the early defect category but does not meet the criterion to be severe. A *severe defect* has *any* of the following:

1. An MD index worse than −12 dB;
2. More than 37 (50%) of the points depressed at the 5% level;
3. More than 20 points depressed at the 1% level;
4. A point in the central 5 degrees with 0-dB sensitivity; **OR**
5. Points closer than 5 degrees of fixation under 15-dB sensitivity in both the upper and lower hemifields.

Another, more complex scoring system is being used in an ongoing clinical trial.[24] It includes 20 levels of severity and is used to classify the stage of the disease on entry to the study; changes in severity are used as evidence of progression.

ARTIFACTS

Edge Artifacts

Edge points are particularly susceptible to artifactual reduction of sensitivity—for example, from an overhanging eyebrow or interference from a lens rim[33] (particularly nasally). A field defect should be particularly suspect if its nature or

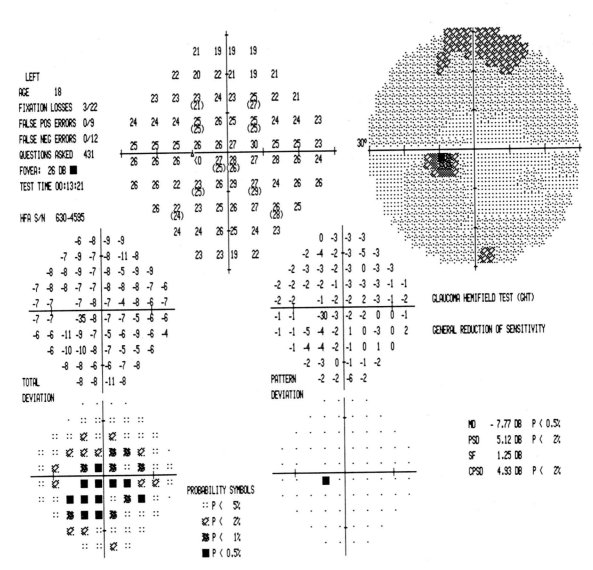

FIG. 7-32. Abnormal CPSD Without Glaucoma. This 18-year-old patient has a generally depressed field. Her congenital cataracts associated with rubella were removed, and she wears aphakic spectacles. The physiologic blind spot is optically displaced 10 degrees inward (see triangle on threshold map) and affects one of the 74 points included in the calculation of the global indices. This accounts for the abnormal CPSD index. There is no cluster of abnormal points on the pattern deviation plot, nor is the GHT abnormal. This example illustrates that none of the criteria for the presence of abnormality can be accepted without thoughtful inspection of the raw data that went into the statistical manipulations.

severity is not in keeping with the constellation of other clinical signs. Lens artifacts are so commonly misinterpreted that a number of examples are provided. In contrast to lens rim artifacts, arcuate glaucomatous defects typically are narrower near the blind spot than nasally. Additionally, if there are both upper and lower arcuate scotomas, they likely will be misaligned nasally to produce a nasal step (strikingly different sensitivities at several adjacent locations just above and below the horizontal nasal meridian) (Fig. 7-37).

Learn to recognize lens rim artifacts.

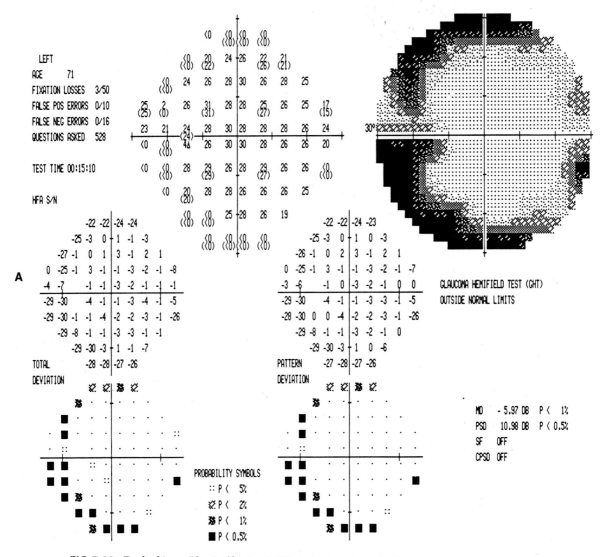

FIG. 7-33. Typical Lens Rim Artifacts. A, When the lens is too far from the eye or not properly centered, its rim can produce a sharply demarcated absolute (0-dB stimulus not seen) defect. As in this example, it need not extend around the entire circumference.

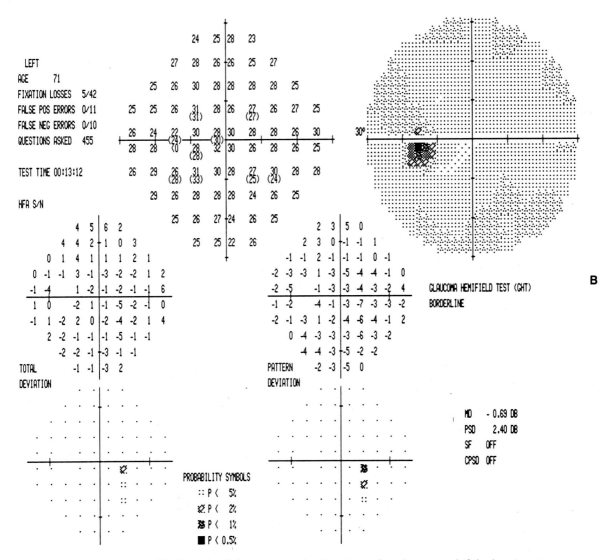

LEFT

AGE   71
FIXATION LOSSES   5/42
FALSE POS ERRORS 0/11
FALSE NEG ERRORS 0/10
QUESTIONS ASKED   455

TEST TIME 00:13:12

HFA S/N

```
                    24  25 |28  23
                27  28  26 +26  25  27
            25  26  30  28 |28  28  28  25
        25  25  26  31  28 |26  27  26  27  25
                      (31)        (27)
        26  24  22  30  28 |30  28  28  26  30
        28  28  (24) 28  28 |32  30  26  28  26  25
                (0)  (28)
        26  29  26  31  30 |28  27  30  28  28
                (28)(33)        (25)(24)
            29  26  28  28 |28  24  26  25
                    25  26  27 +24  26  25
                    25  25  22  26
```

30°

TOTAL DEVIATION
```
        4   5   6   2
      4   4   2 + 1   0   3
    0   1   4   1 | 1   1   2   1
  0  -1  -1   3  -1 |-3  -2  -2   1   2
 -1  -4       1  -2 |-1  -2  -1  -1   6
  1   0      -2   1 |-1  -5  -2  -1   0
 -1   1  -2   2   0 |-2  -4  -2   1   4
    2  -2  -1  -1 |-1  -5  -1  -1
     -2  -2  -1 +-3  -1  -1
          -1  -1 |-3   2
```

PATTERN DEVIATION
```
                    2   3 | 5   0
                  2   3   0 +-1  -1   1
               -1  -1   2  -1 |-1  -1   0  -1
             -2  -3  -3   1  -3 |-5  -4  -4  -1   0
             -2  -5      -1  -3 |-3  -4  -3  -2   4
             -1  -2      -4  -1 |-3  -7  -3  -3  -2
             -2  -1  -3   1  -2 |-4  -6  -4  -1   2
                 0  -4  -3  -3 |-3  -6  -3  -2
                  -4  -4  -3 +-5  -2  -2
                      -2  -3 |-5   0
```

GLAUCOMA HEMIFIELD TEST (GHT)
BORDERLINE

MD   - 0.69 DB
PSD   2.40 DB
SF   OFF
CPSD   OFF

PROBABILITY SYMBOLS
:: P < 5%
▨ P < 2%
▩ P < 1%
■ P < 0.5%
```

**FIG. 7-33, cont'd. B,** During follow-up examination, the artifact disappeared. If the lens is not centered, there is a tendency to crowd the nasal side of the field and mimic nasal depression.
```

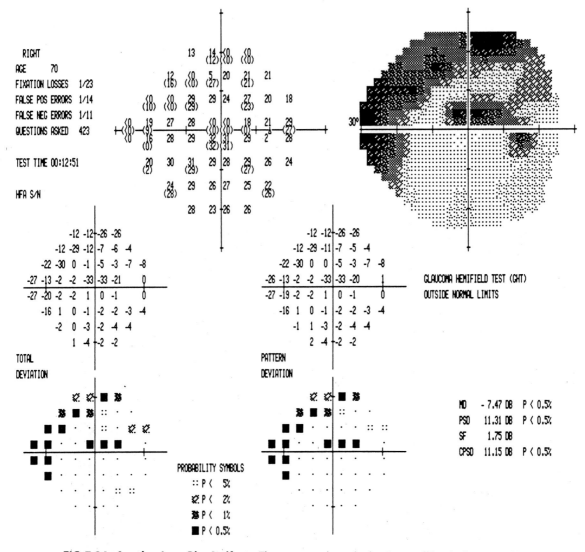

RIGHT

AGE 70

FIXATION LOSSES 1/23

FALSE POS ERRORS 1/14

FALSE NEG ERRORS 1/11

QUESTIONS ASKED 423

TEST TIME 00:12:51

HFA S/N

```
                                    13   14  (8)  (8)
                                        (12) (8) (8)
                              12   (8)   5   20  21   21
                             (16) (8) (27)    (21)
                    (8)  (8)  29   29   24   27   20   18
                   (18) (8) (29)            (23)
          (8)  19   27   28  (8) (8)  18   21   29
          (8) (9)            (8)(8)       2     (27)
          (0)  16   28   29  (32)(31) 29       28
                    20   30   31   29   28   29   26   24
                   (2)      (31)             (27)
                    24   29   26  27   25   22
                   (28)                    (26)
                         28   23  26   26
```

```
         -12 -12 -26 -26
     -12 -29 -12  -7  -6  -4
 -22 -30   0  -1  -5  -3  -7  -8
 -27 -13  -2  -2 -33 -33 -21      0
 -27 -20  -2  -2   1   0  -1      0
 -16   1   0  -1  -2  -2  -3  -4
      -2   0  -3  -2  -4  -4
           1  -4  -2  -2
```

TOTAL
DEVIATION

```
         -12 -12 -26 -26
     -12 -29 -11  -7  -5  -4
 -22 -30   0   0  -5  -3  -7  -8
 -26 -13  -2  -2 -33 -33 -20      1
 -27 -19  -2  -2   1   0  -1      0
 -16   1   0  -1  -2  -2  -3  -4
      -1   1  -3  -2  -4  -4
           2  -4  -2  -2
```

PATTERN
DEVIATION

GLAUCOMA HEMIFIELD TEST (GHT)
OUTSIDE NORMAL LIMITS

PROBABILITY SYMBOLS

∷ P < 5%

⌘ P < 2%

▨ P < 1%

■ P < 0.5%

MD   - 7.47 DB   P < 0.5%

PSD   11.31 DB   P < 0.5%

SF   1.75 DB

CPSD 11.15 DB   P < 0.5%

FIG. 7-34. Another Lens Rim Artifact. The upper and nasal edge is cut off by the lens rim. This artifactual nasal defect disappeared on repeat examination but the real arcuate defect impinging on fixation remained. Typical lens rim artifacts are easily recognized because they tend to be absolute and sharply demarcated.

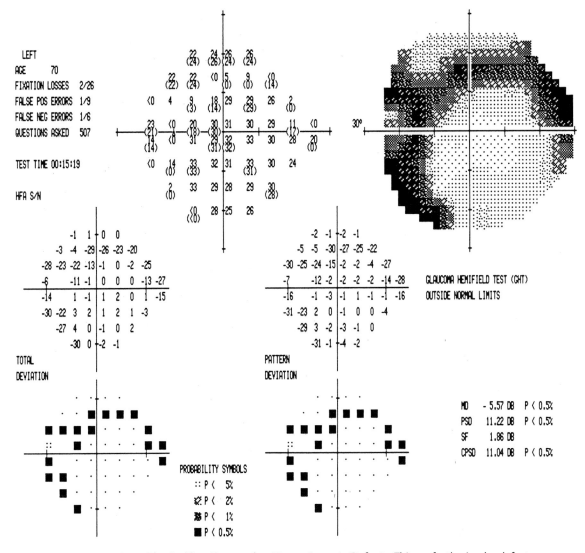

LEFT
AGE   70
FIXATION LOSSES   2/26
FALSE POS ERRORS 1/9
FALSE NEG ERRORS 1/6
QUESTIONS ASKED   507

TEST TIME 00:15:19

HFA S/N

```
                          22   24  26    26
                         (24) (26)(24) (24)
                          22   22  <0 |5   9    <9
                         (22) (24)     (0) (0) (14)
                   <0   4   9   |18  29   28   26    2
                          (3) (14)         (28)        (0)
                   23  <0  20  |30 |31   30   29   11    <0
                  (21)(0) (30)|(32)                (28)  (0)
                   14  <0  30  |32 |33   33   30   20
                  (14)    (31)|(32)                     (0)
             <0   14  33   32 |31   33   30   24
             (0) (33)           (31)
                   2   33   29 |28   29   28
                  (0)                    (28)
                   <9   28 |25   26
                  (0)
```

```
              -1   1 |0   0
          -3  -4 -29|-26 -23 -20
     -28 -23 -22 -13|-1  0  -2  -25
     -6      -11 -1 |0   0   0  -13 -27
     -14      1  -1 |1   2   0      -15
     -30 -22  3   2 |1   2   1  -3
         -27  4   0 |-1  0   2
              -30  0|-2  -1
```

TOTAL
DEVIATION

```
              -2  -1 |-2  -1
          -5  -5 -30|-27 -25 -22
     -30 -25 -24 -15|-2  -2  -4  -27
     -7      -12 -2 |-2  -2  -2  -14 -28
     -16     -1  -3 |-1  1  -1  -1  -16
     -31 -23  2   0 |-1  0   0  -4
         -29  3  -2 |-3  -1  0
              -31 -1|-4  -2
```

PATTERN
DEVIATION

GLAUCOMA HEMIFIELD TEST (GHT)
OUTSIDE NORMAL LIMITS

MD   - 5.57 DB   P < 0.5%
PSD   11.22 DB   P < 0.5%
SF   1.86 DB
CPSD   11.04 DB   P < 0.5%

PROBABILITY SYMBOLS
    :: P < 5%
    ▨ P < 2%
    ▩ P < 1%
    ■ P < 0.5%

FIG. 7-35. Lens Rim Artifact Suggesting Upper Arcuate Defect. This perfectly circular defect passes through the physiologic blind spot, does not widen on the nasal side of its arcuate course (which would be typical in glaucoma), and disappeared on subsequent testing with appropriate positioning of the lens.

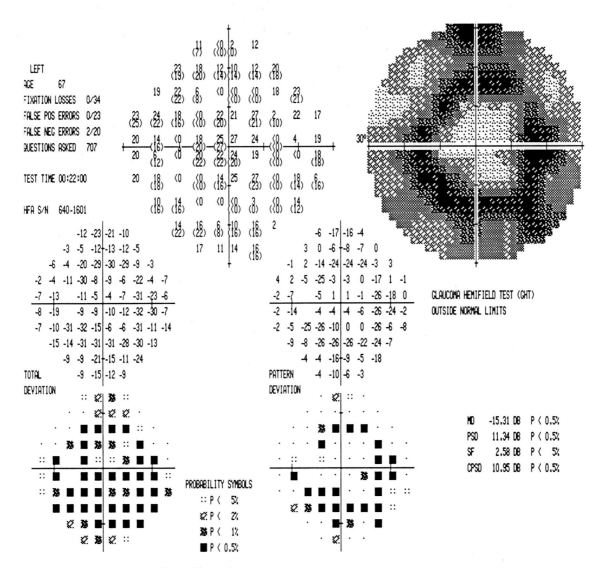

FIG. 7-36. Lens Rim Artifact Mimicking Double Arcuate Scotoma. The lens was not placed sufficiently close to the eye. No defects were present on repeat examination.

LEFT
AGE   55
FIXATION LOSSES   0/35
FALSE POS ERRORS   0/20
FALSE NEG ERRORS   2/21
QUESTIONS ASKED   720
FOVEA: 25 DB ■
TEST TIME 21:40

HFA S/N   630-6803

```
                27   23 |22  12
               (25) (23)|
        27   28  (18)(20) (8) (6)
       (29) (28) (18)(20)(12)(16)
     23  24  18  (0 (0  (8
    (23)(28)(18)    (0)(8)   2   (0
 29  28  22  (0  24 (19  23  14   6   (0
   (28)(22)(0) (22)(21)(9) (0)
32 26 (0 30 -31 31 -30 29 24 -14
   (28)(0) (32)(33)(33)(32)(31)(20)(14)
32 (30   31  35 32 (0 (0
   (30)  (31)(35)(32)(0) (0)
30 30 (0 17 30 19 21 (0  (0  (0
   (32)(0)(11)(28)   (15)(0)
   26  8  (0 (0 (0  (8  (0
  (28)(10)(0)(0) (0) (8)
   30 (0 8 (0  (0  (0
  (30)(14)(0)
   26  22 (0
  (25)(13)(8)
   26 (0
```

```
     4   1  -2 -11
   3   2 -14 -5 -16 -14
 3  -1 -11 -30 -31 -30 -26 -29
2  0  -8 -31 -7 -11 -15 -23 -22 -27
4 -2    1  0  0  0  0 -6 -12
3  1    0  2  0 -34 -33 -31 -28
2  2 -32 -17 -2 -12 -13 -32 -30 -28
  -2 -21 -32 -32 -32 -32 -31 -29
    2 -17 -26 -31 -30 -29
```

TOTAL   -1 -7 -19 -28
DEVIATION

```
     4   1  -2 -11
   3   2 -14 -5 -16 -15
 2  -1 -11 -30 -31 -30 -26 -28
2  0  -8 -31 -7 -11 -15 -23 -22 -27
4 -2    0  0  0 -1  0 -6 -12
3  0    0  2  0 -34 -33 -31 -29
2  2 -32 -17 -2 -12 -13 -32 -30 -28
  -2 -21 -32 -32 -32 -32 -31 -29
    1 -17 -26 -31 -30 -29
```

PATTERN   -1 -8 -19 -28
DEVIATION

GLAUCOMA HEMIFIELD TEST (GHT)
OUTSIDE NORMAL LIMITS

PROBABILITY SYMBOLS

:: P < 5%
⊠ P < 2%
⊠ P < 1%
■ P < 0.5%

MD   -14.33 DB   P < 0.5%
PSD   15.55 DB   P < 0.5%
SF   4.64 DB   P < 1%
CPSD   14.63 DB   P < 0.5%

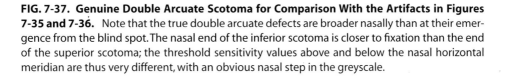

FIG. 7-37. Genuine Double Arcuate Scotoma for Comparison With the Artifacts in Figures 7-35 and 7-36. Note that the true double arcuate defects are broader nasally than at their emergence from the blind spot. The nasal end of the inferior scotoma is closer to fixation than the end of the superior scotoma; the threshold sensitivity values above and below the nasal horizontal meridian are thus very different, with an obvious nasal step in the greyscale.

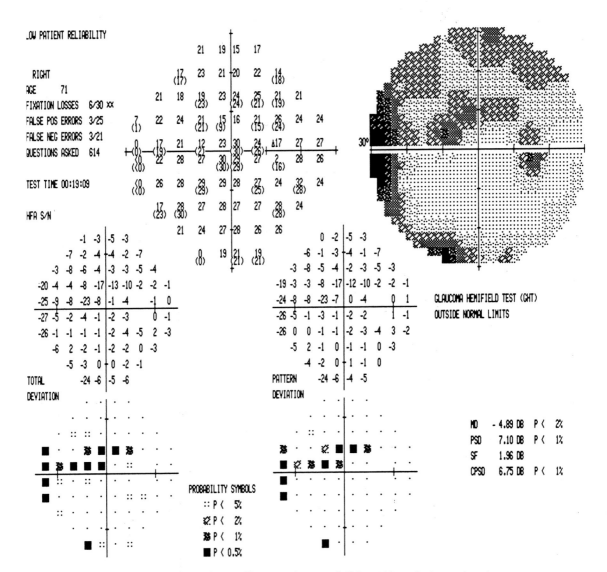

FIG. 7-38. Possible Lens Rim Artifact On the Nasal Side. Although the patient has a true upper arcuate defect, the absolute loss crowding both the superior and inferior nasal edge of the field could be a superimposed lens rim artifact. Only repeat testing with careful attention to lens position can make the distinction.

Look at the patient's face.

The upper portion of the visual field normally is less sensitive than the lower portion, even with the eyes wide open. However, partial obstruction by the eyelid or eyebrow can add depression superiorly, especially if the patient leans forward slightly during perimetry, producing a forward head tilt. Although this superimposed depression at the upper edge of the field usually can be eliminated by attention to positioning of the head (see Chapter 11, Fig. 11-3), artificial depression of the upper edge of the field is so common that even profound loss of sensitivity in the upper row of points usually is not assigned much significance. Inspection of the patient's facial features helps you identify artifacts of the superior hemifield.

Refraction scotomas

Another localized defect that can be a pitfall in diagnostic interpretation is the refraction scotoma,[34-44] which also has been called the *tilted disc syndrome*. In mild form it is fairly common. It may appear as either a scotoma or a localized depression, typically within a wedge-shaped zone above the physiologic blind spot. A refraction scotoma can be mistaken for an arcuate scotoma or an upper temporal hemianopia, perhaps typically in both eyes, falsely suggesting a bitemporal hemianopia.

In a normally configured eye, the lens that provides the best visual acuity by bringing the fovea into focus also brings the rest of the retina into focus. A refraction scotoma results when this is not the case and the lens required to focus an eccentric stimulus on the retina away from the fovea is different from the one required to focus the fixation point on the fovea. Typically this occurs with some degree of astigmatism or myopia, when the back of the eye is not symmetric but has bulges around (and especially below) the optic nerve. The refraction scotoma appears in the zone of the visual field that corresponds to the part of the retina not in proper focus because a blurred stimulus is not as visible as a focused one. The optic disc is tilted, and the fundus color (retinal pigment epithelium and choroid) often is pale in the region of the ocular coat that bulges outward.

If a specific scotoma is suspected of being a refraction scotoma, the lens being used for the field testing can be varied by several diopters. If the raw threshold values improve in the region of the scotoma, there must be an improved focusing of the stimulus on the retina. If the stimulus already was in focus and the defect is a true scotoma, the scotoma remains the same or becomes deeper because changing the lens can only serve to make the stimulus less visible. Another approach is to test with a size-V stimulus, which is influenced less by blurring of the stimulus.

These maneuvers are rarely undertaken because once the artifact is suspected, the defect usually is recognized by its typical features. There is a shallow depression of sensitivity in a wedge-shaped region that extends upward from the blind spot. It usually does not cross into the nasal field in an arcuate fashion, but it may cross the midline slightly or at least have a boundary that cannot be said to end distinctly at the vertical meridian, in contrast to the sharp boundary at the vertical midline that is typical of a hemianopia.

At least some refraction scotomas have been recognized to correlate with the presence of a tilted disc or a wedge of pale color in the lower nasal retina emanating from the optic disc. Such defects may be an exaggeration of the physiologic, superior "baring of the blind spot" of kinetic perimetry, in which visual sensation is reduced slightly above the blind spot so that the isopter curves around the blind spot without enclosing the region just above it.

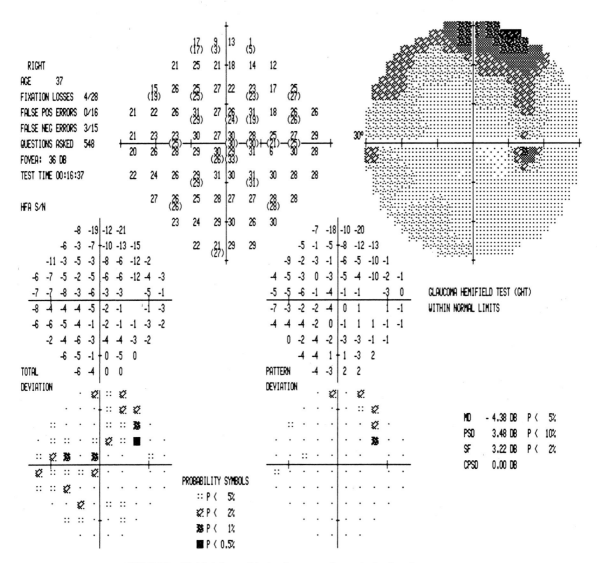

FIG. 7-39. Field defect with the features of a typical refraction scotoma.

Incorrect fixation

Sometimes after the foveal threshold has been determined, the patient continues to maintain his gaze toward the special fixation target 10 degrees below fixation. When this occurs, the physiologic blind spot is represented as a scotoma about 10 degrees below the horizontal meridian. Typically there would be a high FL index because stimuli presented in the proper blind spot location are seen (Fig. 7-41). An exception would be a dense visual field defect in the upper field above the blind spot (Fig. 7-42).

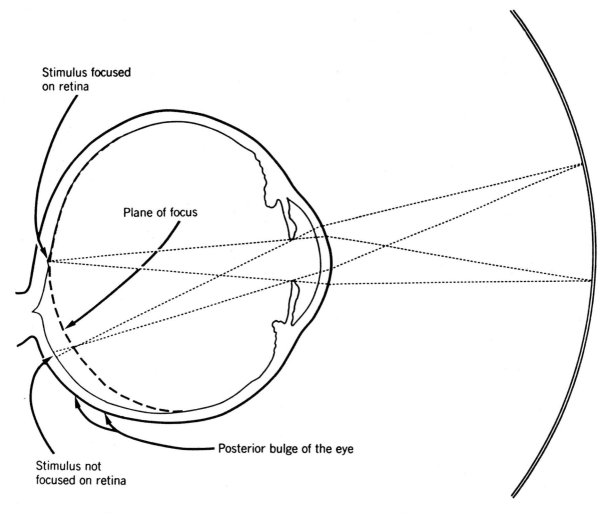

FIG. 7-40. Anatomic Cause of a Refraction Scotoma. (Illustration by Leona M. Allison.)

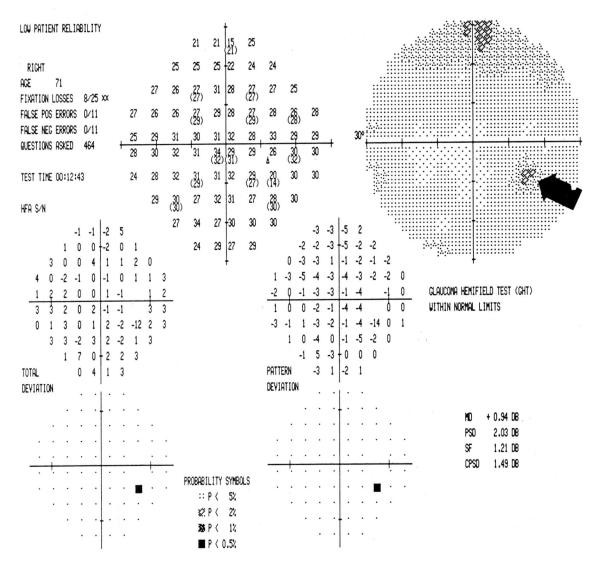

LOW PATIENT RELIABILITY

```
                                21   21 │15   25
                                        │(21)
  RIGHT                    25   25   25 │22   24   24
AGE      71
                     27   26   27   31 │28   27   27   25
FIXATION LOSSES  8/25 xx             (27)         (27)
FALSE POS ERRORS 0/11    27   26   26   27 │29 28   27   28   28   28
FALSE NEG ERRORS 0/11                (29)         (29)   (28)
QUESTIONS ASKED  464     25   29   31   30 │31 32   28   33   29   29
                         28   30   32   31 │34  29  29   26   30   30
                                           (32)(31)           (32)
TEST TIME 00:12:43       24   28   32   31 │31 32   29   20   30   30
                                        (29)         (27)  (14)
HFA S/N                       29   30   27   32 │31  27   28   30
                                     (30)                 (30)
                                   27   34   27 │30   30   30
```

```
          -1  -1 │-2   5                    -3  -3 │-5   2
       1   0   0 │-2   0   1                -2  -2  -3│-5  -2  -2
   3   0   0   4 │ 1   1   2   0          0  -3  -3   1 │-1  -2  -1  -2
 4 0  -2  -1   0 │-1   0   1   1   3      1  -3  -5  -4  -3 │-4  -3  -2  -2   0
 1 2   2   0   0 │ 1  -1       1   2     -2   0  -1  -3  -3 │-1  -4       -1   0
 3 3   2   0   2 │-1  -1       3   3      1   0   0  -2  -1 │-4  -4        0   0
 0 1   3   0   1 │ 2  -2 -12   2   3     -3  -1   1  -3  -2 │-1  -4 -14   0   1
   3   3  -2   3 │ 2  -2   1   3           1   0  -4   0 │-1  -5  -2   0
       1   7   0 │ 2   2   3                -1   5  -3 │ 0   0   0
TOTAL          0   4 │ 1   3         PATTERN     -3   1 │-2   1
DEVIATION                            DEVIATION
```

```
                                27   34   27 │30  30   30

                                24   29 │27   29
```

GLAUCOMA HEMIFIELD TEST (GHT)
WITHIN NORMAL LIMITS

```
MD    + 0.94 DB
PSD     2.03 DB
SF      1.21 DB
CPSD    1.49 DB
```

PROBABILITY SYMBOLS
:: P < 5%
▨ P < 2%
▩ P < 1%
■ P < 0.5%

FIG. 7-41. Incorrect Fixation. Because the patient maintained fixation on the inferior fixation target, the physiologic blind spot is represented as a scotoma in the lower temporal region *(arrow).* The upper field is more depressed than is usual, and a high FL is reported.

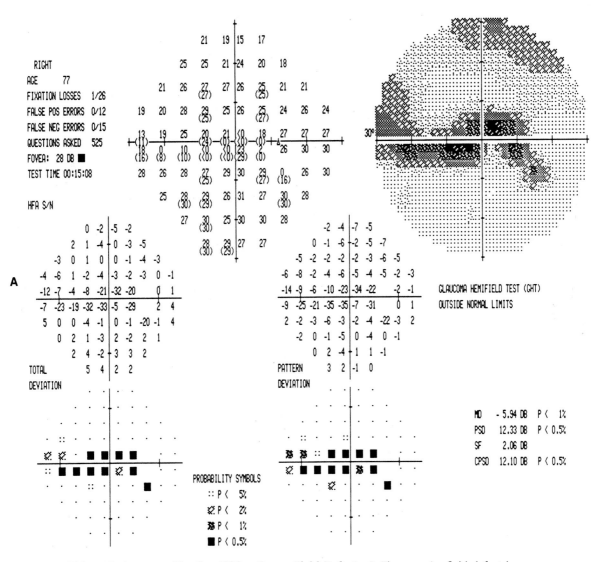

FIG. 7-42. Incorrect Fixation With a Dense Field Defect. A, The superior field defect has a sharp horizontal boundary that is below the horizontal meridian. Stimuli in the normal position of the blind spot are not seen; thus, the FL rate is low.

Continued

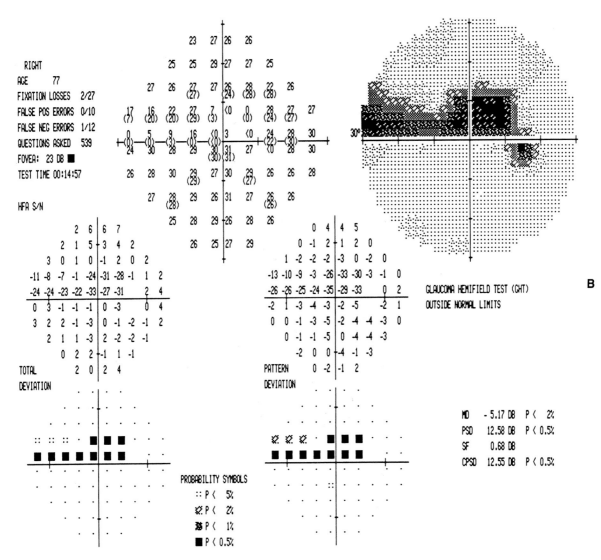

FIG. 7-42, cont'd. B, Repeat field with correct fixation.

Dim light bulb

When the perimeter is functioning properly, threshold values are listed as <0 when the strongest (10,000 asb) stimulus is not seen. A puzzling printout is one that shows threshold values as less than some number other than 0 (such as < 1 or < 7). These values occur when the light bulb is dim, usually because it is old and should be replaced. The less than 1 or less than 7 designations, for example, mean that the 1- or 7-dB stimulus was the strongest intensity that could be achieved (as determined during the automatic calibration procedure), and that those stimuli were not seen by the patient. Such test results are perfectly valid except that there is some loss of information as to the exact depth of the scotomas in question. Replacement of the light bulb likely will remedy this loss of brightness range. An example is shown in Figure 7-43.

Inexperienced patient

A degree of learning occurs when a patient undergoes psychophysical testing. Most patients learn perimetry quickly after the first few stimulus presentations, so that in fact the first test is accurate. A few do not perform their best until the second time they undergo field testing. Some individuals improve over a series of several fields. Apart from learning to respond consistently (reducing the FP and FN rates, as well as improving SF), it appears that with experience patients respond more readily to dim, marginally visible stimuli and more often to dim stimuli farther from the point of fixation (see section on learning effect in Chapter 9). Therefore the usual artifact on the first field test is that overall the recorded sensitivity is low (low MD). The sensitivity is perhaps reduced at some locations more than at others, and the central 10 degrees is affected less than the outer region closer to the edge.[45-49] In extreme cases, the first field may look like that in Figure 7-9 but may be quite normal when repeated. Effects of inexperience and learning are shown in Figures 7-44 through 7-49.

Text continues on p. 188

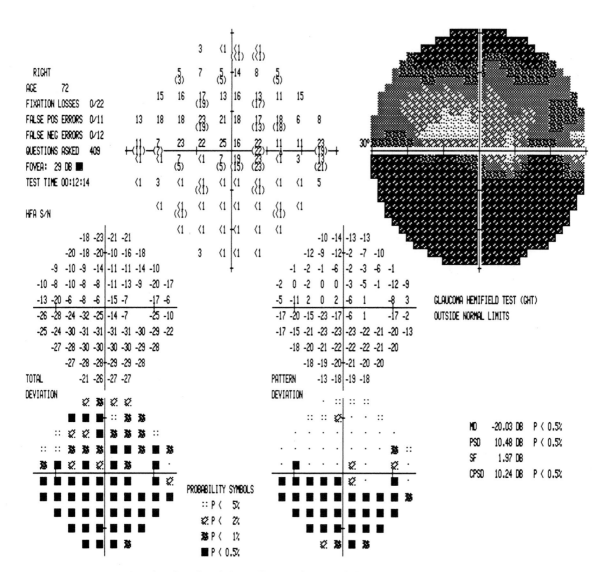

FIG. 7-43. Result Of a Dim Light Bulb. Results are valid except that the maximum available stimulus intensity is, in this case, 1 dB instead of the usual 0 dB.

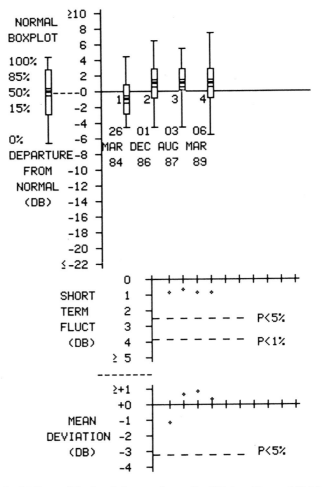

FIG. 7-44. Typical Effect of Patient's Inexperience On MD In a Normal Field. The graph of MD over time *(bottom)* shows that the first test has less sensitivity overall than the others. The box plots *(top)* show the median sensitivity as well as the 15th-85th percentile box to be depressed on the first test of the right eye.

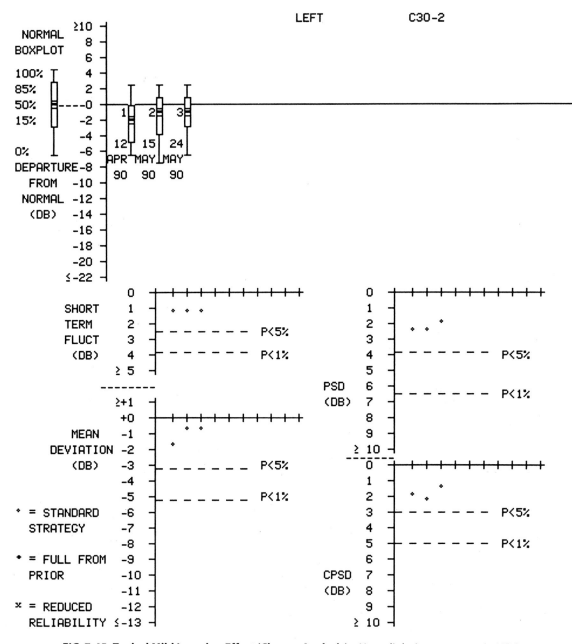

FIG. 7-45 Typical Mild Learning Effect (Change Analysis). Note slight improvement in MD in the second and third fields, as well as a rise in the position of both the median value and the portion of the boxplot.

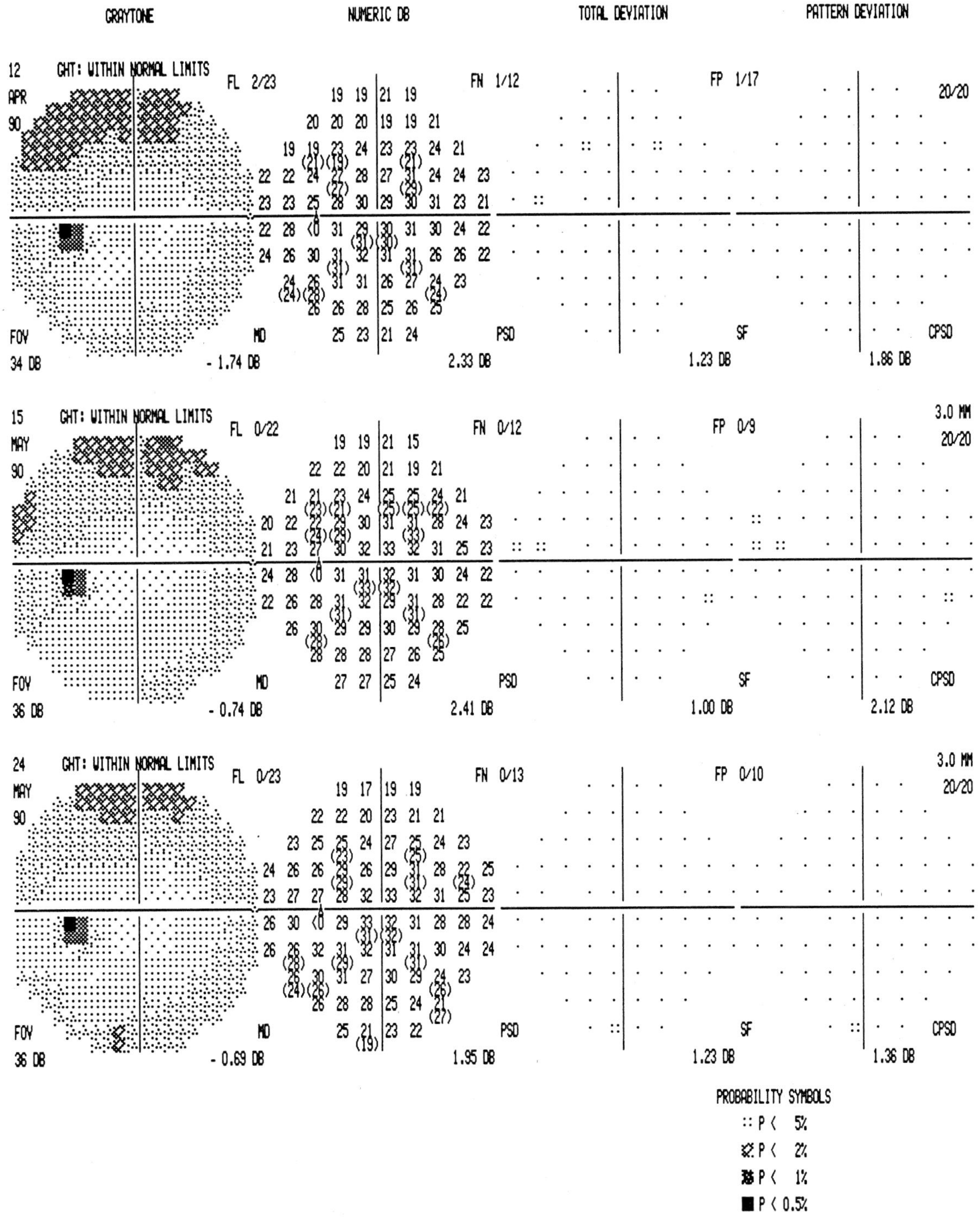

FIG. 7-46. Learning Effect (Overview). Same patient as in Figure 7-45. Note that the four points around fixation rose from 29 to 30 dB to 32 to 33 dB.

183

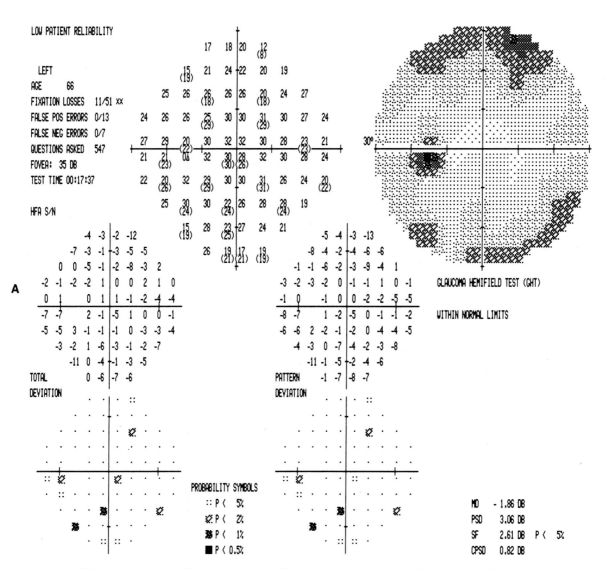

FIG. 7-47. Learning Effect. A, In the first field the sensitivity is generally reduced, perhaps more markedly toward the edge of the field, with some inconsistency represented by frequent duplicate determinations and an elevated SF value.

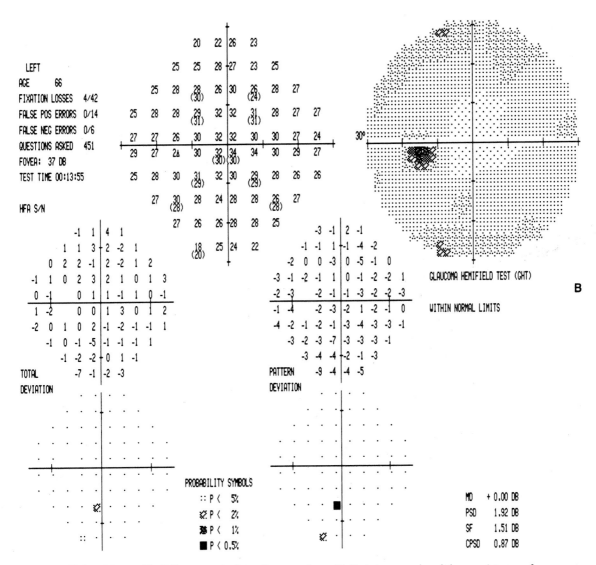

```
                              20  22 │26  23
    LEFT                 25  25  28 ┼27  23  25
    AGE      66      25  28  28  26  30  26  28  27
    FIXATION LOSSES  4/42    (30)        (24)
    FALSE POS ERRORS  0/14    25  28  28  29  32  32  31  28  27  27
    FALSE NEG ERRORS  0/6             (31)     (31)
    QUESTIONS ASKED   451  27  27  26  30  32  32  30  30  27  24
    FOVEA:  37 DB          29  27  28  30  32  34  34  30  29  27
    TEST TIME 00:13:55             (30)(30)
                          25  28  30  31  32  30  28  28  26  26
    HFA S/N                       (29)        (29)
                              27  30  28  24 28  28  26  27
                                 (28)            (28)
                              27  26  26 ┼28  28  25
```

```
              -1  1 │4  1
         1  1  3 ┼2 -2  1          18  25 24  22
      0  2  2 -1  2 -2  1  2      (20)
   -1  1  0  2  3  2  1  0  1  3
    0 -1     0  1  1 -1  1  0 -1
    1 -2     0  0  1  3  0  1  2
   -2  0  1  0  2 -1 -2 -1 -1  1
     -1  0 -1 -5 -1 -1 -1  1
        -1 -2 -2 │0  1 -1

    TOTAL        -7 -1 │-2 -3
    DEVIATION
```

```
                      -3 -1 │2 -1
                  -1 -1  1 ┼-1 -4 -2
              -2  0  0 -3  0 -5 -1  0
          -3 -1 -2 -1  1  0 -1 -2 -2  1
          -2 -3    -2 -1 -1 -3 -2 -2 -3
          -1 -4    -2 -3 -2  1 -2 -1  0
          -4 -2 -1 -2 -1 -3 -4 -3 -3 -1
             -3 -2 -3 -7 -3 -3 -3 -1
                -3 -4 -4 ┼-2 -1 -3

    PATTERN      -9 -4 │-4 -5
    DEVIATION
```

GLAUCOMA HEMIFIELD TEST (GHT)

WITHIN NORMAL LIMITS

B

PROBABILITY SYMBOLS

:: P < 5%

▨ P < 2%

▩ P < 1%

■ P < 0.5%

MD   + 0.00 DB
PSD   1.92 DB
SF   1.51 DB
CPSD   0.87 DB

FIG. 7-47, cont'd. B, Two months later the overall sensitivity is improved and the consistency of responses is better. (Courtesy of Anders Heijl, MD)

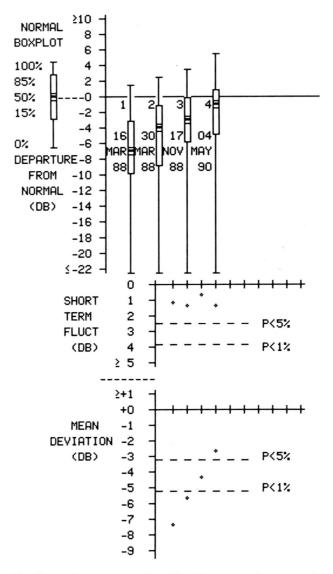

FIG. 7-48. Rare Persistent Improvement Resulting From Learning Over Time. Progressive learning may be more common in individuals with abnormal fields, perhaps because there is more room for improvement.

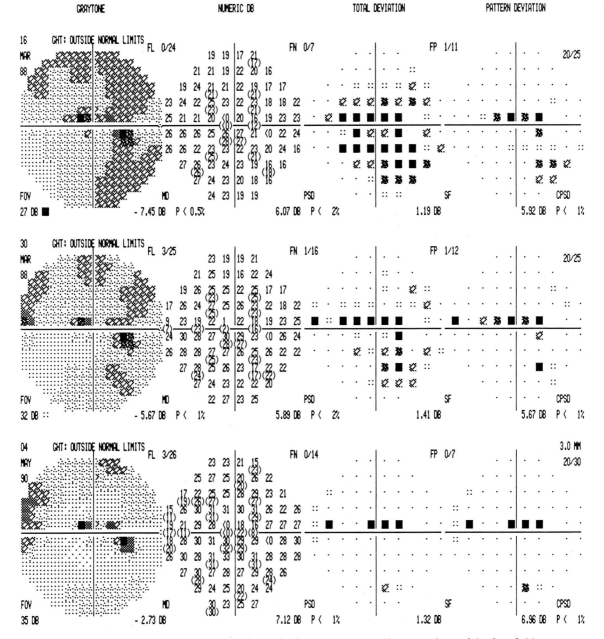

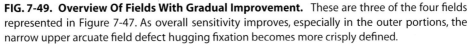

FIG. 7-49. Overview Of Fields With Gradual Improvement. These are three of the four fields represented in Figure 7-47. As overall sensitivity improves, especially in the outer portions, the narrow upper arcuate field defect hugging fixation becomes more crisply defined.

CONFIRMATION OF EQUIVOCAL FINDINGS

Generally, any isolated clinical sign is suspect, and this is true of visual field findings. Any number of unpredictable technical problems may confound the examination; for example, the inadvertent use of a −2.00-D lens instead of a +2.00-D lens may cause a peculiar field defect. All abnormalities need confirmation.

The confirmation may be in the form of an associated clinical sign, such as excavation at the inferior rim of the disc in association with an upper arcuate visual field defect. If such corroborating evidence is absent or equivocal, and the field defect is either unexpected or of an unexpected nature, a repeat visual field examination should be undertaken to confirm the abnormality. A true but mild abnormality usually is present on such a repeat examination. However, equivocal findings that are a statistical deviation and those caused by an artifact are less likely to be present on a second examination. Insistence on duplicate positive tests greatly reduces false diagnoses due to statistical accidents while only slightly reducing the sensitivity in finding disease. Most of the lost sensitivity is regained if a third test is performed to break the tie when a positive test is followed by a negative repeat test.

At times, a different test is selected for the repeat visual field examination; for example, a closer grid of points in the suspect area. A complimentary pattern (such as the Central 30-1 test, Fig. 8-17) with a different set of test points has been used for the purposes of confirmation; however, a repeat of the same examination usually is a wiser choice.

UNSUSPECTED DISEASE

The examiner always should be sure that the confirmed visual field abnormality is caused by the disease under consideration. Subtle generalized depression may be caused by glaucoma, early changes in the media, or nonglaucomatous prechiasmal or preretinal causes. Well-established pure generalized depression is for practical purposes always nonglaucomatous. Localized defects that resemble glaucoma can be produced by such conditions as branch retinal vascular occlusions, ischemic optic neuropathy, or giant drusen of the optic disc. For these localized prechiasmal field defects, which include glaucoma and its differential diagnoses, thoughtful consideration of the clinical setting, including ophthalmoscopic findings, usually is more helpful in making the diagnosis than isolated study of the visual field test result. For diagnosis of chiasmal and postchiasmal field defects, both the character of the field defect and the accompanying neurologic signs must be considered.

REFERENCES

1. Johnson LN: Visual field interpretation with empiric probability maps, *Arch Ophthalmol* 107:1423, 1989.
2. Heijl A, Lindgren G, Olsson J: Reliability parameters in computerized perimetry, *Doc Ophthalmol Proc Ser* 49:593-600, 1987.
3. Katz J, Sommer A: Reliability indexes of automated perimetric tests, *Arch Ophthalmol* 106:1252-1254, 1988.

4. Katz J, Sommer A, Witt K: Reliability of visual field results over repeated testing, *Ophthalmology* 98:70-75, 1991.

5. Donovan HC, Weale RA, Wheeler C: The perimeter as a monitor of glaucomatous changes, *Br J Ophthalmol* 62:705-708, 1978.

6. Heijl A, Lindgren G, Olsson J: Reliability parameters in computerized perimetry, *Doc Ophthalmol Proc Ser* 49:593-600, 1987.

7. Heijl A, Drance SM: Changes in differential threshold in patients with glaucoma during prolonged perimetry, *Br J Ophthalmol* 67:512-516, 1983.

8. Werner EB, Drance SM: Early visual field disturbances in glaucoma, *Arch Ophthalmol* 95:1173-1175, 1977.

9. Flammer J, Drance SM, Zulauf M: Differential light threshold. Short- and long-term fluctuation in patients with glaucoma, normal controls, and patients with suspected glaucoma, *Arch Ophthalmol* 102:704-706, 1984.

10. Werner EB, Drance SM: Increased scatter of responses as a precursor of visual field changes in glaucoma, *Can J Ophthalmol* 12:140-142, 1977.

11. Werner EB, Saheb N, Thomas D: Variability of static visual threshold responses in patients with elevated IOPs, *Arch Ophthalmol* 100:1627-1631, 1982.

12. Katz J, Sommer A, Witt K: Reliability of visual field results over repeated testing, *Ophthalmology* 98:70-75, 1991.

13. Bickler-Bluth M, Trick GL, Kolker AE, Cooper DG: Assessing the utility of reliability indices for automated visual fields testing ocular hypertensives, *Ophthalmology* 96:616-619, 1989.

14. Nelson-Quigg JM, Twelker JD, Johnson CA: Response properties of normal observers and patients during automated perimetry, *Arch Ophthalmol* 107:1612-1615, 1989.

15. Katz J, Sommer A: Reliability indexes of automated perimetric tests, *Arch Ophthalmol* 106:1252-1254, 1988.

16. Johnson CA, Nelson-Quigg JM: In reply, *Arch Ophthalmol* 108:778, 1990.

17. Hardage L, Stamper RL: Reliability indices for automated visual fields, *Ophthalmology* 96:1810, 1989.

18. Sanabria O, Feuer WJ, Anderson DR: Pseudo-loss of fixation in automated perimetry, *Ophthalmology* 98:76-78, 1991.

19. Feuer WJ, Anderson DR: Static threshold asymmetry in early glaucomatous visual field loss, *Ophthalmology* 96:1285-1297, 1989.

20. Brenton RS, Phelps CD, Rojas P, Woolson RF: Interocular differences of the visual field in normal subjects, *Invest Ophthalmol Vis Sci* 27:799-805, 1986.

21. Heijl A, Lindgren G, Olsson J, Asman P: Visual field interpretation with empiric probability maps, *Arch Ophthalmol 107:204-208, 1989.*

22. Heijl A, Asman P: Clustering of depressed points in the normal visual field. In Heijl A, editor: *Perimetry update 1988/89, Proceedings of the VIIIth International Perimetric Society Meeting, Vancouver, 1988,* pp 185-189, Berkeley, CA, 1989, Kugler and Ghedini.

23. Katz J, Sommer A, Gaasterland DE, Anderson DR: A comparison of analytic algorithms for detecting glaucomatous visual field loss, *Arch Ophthalmol* 109:1017-1025, 1991.

24. The Advanced Glaucoma Intervention Study Investigators. The Advanced Glaucoma Intervention Study: 2. Visual field test scoring and reliability, *Ophthalmology* 101:1445-1455, 1994.

25. Sommer A, Enger C, Witt K: Screening for glaucomatous visual field loss with automated threshold perimetry, *Am J Ophthalmol* 103:681-684, 1987.

26. Duggan C, Sommer A, Auer C, Burkhard K: Automated differential threshold perimetry for detecting glaucomatous visual field loss, *Am J Ophthalmol* 100:420-423, 1985.

27. Katz J, Sommer A: Screening for glaucomatous visual field loss, *Ophthalmology* 97:1032-1037, 1990.

28. Enger C, Sommer A: Recognizing glaucomatous field loss with the Humphrey Statpac, *Arch Ophthalmol* 105:1355-1357, 1987.

29. Katz J, Sommer A: Screening for glaucomatous visual field loss: The effect of patient reliability, *Ophthalmology* 97:1032-1037, 1990.

30. Heijl A, Lindgren G, Olsson J: Reliability parameters in computerized perimetry. In Greve EL, Heijl A, editors: *Seventh International Visual Field Syposium, Amsterdam, Sept 1986.* pp 593-600, Boston, Martinus Nijhof/Dr. W Junk Publishers, 1987 [*Doc Ophthalmol Proc Ser* 49:593-600, 1987].

31. Sponsel WE, Ritch R, Stamper R, et al for the Prevent Blindness America Glaucoma Advisory Committee: Prevent Blindness America visual field screening study, *Am J Ophthalmol* 120:699-708, 1995.

32. Hodapp E, Parrish RK, Anderson DR: *Clinical decisions in glaucoma,* p 52, St Louis, 1993, Mosby.

33. Zalta AH: Lens rim artifact in automated threshold perimetry, *Ophthalmology* 96:1302-1311, 1989.

34. Aulhorn E: Visual field defects in sellar and parasellar processes, *Annee Ther Clin Ophthalmol* 25:424-434, 1974.

35. Dimitrakos SA, Safran AB: La dysversion papillaire. Diagnostic differentiel du syndrome chiasmatique, *Ophthalmologica* 184:30-39, 1982.

36. Fankhauser F, Enoch JM: The effects of blur upon perimetric thresholds: A method for determining a quantitative estimate of retinal contour, *Arch Ophthalmol* 68:240-251, 1962.

37. Goldmann H: Lichtsinn mit besonderer Berucksichtigung der Perimetrie, *Ophthalmologica* 158:362-386, 1969.

38. Kommerell G: Binasale Refraktionsskotome, *Klin Monatsbl Augenheilkd* 154:85-88, 1969.

39. Manor RS: Will we master the Humphrey perimeter or will it master us? *Arch Ophthalmol* 107:1565-1566 (correction in *Arch Ophthalmol* 108:496, 1990), 1989.

40. Riise D: The nasal fundus ectasia, *Acta Ophthalmol* (Suppl)126:4-108, 1975.

41. Rucker CW: Bitemporal defects in the visual fields resulting from developmental anomalies of the optic disks, *Arch Ophthalmol* 35:546-554, 1946.

42. Schmidt T: Kurzes Repetitorium der klinischen Perimetrie, *Ophthalmologica* 149:250-265, 1965.

43. Schmidt T: Perimetrie relativer Skotome, *Ophthalmologica* 129:303-315, 1955.

44. Young SE, Walsh FB, Knox DL: The tilted disk syndrome, *Am J Ophthalmol* 82:16-23, 1976.

45. Wood JM, Wild JM, Hussey MK, Crews SJ: Serial examination of the normal visual field using Octopus automated projection perimetry. Evidence for a learning effect, *Acta Ophthalmol* 65:326-333, 1987.

46. Werner EB, Adelson A, Krupin T: Effect of patient experience on the results of automated perimetry in clinically stable glaucoma patients, *Ophthalmology* 95:764-767, 1988.

47. Autzen T, Work K: The effect of learning and age on short-term fluctuation and mean sensitivity of automated static perimetry, *Acta Ophthalmol* 68:327-330, 1990.

48. Heijl A, Lindgren G, Olsson J: The effect of perimetric experience in normal subjects, *Arch Ophthalmol* 107:81-86, 1989.

49. Wild JM, Dengler-Harles M, Searle AET, et al: The influence of the learning effect on automated perimetry in patients with suspected glaucoma, *Acta Ophthalmol* 67:537-545, 1989.

CHAPTER 8

Selection of automated tests

Most needs are met by a few select alternatives to supplement the standard 30-2 or 24-2 size-III white stimulus.

The 30-2 central threshold test with a white size-III stimulus, as described in the previous three chapters, has for some years been the fundamental standard program. This chapter identifies the best times to use this test and also concentrates on departures from the standard program, including modifications of the standard test and other options that are available. Some of these options are valuable for specific clinical purposes, but nearly all clinical needs are well satisfied by a few select alternatives. It is best not to become too innovative or to deviate too widely into the dozens, if not hundreds, of possible combinations of strategies, test patterns, and stimulus modifications available. The normal database and the statistical analyses that depend on it are available only for standard programs. A standard selection is especially handy if the patient moves from one community to another.

GLAUCOMA DIAGNOSIS IN THE OFFICE

Standard office testing

The selection of the central 30-2 static threshold program for routine use in glaucoma (both to detect defects and to follow for progression) is derived from two axioms that are widely, but not universally, accepted: (1) Threshold tests should be used rather than suprathreshold tests; and (2) testing of 76 points over the central 30-degree region is a reasonable balance between time expenditure on one hand and the need both for detection and for a quantitative baseline on the other hand.

Shorter alternatives are attractive. There is a fixed set-up time unaffected by the length of the test time, but any other increment of savings in time is an increment of savings in cost to administer. Perhaps more important is that a shorter time of intense concentration makes the test more pleasant for the patient and at times more reliable. The test time can be shortened by selecting a shorter thresholding algorithm, by use of suprathreshold testing, and by testing fewer locations in the visual field.

Most Humphrey perimeters are now equipped with software allowing selection from among 2 to 4 alternative types of thresholding algorithms: Full Threshold,

The two Sita algorithms should be used when available.

Sita Standard, Fastpac, or Sita Fast (see Chapter 5). When possible, it probably is best to use the Full Threshold or Sita Standard because both seem highly reliable and somewhat more sensitive to early subtle loss. However, with elderly or easily fatigued patients, the shorter algorithm (either Sita Fast or Fastpac, depending on availability) may provide a clearer diagnostic picture. When detection of early loss is the goal, a disadvantage of Fastpac is that a statistical database that permits use of the Glaucoma Hemifield Test (GHT) is not available (although it is available for both types of Sita tests). Overall, the two Sita algorithms have some clear advantages and should be used in preference to the older methods when all four alternatives are available.

Another method that achieves a shorter test time is suprathreshold testing. It is a sensible choice when evidence of a clinically significant disease of low prevalence is sought in population screening for glaucoma; however, for the office setting, professional consensus is that a threshold test is worth the extra time (and expense). For the purpose of detection, it is helpful to compare threshold values with a baseline threshold test in addition to making a comparison with normal values. After diagnosis, when following the course of glaucoma, a series of suprathreshold tests will only reveal broadening of the area of involvement; the threshold method also allows recognition of the deepening of defective areas. Thus, for both diagnosis and long-term evaluation, the threshold methods are standard.

When time must be shortened, it is better to reduce the number of test locations than to use suprathreshold testing. The 24-2 test pattern (Fig. 8-1) has become a widely used shorter alternative to the 30-2 pattern. The 24-2 pattern omits the outer ring of points of the 30-2 pattern, except that the two most nasal edge points are retained. Not only do most patients with established cases of glaucoma have abnormalities at points represented in the 24-2 pattern (Fig. 8-2), but if an abnormality is revealed only in the outer ring of points in the central 30-2 pattern, the finding often is ignored as nonspecific (see the diagnostic criteria given in Chapter 7). If isolated findings at the edge locations are equivocal, there is little reason to test these locations. The counter-argument is that at the conclusion of the 24-2 examination, there is a new rim of edge points that may have isolated, and therefore uncertain, abnormalities. If a 30-2 had been done instead, reduced threshold sensitivity at adjacent points in the outer ring of the 30-2 pattern would have confirmed an equivocal finding in the outermost circle of the 24-2 pattern. A further counter-argument is that the availability of the faster Sita strategies (see Chapter 5) reduces the time enough to make testing the full central 30 degrees practical. Finally, in cases of moderately advanced disease in the paracentral region, the points temporal to the physiologic blind spot may provide valuable baseline information for following the course of the disease in the remaining visual field.

All things considered, we still prefer the 30-2 as our primary testing pattern, but use the 24-2 for situations in which a very short threshold test is required. Fortunately, the statistical programs for analysis of a series of field examinations accept a mixture of 24-2 and 30-2 programs. When the series of field examinations includes both central 30-2 and central 24-2 threshold tests, data from the extra 22 points in the 30-2 pattern are not used for the statistics.

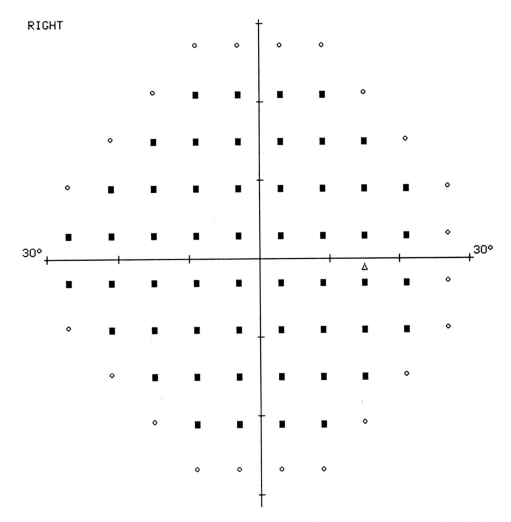

RIGHT

30°   30°

FIG. 8-1. Comparison of the 24-2 and 30-2 Patterns. The 24-2 pattern, indicated by black squares, includes all points within 24 degrees, plus two points on the nasal side. The 30-2 pattern also includes the locations indicated by small circles—76 points in all.

Interestingly, although some examiners confine their attention to the central 24 degrees to save time, a minority do the opposite because they are uncomfortable not exploring the peripheral field outside 30 degrees.[1-6] The region from 30 degrees to 60 degrees can be quantified with a 60-2 pattern threshold test of the original Humphrey perimeter or the 60-4 pattern of the Humphrey HFA-2. (The 60-4 pattern is identical to the 60-2, except that a few of the superior and inferior points that frequently are outside the area of normal vision have been removed.) This area is large, and although the tested points are more widely spaced apart (12 degrees), the test is as lengthy as the 30-2 and testing both the central and peripheral field doubles the test time.

The nasal-step program, an optional method of testing the peripheral field, thresholds only selected locations above and below the horizontal meridian outside the central 30 degrees; this saves time by ignoring the superior, inferior, and temporal sectors. Another option is to make a superficial effort to examine the

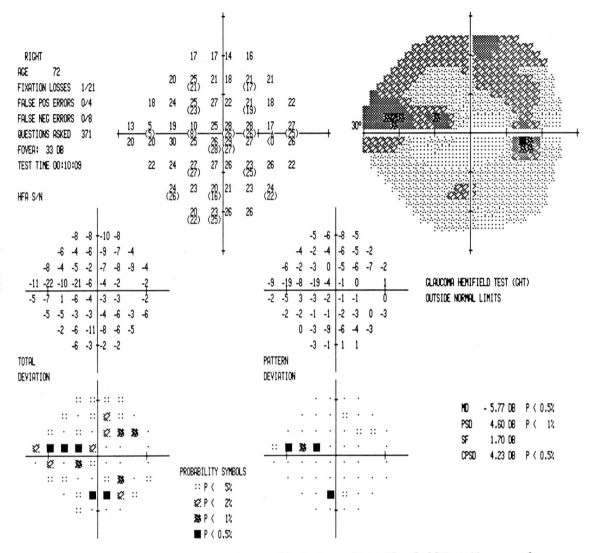

FIG. 8-2. Glaucomatous Defect Shown with the Central 24-2 Threshold Test. (Courtesy of Harry Quigley, MD)

With rare exceptions we have continued to concentrate exclusively on the central field in automated perimetry.

periphery with suprathreshold methods (e.g., the P68 screening program), or to plot a kinetic isopter in the periphery. However, we have continued to concentrate only on the central field in automated perimetry; there is no clear report of much significant diagnostic yield from efforts to screen the peripheral field, especially with the improved methods currently available for the central field.

However, there may be two reasons to test the peripheral field. When detection is the goal and the central field test is unrevealing, the peripheral field may be tested if clinical signs suggest that an abnormality should be present and may be limited to the peripheral region not yet tested; nasal cupping of the disc may suggest that a temporal wedge defect that was not revealed by a central 24-2 threshold test is present. Very infrequently there also may be cases of advanced disease in which the central field has so little remaining vision that the only way to monitor the continued course of the disease is to test the temporal peripheral field.

In summary, with various combinations of test patterns, stimulus sizes, and strategies available, the practitioner can tailor the test to the situation at hand. Although there is latitude in choosing testing protocols for threshold perimetry, 30-2 or 24-2 white size-III testing with Sita Standard when available (or Full Threshold, when Sita Standard is unavailable) may be considered appropriate for almost all situations. When a short test is needed, 24-2 testing with Sita Fast when available (or Fastpac, when Sita Fast is unavailable) may be chosen. The best way to achieve test brevity may depend on the clinical situation:

- For detection of early disease, Fastpac does not provide the GHT analysis to help discern subtle abnormality; therefore, use of the 24-2 test pattern, a Sita strategy, or both, may be the best way to shorten the test time for initial diagnosis.

- For following a disease, the 24-2 pattern provides fewer locations as a baseline and for following a series of fields to detect progression; thus, the 30-2 pattern may be preferable. Fastpac may be used to make the test briefer because the GHT analysis is not needed to follow progression; however, Sita is a better choice, if available. The ranges of test times typical for testing the central field with these alternatives were illustrated in a previous chapter (see Fig. 5-7).

Keep in mind that it is common for longer tests to show somewhat deeper or more extensive defects than shorter tests. Longer tests may produce psychophysical fatigue effects and act as a visual stress test; defects therefore are more pronounced with the full-threshold method than with Fastpac or Sita (Figs. 8-3 and 8-4). Of particular note is that with Sita strategies, the defect depths measured in decibels are generally shallower. However, the range of normal threshold values is narrower (intersubject variability is less), with the net result that in the Total Deviation and Pattern Deviation probability plots, with both the Sita-Fast and the Sita-Standard strategies, uncover milder defects than the Standard Full Threshold algorithm. The differences among tests also must be considered when comparing tests with different strategies to judge progression (see Chapter 9). Shallower defects may be more reproducible and give a longer range over which progression can be monitored, both of which are advantages when monitoring the course of the disease.

Use of blue-yellow testing (Swap)

Short Wavelength Automated Perimetry (Swap) also is known as blue-yellow perimetry. Swap testing (described in Chapter 2) recently has become a practical reality and is an available option on newer Humphrey perimeters. Although the procedure has been available for some time, it was not until its normative Statpac significance limits were developed that the test results could be interpreted properly and clinical experience could be accumulated.

Two longitudinal studies reported that Swap performs better in the detection of early glaucomatous field damage than standard computerized perimetry.[7,8] Swap also was shown to be effective in managing ocular hypertension and in detecting

Text continued on p. 199

195

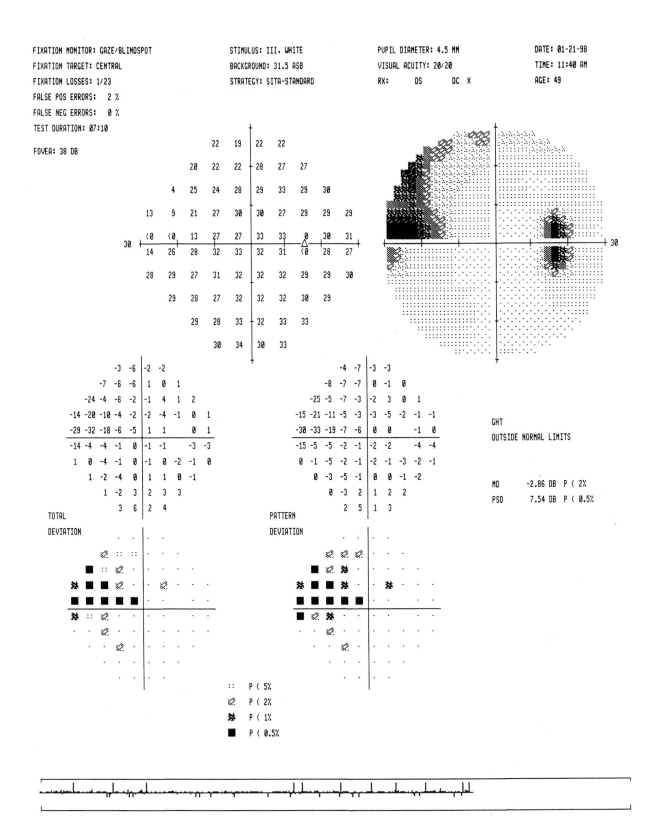

FIXATION MONITOR: GAZE/BLINDSPOT
FIXATION TARGET: CENTRAL
FIXATION LOSSES: 1/23
FALSE POS ERRORS: 2 %
FALSE NEG ERRORS: 0 %
TEST DURATION: 07:10

FOVEA: 38 DB

STIMULUS: III, WHITE
BACKGROUND: 31.5 ASB
STRATEGY: SITA-STANDARD

PUPIL DIAMETER: 4.5 MM
VISUAL ACUITY: 20/20
RX: DS   DC X

DATE: 01-21-98
TIME: 11:40 AM
AGE: 49

GHT
OUTSIDE NORMAL LIMITS

MD   -2.86 DB P < 2%
PSD   7.54 DB P < 0.5%

TOTAL
DEVIATION

PATTERN
DEVIATION

::   P < 5%
⊠   P < 2%
⊞   P < 1%
■   P < 0.5%

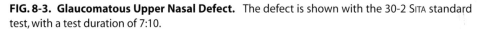

FIG. 8-3. Glaucomatous Upper Nasal Defect. The defect is shown with the 30-2 SITA standard test, with a test duration of 7:10.

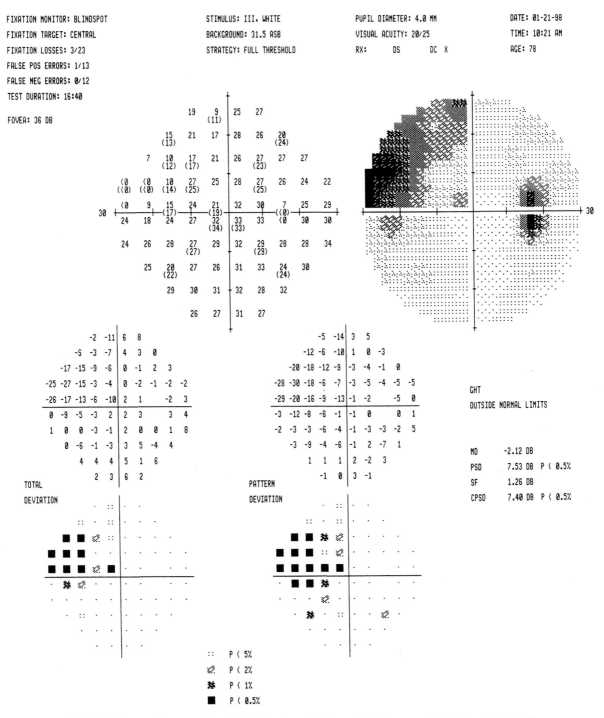

FIXATION MONITOR: BLINDSPOT
FIXATION TARGET: CENTRAL
FIXATION LOSSES: 3/23
FALSE POS ERRORS: 1/13
FALSE NEG ERRORS: 0/12
TEST DURATION: 16:40

FOVEA: 36 DB

STIMULUS: III, WHITE
BACKGROUND: 31.5 ASB
STRATEGY: FULL THRESHOLD

PUPIL DIAMETER: 4.0 MM
VISUAL ACUITY: 20/25
RX: DS   DC X

DATE: 01-21-98
TIME: 10:21 AM
AGE: 78

GHT
OUTSIDE NORMAL LIMITS

MD   -2.12 DB
PSD   7.53 DB P < 0.5%
SF   1.26 DB
CPSD   7.40 DB P < 0.5%

TOTAL
DEVIATION

PATTERN
DEVIATION

:: P < 5%
⊠ P < 2%
✻ P < 1%
■ P < 0.5%

FIG. 8-4. Same Glaucomatous Defect as Seen in Figure 8-3, Documented with a 30-2 Full Threshold Test an Hour Earlier, with a Test Duration of 16:40. Although the threshold values and greyscale tend to be worse in the affected area than in Figure 8-3, the normal range is smaller with SITA and therefore the probability plots indicating the area of disease involvement are very similar.

neurologic disease.[9,10] It has been reported that SWAP detects progression of established visual field defects earlier than white-on-white perimetry.[11,12]

Early SWAP research protocols required measurement of the yellowness of ocular media to correct the height of the hill of vision for media absorption. Such measurements are too time consuming for clinical use, and some data suggest that the correction for the media may be unnecessary because it adds little diagnostic information.[13] Even without making such corrections for the media, SWAP is a somewhat lengthier and more difficult test for the patient than standard white testing.

Based on current and accumulating data, including refinements in the normative database, there is an evolving and diverse spectrum of opinion as to when SWAP should be performed. Some suggest that SWAP could supplant current conventional testing; others suggest a more limited role. Until further data are collected and statistical analyses are refined, perhaps the following considerations will serve to guide the practitioner in the use of SWAP:

1. Patients with significant cataract may produce profoundly depressed fields that are difficult to interpret. In advanced cases, general depression of the field may be severe enough to mask localized defects. However, mild to moderate cataracts do not prevent useful SWAP testing.

2. The test itself takes about 15% longer than standard white testing. Patients frequently report that SWAP testing is more fatiguing than white testing, not only because the test time is longer but also because the stimuli are more difficult to discern with certainty.

3. The mean normal SWAP threshold values expressed in decibels are lower than for white stimuli; thus the SWAP greyscale is darker in appearance and may mislead clinicians accustomed to the greyscale for white-on-white testing. The probability plots are important, just as they are for standard white testing.

4. The *range* of normal is more extensive than for white-on-white perimetry, especially when individual correction is not made for the media.[14,15] The practitioner must rely on the SWAP Statpac probability plots that take this fact into account. The $p < 0.5\%$ symbol means, as it does in white testing, that fewer than 0.5% of normal subjects are expected to produce the threshold value obtained; with attention to such statistics, false-positive diagnoses should be no more frequent than with standard white-on-white testing. It is not yet known whether sensitivity to detection of early defects changes when the criteria are altered to confine specificity to the same limit as used for white-on-white.

5. SWAP results are only part of the diagnostic picture; the clinical goal remains the same: thoughtful resolution of sometimes contradictory pieces of information into a diagnostic whole. If, for example, white testing is normal in a patient with elevated intraocular pressure and a family history of glaucoma, but SWAP results show a defect closely corresponding to observed optic nerve abnormalities, then a diagnosis of mild glaucoma may be justified. If SWAP testing is abnormal in a patient who lacks other signs of disease, then perhaps judgment should be deferred.

When should SWAP be performed?

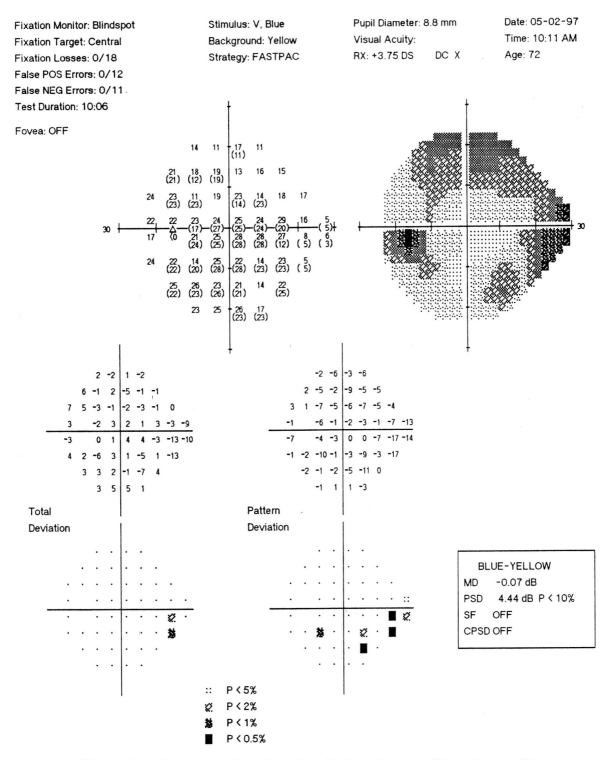

Fixation Monitor: Blindspot
Fixation Target: Central
Fixation Losses: 0/18
False POS Errors: 0/12
False NEG Errors: 0/11
Test Duration: 10:06

Fovea: OFF

Stimulus: V, Blue
Background: Yellow
Strategy: FASTPAC

Pupil Diameter: 8.8 mm
Visual Acuity:
RX: +3.75 DS   DC X

Date: 05-02-97
Time: 10:11 AM
Age: 72

Total Deviation

Pattern Deviation

:: P < 5%
⊠ P < 2%
▒ P < 1%
■ P < 0.5%

BLUE-YELLOW
MD   -0.07 dB
PSD   4.44 dB P < 10%
SF   OFF
CPSD OFF

FIG. 8-5. Early Glaucomatous Defect Revealed with Swap. (Courtesy of Murray Fingeret, OD)

SWAP is best used in patients who have signs or risk of glaucoma but normal white fields.

6. The most obvious place to start using SWAP in situations in which conventional tests have yielded equivocal or contradictory results. Under this approach, SWAP should be used in pursuing a diagnosis in those patients who have significant signs of and risk factors for glaucoma—including race, suspicious optic discs, and/or elevated pressures—but who have normal standard white fields.

Use of suprathreshold tests in clinical office settings

Although threshold testing remains the gold standard for perimetry, there still are infrequent situations in which suprathreshold strategies are appropriate. In normal areas of the visual field most suprathreshold stimuli are seen easily, and suprathreshold tests can be even shorter than the most efficient thresholding tests. They demand less test-taking skill and may be a good choice for the rare occasions when young children and very elderly patients cannot undergo the briefest available threshold test.

Principles. Suprathreshold tests are of limited use when looking for very early glaucomatous loss.[16] They may be suitable for situations in which detection of subtle defects is either unimportant or impractical (e.g., population screening programs, to be discussed later); the goal of suprathreshold tests is to establish the absence of moderate or severe field loss in cases in which the presence of disease is possible but unlikely.

Apart from insensitivity to mild defects, the use of suprathreshold tests in the office has two other disadvantages in the context of glaucoma. First, if many spots are abnormal, the test becomes lengthy because abnormal locations undergo double or triple testing with suprathreshold stimuli or thresholding by the inefficient strategy necessarily used in these tests. The SITA Fast 24-2 threshold test, for example, may be both more informative and faster. Second, suprathreshold tests do not provide a quantitative baseline for following the course of the disease.

Options available. When it is necessary to use a suprathreshold test and it is not already known that there are many abnormal points, our preference in the context of glaucoma is the Central 64-point test, run in the Age-Corrected test mode. This pattern is standard on the HFA-2 and can be accessed on the HFA-1 by running the full-field 120-point test and then stopping the test after the central section has been completed. The 64-point pattern concentrates on the nasal field and thus is fairly sensitive to glaucomatous loss. It also is less prone to trial lens artifact because it has few points near the edge of the 30-degree central field.

If the briefest of screening tests is required, the 40-point test seems best—again, with the quantify-defects strategy in the Age-Corrected mode. It can be completed in 1 to 2 minutes and usually gives considerably more information than can be obtained from a confrontation test. With either test pattern, the Quantify-Defects strategy is helpful in evaluating small defects. If the field turns out to be normal, no time is lost by using the Quantify-Defect strategy and the test can be completed in only 2 or 3 minutes; if field loss is detected at a few locations, knowing the depth of the defect(s) can help in deciding whether the loss is genuine and of significant depth. The time-saving advantage is lost if many locations are abnormal and each of them is thresholded; therefore the perimetrist would be wise to terminate the test when it becomes prolonged, especially if the diagnostic purpose of testing (determining that a defect exists) has been satisfied.

Optionally, if a large defect is suspected and the purpose is to document its presence as well as characterize its topography, the Two-Zone and Three-Zone strategies offer time-saving advantages because thresholding of numerous locations is not performed. In cases such as these, a cluster of abnormal points in a diagnostically typical location serves the purpose of giving confidence that the defect is real, whereas with small defects this assurance derives from the depth determined by the Quantify-Defect mode. Nonetheless, if it is available, the SITA Fast test may be more informative than any of the suprathreshold tests and just as brief in many cases, with defects covering a sizable area.

POPULATION SCREENING FOR GLAUCOMA

Because the practicing clinician may be consulted by those who wish to undertake community screening programs, he should realize that the tests most commonly used for office diagnosis probably are not suitable for screening a large number of people—of whom only a minority will prove to have glaucoma. Conversely, most tests used for community screening are neither sensitive enough nor quantitative enough to be used in the office.

Principles

The first issue addressed in detection is the amount of time that can be devoted to each person screened or to each case detected.[17] Office examinations of high-risk patients have a high yield of detection and diagnosis, so it is proper to devote more time to diagnosis and establishing a basis for follow-up. The time that can and should be devoted to each person participating in a general screening of a relatively low-risk population is of necessity much shorter.

Second is the related issue of sensitivity versus specificity. In an office, visual field examinations are performed on patients who are more likely to have glaucoma than the general population. Consequently, the in-office emphasis is on sensitivity to mild damage in a group likely to have some abnormality and on a quantitative baseline in a group that is normal. Thus, both the tests used and the interpretative criteria applied should not be biased toward extremely high specificity at the expense of sensitivity.

In general screening of a large group for glaucoma, the emphasis must shift toward a higher level of specificity and toward screening high-risk segments of the population.[18] Otherwise, false-positive results will vastly outnumber the true cases of glaucoma. For example, a test that is 80% specific, applied to a population having a 0.5% prevalence of glaucoma, will by definition falsely identify 40 normals in each group of 200 individuals tested in which there is one afflicted person. Within the group of 41 individuals who test positive, the prevalence of actual glaucoma will be only 1 in 41, or 2.5%. The necessary follow-up examinations will be numerous and low in yield. By comparison, if screening can be restricted to a subset of the population having, for example, a 2% prevalence of glaucoma, and if criteria can be applied that are 96% specific, the test will falsely identify only two normals for every true case of glaucoma. The prevalence of true disease in the screened positive group then will be 33%, and the number of follow-up examinations will be only 7% as large as in the other scenario.

Effective population screening: *specific* tests applied to *high-risk* groups

Therefore mass glaucoma screenings must be aimed at groups having a significantly higher prevalence of the disease than does the general population; additionally, highly specific test strategies and criteria for abnormality must be used. The unfortunate and unavoidable side effect of using highly specific tests is that examiners must be resigned to missing cases with mild defects. However, there really is no choice if the screening is to pick up the established cases that are in greatest need of detection. For selection of screening tests, Prevent Blindness America[18a] has set its standards at 95% to 98% specificity, 85% sensitivity for moderate and severe glaucoma (and other optic neuropathies), 95% sensitivity for hemianopias, and testing of both eyes at a rate of 9 to 10 patients per hour.[18a] Test time is an important consideration.[19,20]

Application

For reasons previously discussed, glaucomatous field defect detection is best accomplished by attention to the central field.[21,22] Inexpensive portable instrumentation with limited or less flexible capabilities focused on screening may be suited for many outreach programs; however, we limit our attention here to the tests that may be used if community screening is done with the standard Humphrey perimeter designed for office use.

Although there is little documentation of the relative strengths of the various tests available, the central 64-point Age-Related test mode described earlier in this chapter probably offers a reasonable trade-off between speed and diagnostic efficiency. As an alternative, SITA Fast with a 24-2 pattern may be time-competitive with suprathreshold screening because testing of normal subjects (the majority of people screened) commonly requires less than 3 minutes per eye with this test. Inexperienced subjects may have more trouble with threshold than with suprathreshold tests but a pilot study[23] has reported reasonable success with a 24-2 Fastpac threshold test. Although use of SITA Fast has not been evaluated for screening, it is faster than Fastpac, and the longer time required compared with suprathreshold testing may be compensated for if a smaller percentage of those screened require retesting because of uncertain results on the initial test. Further data are needed on this and other methods of population screening.

Interpretive criteria

Effectiveness of screening depends not only on the test used but also on the criteria that constitute reason to send the person for more definitive diagnostic evaluation. There is little in the literature to suggest specific guidelines as to which test results in a mass screening should be labeled abnormal,[20] and interpretive criteria must be defined in pilot studies that are suited for the particular population being screened. If the Quantify-Defect screening strategy is used in Age-Related mode, a criterion such as that used for clinical threshold testing might be adopted. It might be required, for example, that defects be found in at least three adjacent test points, one of which should be at least 10 dB deep and/or a defect in a single nonedge point that is at least 15 dB deep. Refinements include requiring a different defect depth centrally versus peripherally or using deviation probability plots for Fastpac or SITA-Fast. False-positive results may be caused by other diseases; whether this is desirable depends on whether it is the intent of the screening project to find other visual problems in addition to glaucoma. Thus perimetric testing should be preceded by a visual acuity check to identify such, unless the goal of the community project is to detect visual loss from any cause. The issues are complex and not yet well studied, so any chosen criteria must be validated in pilot studies—and probably modified—before use.

FOLLOWING PATIENTS WITH GLAUCOMA

Typical patients

A 30-2 threshold test usually is the most suitable option for in-office detection of field defects caused by chronic glaucoma. Alternatively, the time saved by using the central 24-2 threshold test may be worth the compromise in information obtained, at least for selected cases. In either case, the same tests will usually serve as a suitable baseline against which to judge whether, and how rapidly, the visual field may be worsening when the same test is performed at some later time.

Three of the four thresholding strategies available in recent Humphrey software versions have (or soon will have) known significance limits for the intertest variability typical of stable glaucomatous fields. These three strategies are Full Threshold, SITA Standard, and SITA Fast. (The variability limits have not been established for Fastpac.) Follow-up visual field tests can be compared with the baseline examination(s), and an analysis can be made of the frequency (probability) that any observed change at one point could occur by chance alone. The information is presented in the form of a Glaucoma Change Probability Analysis (see Chapter 9).

Research to date suggests that the intertest variability of the quickest strategy, SITA Fast, is approximately the same as Full Threshold and SITA Standard. Testing time for SITA Fast is approximately one third that of Full Threshold, and two thirds that of SITA Standard. Thus although the two slower strategies may be more sensitive for detecting early loss, SITA Fast may well prove to be quite suitable for use in follow-up testing.

Combining SITA Fast with the 24-2 pattern can further reduce the test time and may be particularly useful with elderly and frail patients. However, if much of the central field is seriously abnormal, the full 30-2 pattern offers a larger number of points by which to judge whether there is progression of the disease. Thus if time is an important consideration in *detecting a defect* in the first place, a 24-2 pattern with a SITA Standard strategy may offer the most sensible balance between time spent and sensitivity. However, for *following a defect,* the 30-2 pattern offers more points to follow, and SITA Fast can be used with it to save time.

Atypical patients

> The central 10-2 test is like a 30-2 pattern scaled down by a factor of three.

Three other options are useful for following the progress of certain patients, especially those with advanced glaucoma: the central 10-2 pattern, the Macula Test, and the size-V stimulus.

The central 10-2 pattern of points (with a threshold strategy) can be used to advantage when most or all of the points in the arcuate region between 10 and 30 degrees have threshold sensitivities of near 0 dB (so that a value of 0 dB on follow-up examination is inconclusive concerning progression). In such cases, it is a waste of time to threshold all the points between 10 and 30 degrees; better is a more thorough examination within the central 10 degrees.[24-26] The 10-2 pattern may be thought of as a 30-2 pattern scaled down in size by a factor of three. Thus, test points in the 10-2 are spaced on a 2-degree grid, compared with the 6-degree spacing of the 30-2. (Actually, the 10-2 has only 68 points, in contrast to the 76 of the 30-2, with 8 points having been removed from the edge to speed testing.) With this pattern, wasteful testing of locations with no measurable vision is avoided and the precious central island is tested more thoroughly. The 10-2 is administered in the same way as the 30-2.

When vision is limited to the central 5 degrees, the Macula Test can be used in a similar way to replace examination of the entire central field. It consists of a square grid of 16 points, 2 degrees apart, centered around the point of fixation. The option of also testing the point of fixation should be used routinely. In the original Humphrey perimeter, each point in the macula pattern was tested three times. In the newer HFA-2 model, the points no longer are tested three times.

The Macula Test also is useful to monitor eyes that have a defect that impinges on fixation, so that further encroachment can be detected with 2-degree resolution rather than 6-degree resolution. If, despite a defect threatening the point of fixation, there are many locations within the central 24 or 30 degrees with measurable threshold sensitivities, the 30-2 or 24-2 test also should be performed. The Macula Test in this case supplements, rather than replaces, an examination of the full extent of the central field.

The third option for severely affected visual fields is to use a size-V stimulus[25,27] with the 30-2, 24-2, 10-2, or Macula Test patterns. Size V is useful whenever most of the points have thresholds close to zero (10 dB or less), which makes the presence or absence of any further deterioration difficult to assess. By switching to a larger stimulus, the sensitivity increases at normal points by 7 or 8 dB.[28] Abnormal points often seem to increase even more, and in such cases the use of a size-V stimulus is of even greater advantage.

The use of these options (the central 10-2 threshold test, the Macula Test, and a size-V stimulus) and their interpretation when following a patient with severe glaucoma are covered further in Chapter 9.

Text continued on p. 216

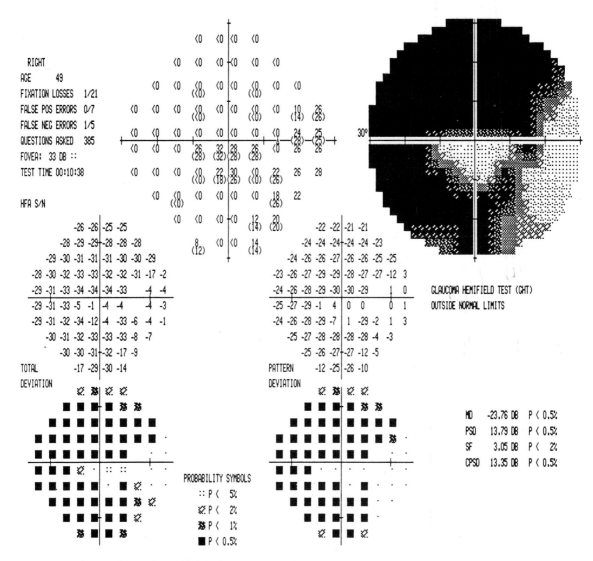

FIG. 8-6. Constricted Field. Region of visibility is limited to within 10 degrees of fixation, as shown with the central 30-2 threshold test.

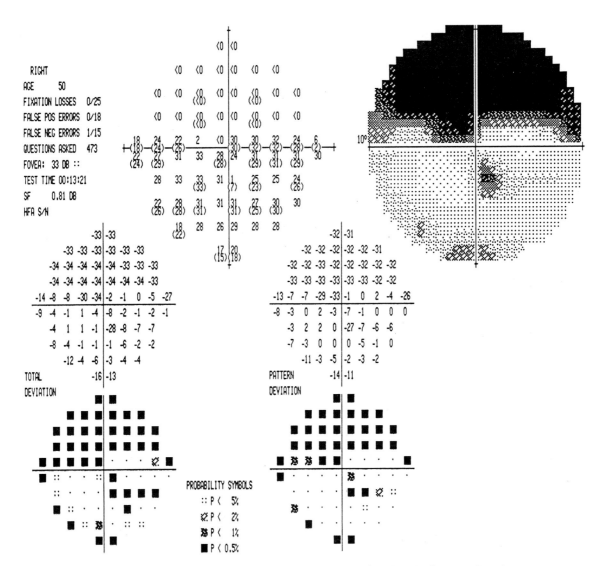

FIG. 8-7. The central 10-2 threshold test concentrates on 68 locations in the central 10 degrees (same patient as Fig. 8-6).

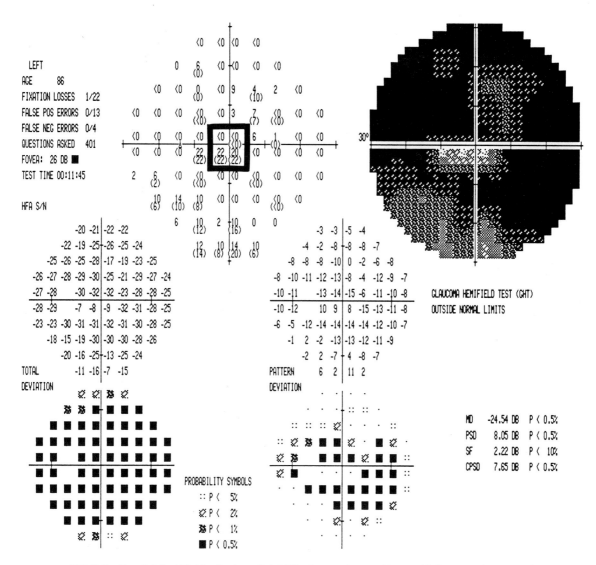

FIG. 8-8. Constricted Field. Region of visibility does not extend beyond 5 degrees when tested with the 30-2 threshold test. The black square shows the region tested with the macula test (see Fig. 8-9), with the four most central points in the 30-2 pattern being the corner points in the 4 × 4 grid of the Macula Test. The test points are 6 degrees apart.

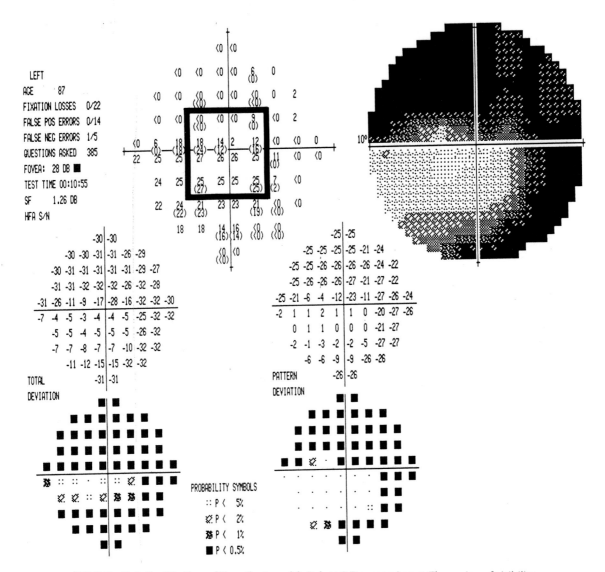

FIG. 8-9. Detailed Testing of Very Center with Points 2 Degrees Apart. The region of visibility is shown here with the central 10-2 test, and the region covered by the Macula Test is outlined by a square (same patient as Fig. 8-8).

Continued

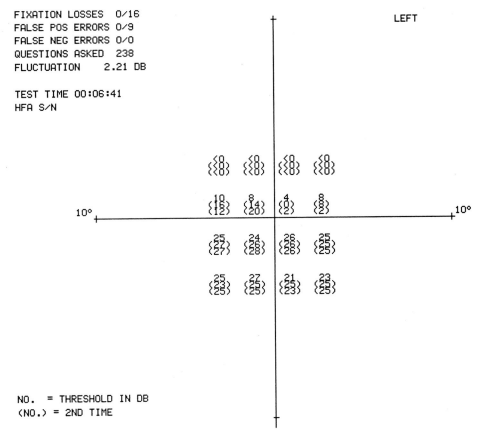

FIXATION LOSSES 0/16
FALSE POS ERRORS 0/9
FALSE NEG ERRORS 0/0
QUESTIONS ASKED 238
FLUCTUATION   2.21 DB

TEST TIME 00:06:41
HFA S/N

LEFT

10°   10°

NO. = THRESHOLD IN DB
(NO.) = 2ND TIME

FIG. 8-9, cont'd. Macula Test. Same patient shown in Fig. 8-8.

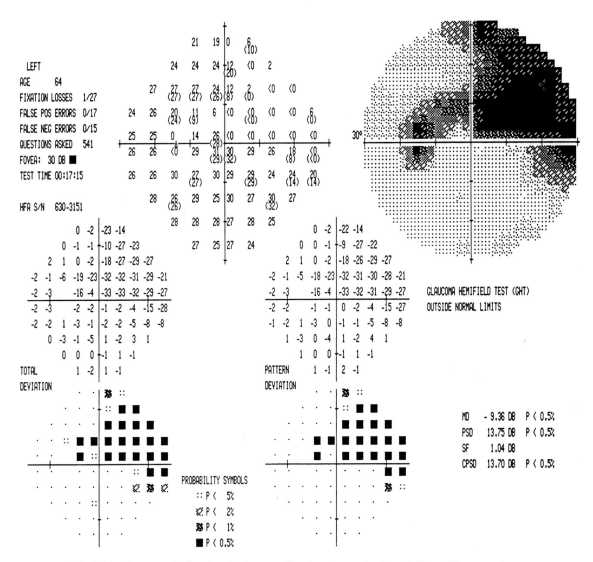

FIG. 8-10. Arcuate Defect Impinging on Fixation From the Nasal Side. The central 30-2 threshold test. *Continued*

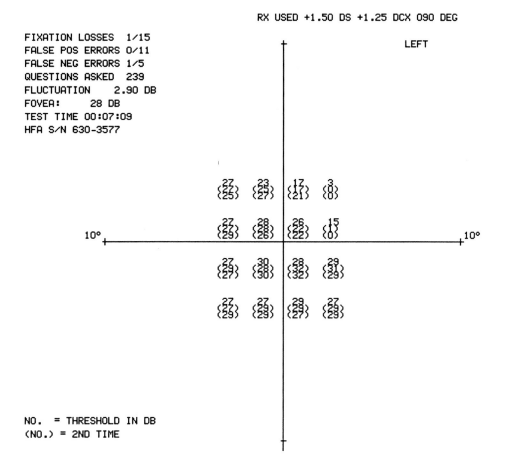

RX USED +1.50 DS +1.25 DCX 090 DEG

LEFT

FIXATION LOSSES 1/15
FALSE POS ERRORS 0/11
FALSE NEG ERRORS 1/5
QUESTIONS ASKED 239
FLUCTUATION   2.90 DB
FOVEA: 28 DB
TEST TIME 00:07:09
HFA S/N 630-3577

27   23   17   3
{25}   {27}   {21}   {8}

27   28   28   15
{29}   {26}   {22}   {0}

27   30   28   29
{27}   {30}   {32}   {29}

27   27   28   27
{29}   {29}   {27}   {29}

10°   10°

NO. = THRESHOLD IN DB
(NO.) = 2ND TIME

FIG. 8-10, cont'd. The macula test of the same eye, defining more carefully the central 5 degrees.

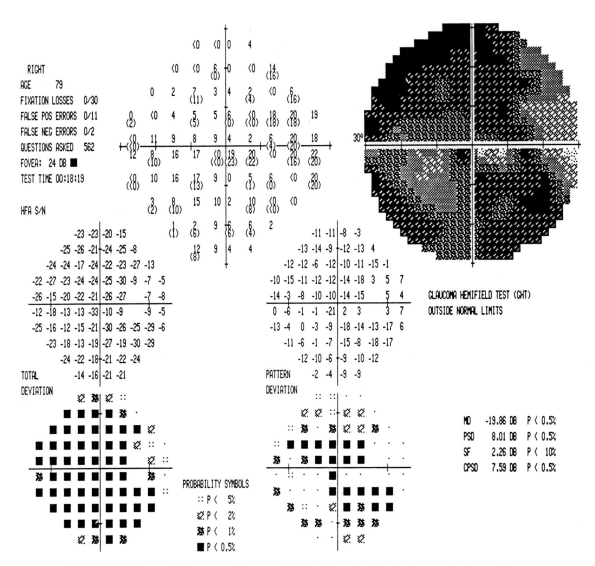

FIG. 8-11. Advanced Glaucoma. The sensitivities with a size-III stimulus are low (central 30-2 test).

Continued

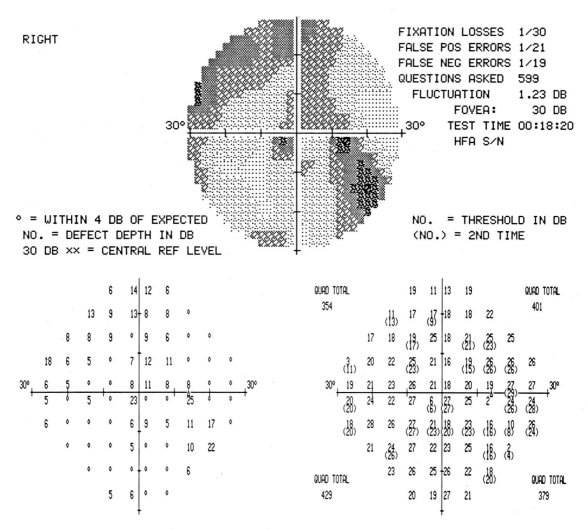

RIGHT

FIXATION LOSSES   1/30
FALSE POS ERRORS 1/21
FALSE NEG ERRORS 1/19
QUESTIONS ASKED   599
  FLUCTUATION   1.23 DB
        FOVEA: 30 DB
   TEST TIME 00:18:20
          HFA S/N

° = WITHIN 4 DB OF EXPECTED
NO. = DEFECT DEPTH IN DB
30 DB ×× = CENTRAL REF LEVEL

NO.   = THRESHOLD IN DB
(NO.) = 2ND TIME

FIG. 8-11, cont'd. In the same patient, with a size-V stimulus, the sensitivities are higher; thus, any subsequent deterioration will be more easily recognized. The threshold values are mapped on the lower right. The Defect Depth is mapped on the lower left (see p. 216 for explanation).

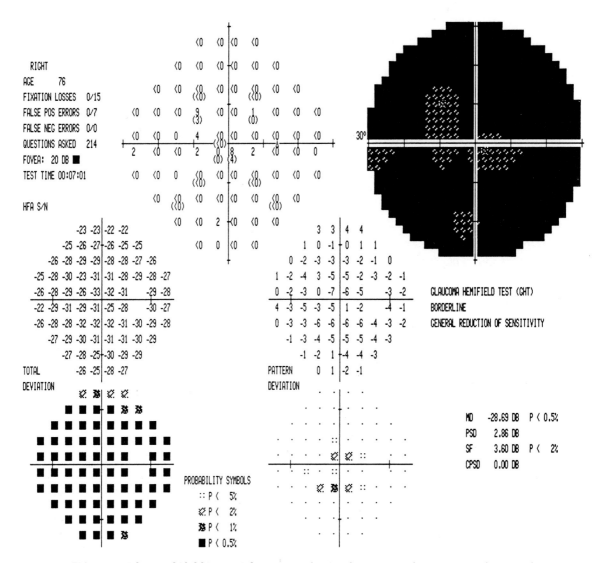

FIG. 8-12. Advanced Field Loss. A few scattered points have minimal sensitivity in the central 30-2 threshold test with a size-III stimulus. *Continued*

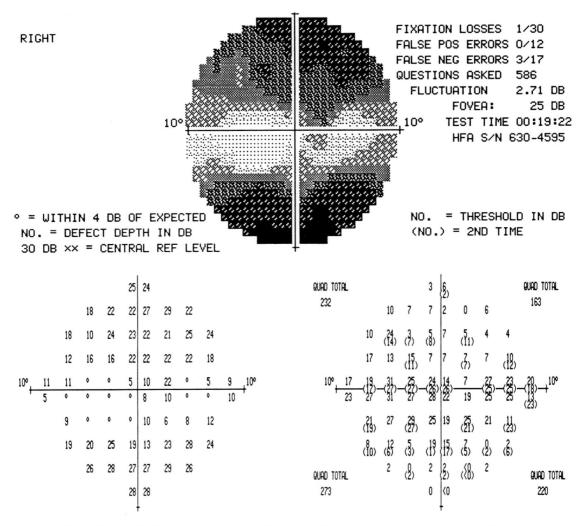

RIGHT

FIXATION LOSSES   1/30
FALSE POS ERRORS 0/12
FALSE NEG ERRORS 3/17
QUESTIONS ASKED   586
 FLUCTUATION   2.71 DB
    FOVEA: 25 DB
 TEST TIME 00:19:22
 HFA S/N 630-4595

° = WITHIN 4 DB OF EXPECTED
NO. = DEFECT DEPTH IN DB
30 DB ×× = CENTRAL REF LEVEL

NO. = THRESHOLD IN DB
(NO.) = 2ND TIME

FIG. 8-12, cont'd. The same case can be followed with the combined use of a central 10-2 test and size-V stimulus. As in Figure 8-11, the printout of a test performed with a size-V stimulus produces the threshold values on the lower right and the Defect Depth grid on the lower left; this example represents only the central 10 degrees.

215

Non-Statpac printouts

The main use of the size-V stimulus is to follow the progress of severe disease.

When a size-V stimulus is used, there is no question about whether the field is normal; a size-V stimulus is used only because the field is already known to be quite abnormal.* Therefore the Statpac Single-Field Analysis, aimed at recognizing and characterizing abnormality, usually is not relevant. In fact, a normal database with a size-V stimulus has not been obtained.

The familiar Statpac Single-Field Analysis printout is used only when a normal database is available. When it is not available, such as for a size-V stimulus, the printout provides the greyscale at the top, the map (value table) of threshold sensitivity values in decibels at the bottom right, and a difference-from-expected plot, called the "Defect Depth Grid (or Plot)," at the bottom left (Figs. 8-11 and 8-12).

The Defect Depth grid resembles the Pattern Deviation plot in calling particular attention to localized defects within widespread abnormality. It does not depend on normal threshold sensitivity data but does depend on the normal shape and slope of the hill of vision.

The Defect Depth grid is derived as follows: the overall height of the hill of vision is determined from the second-most sensitive of the four primary points[†] and the point of fixation, if it was tested. An extrapolation is performed to yield the so-called *Central Reference Level*.[‡] The second highest sensitivity is used as the basis for extrapolation because the point with the *highest* sensitivity is in some patients falsely high because of false-positive button pushes.

The Central Reference Level is used to calculate an expected threshold value for every point in the field based on its eccentricity from the point of fixation. It is the difference between this expected value and the observed value obtained that is

---

*A common technical error is to assume that if the acuity is poor, a size-V stimulus should be used. In nearly all cases, it is best if the first field test be done with a size-III stimulus. If the reduced acuity is due to a localized central defect, fixation may be steady (perhaps with use of the larger fixation target if necessary), and many points in the central field may have normal values with a size-III stimulus. The opportunity to document the normalcy or to quantify the degree of abnormality at each location is lost if size III is not used. Thus size V has limitations for initial diagnosis, and the main use for size V is to follow the progress of severe disease.

[†]Recall that primary points are the four points, one in each quadrant, at which threshold initially is determined at the beginning of a threshold test (after the foveal threshold is determined) and at the beginning of a threshold-related suprathreshold test (see Chapter 5).

[‡]The Central Reference Level is not the foveal threshold. It is a reference value representing a linear extrapolation of threshold at nonfoveal points back to the center of the field—not taking into account that the foveal peak is nonlinearly more sensitive than the surrounding regions. However, the reference level is not permitted to be set below a minimal value that is approximately the 99th percentile value for central reference level in healthy individuals older than 70 years of age; that is, 99% of elderly controls would be expected to have a Central Reference Level higher than the minimum. The minimal values are 19 dB, 23 dB, 26 dB, 28 dB, and 30 dB, respectively, for stimulus sizes I through V. (In SWAP testing, there is a much larger normal range for the height of the hill of vision than is found in standard white testing. For this reason, no minimum Central Reference Level is imposed in non-Statpac analyses of SWAP results.) In addition to its use in the Defect Depth grid, a Central Reference Level is assigned according to the patient's age for age-related suprathreshold tests, and the stimulus intensity presented during the test depends on the test location and the reference level being used. For the threshold-related suprathreshold strategy, test stimuli are based on a reference level that is selected for the individual—not according to age but in the same way as described for determining an estimated defect depth in non-Statpac printouts of threshold tests.

printed (similar to the fact that the total deviation is the difference between normal values and the observed value). The numerical conventions of this plot differ from those of the total and pattern deviation plots in that values are given as positive numbers if the observed sensitivity is less than expected and the differences are given only when they exceed 4 dB.

The Central Reference Level is intended to provide some adjustment for variations in overall sensitivity from one individual to another and to correct for mild generalized depression as a result of media opacity—thus causing the Defect Depth plot to highlight localized defects in the same way that the *Pattern* Deviation plot of Statpac does. Because there is a minimal permitted reference value, deviation values may be given for all the points if the entire field is sufficiently depressed; when this happens, the Defect Depth plot more closely resembles the character of the Statpac *Total* Deviation plot. Although these representations of the threshold data help characterize the diagnostic nature of the field defect, they are irrelevant if the reason for using a size-V stimulus was to provide higher threshold values and a larger range over which progression can be monitored.

The Defect Depth representation was developed before the normal database and Statpac Single-Field Analyses became available. It is retained for those tests for which the normal database (and Statpac analysis) does not apply—for example, when a nonstandard stimulus size is used, for printouts of master files or average files (see Fig. 9-10), and for the Fast Threshold printout (see Fig. 9-14).

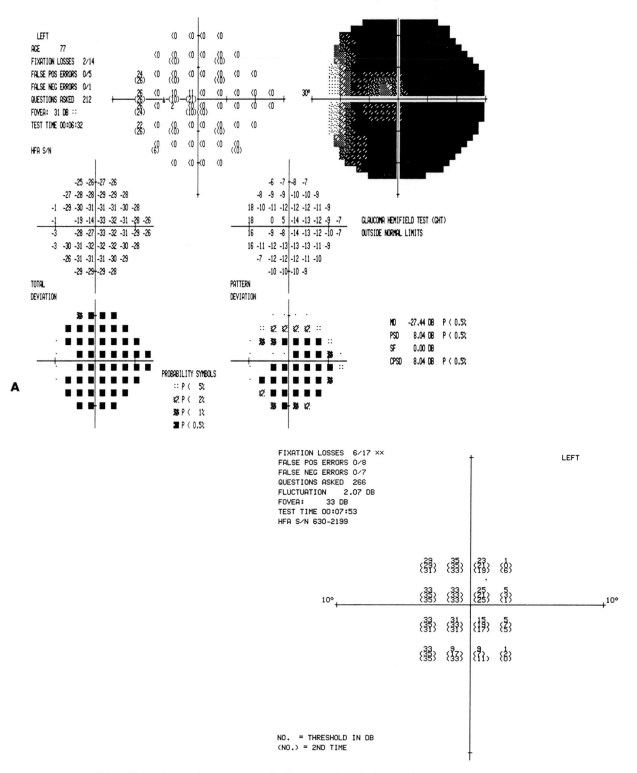

FIG. 8-13. Advanced Glaucoma. A, The central 24-2 threshold test of the left eye *(above)* shows a small central island of remaining vision and another zone of visibility temporal to the blind spot. A 30-2 pattern would permit better monitoring of the temporal portion of the central field. The macula test can be used to follow the central island, and although rarely used, superthreshold testing **(B)** can be used to follow the boundary of the temporal island.

Continued

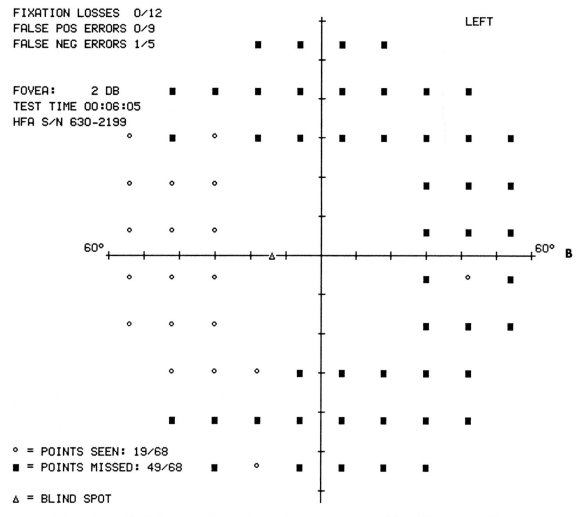

FIXATION LOSSES 0/12
FALSE POS ERRORS 0/9
FALSE NEG ERRORS 1/5

FOVEA: 2 DB
TEST TIME 00:06:05
HFA S/N 630-2199

60°

60° B

LEFT

○ = POINTS SEEN: 19/68
■ = POINTS MISSED: 49/68

Δ = BLIND SPOT

FIG. 8-13, cont'd. B, A threshold-related screening strategy between 30 and 60 degrees outlines the temporal island, but not its full extent.

NEUROLOGIC CONDITIONS

It is rare for a neurologic field defect to affect only the area outside 30 degrees.

The central 30-2 threshold test often is used as a general test for any visual field application. As a thorough test of the central 30 degrees, it reveals almost any visual field defect. As with glaucoma, it truly is rare for a visual field defect caused by a neurologic problem to be represented only in the peripheral field.

Many patients with neurologic disease are not well enough to undergo the rigors of a lengthy, fully quantitative field examination such as the 30-2 Full Threshold test. For this reason, it may be advantageous to use the 24-2 pattern and shorter threshold algorithms instead. It is appropriate to consider whether a threshold test of any sort always is necessary. Thoughtful selection of a visual field examination may save time and sharpen diagnostic acumen. The manner of clinical presentation should be considered and the goal of performing the examination clearly defined.

For many purposes in a neuro-ophthalmic context, a general screen of the central 30 degrees with suprathreshold testing may serve to reveal and characterize hemianopias caused by lesions severe enough that the patient has sought medical attention for visual or neurologic symptoms.[29-31] The test may be shortened without compromising diagnostic effectiveness by using the age-related, Two-Zone screening strategy,* which presents stimuli at a level very close to those evaluated by Siatkowski and coworkers,[32] who found that this test had a sensitivity and specificity of 87% and 85%, respectively (compared with 93% and 91% for the 30-2 Full Threshold test). It is assumed that the defect of interest in this setting will not be tiny and the emphasis is on characterizing the diagnostic geography of the defect. In this way the goal differs from that of glaucoma screening, for which the Quantify-Defects mode was recommended to detect and verify the presence of slight glaucomatous abnormality, rather than to detect broader field defects of various etiologies and characterize them.

The extra time required by a full-threshold examination or assessment of the peripheral field should be taken only in selected cases in which a high index of suspicion remains despite a negative screening examination. The clinician also might ask whether other diagnostic tests, such as neuroradiologic imaging or a neurologic physical examination, would be more helpful in solving the clinical problem in some circumstances.

Another clinical need *not* well served by a suprathreshold test is to follow the progress of a field defect, for example, to detect further tumor growth or to monitor patients with pseudotumor. The clinical problem in such patients essentially is identical with that of following glaucoma patients. Keep in mind that the variability of test-retest variability in neurologic field defects may or may not be

---

*This method has been among the available options of the software for several years. The automated option uses a Central Reference Level of 34 dB from ages 5 to 39 years, 33 dB to age 49 years, 32 dB to age 69 years, 31 dB to age 89 years, and 30 dB for ages 90 to 104 years. On the earlier software versions, to choose this method, enter the change parameters menu of the screening test selected, choose "central reference level," and specify a level. Siatkowski et al[32] found 2 dB below the median for age to be effective. Such a selection for size-III stimulus would be 35 dB up to age 30 years, 34 dB to age 45 years, 33 dB to age 65 years, 32 dB to age 80 years, and 31 dB above 80 years of age.

the same as for glaucomatous field defects (this has not been scientifically determined either way). Therefore the *Glaucoma Change Probability* analysis may not be valid for conditions other than glaucoma—note that it is called the *Glaucoma Change Probability* analysis.

To screen for hemianopias, the central 76-point screening test may be a useful standard, with test points that coincide with those of the standard 30-2 threshold test. An advantage is that a pointwise correlation can be made with a threshold test if it is performed later. However, the central 80-point screening test also is suitable. No time is wasted on the region immediately surrounding the blind spot, effort is concentrated along the vertical meridian as well as the nasal horizontal meridian, and the region between 25 and 30 degrees receives less emphasis.

Text continued on p. 230

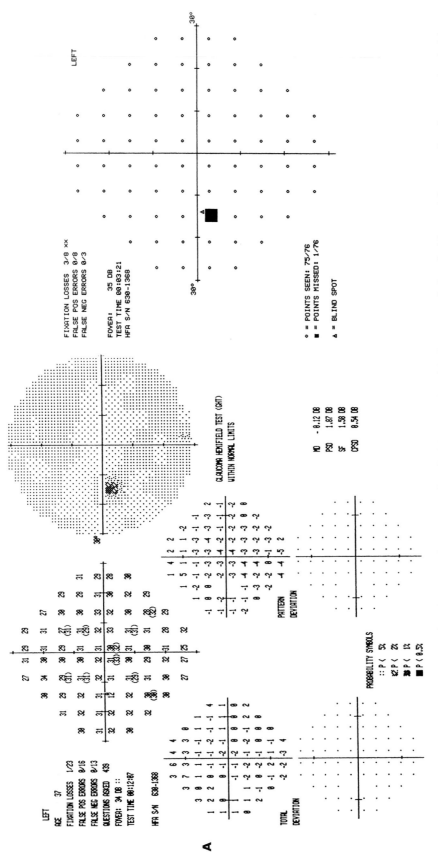

FIG. 8-14. Eight Sample Fields Comparing the Age-Related Suprathreshold Test (*right*) **with the 30-2 Full Threshold Test** (*left*). Note that the suprathreshold test closely resembles the pattern deviation probability plot of the threshold test. Note that any diagnostic uncertainty of a defect configuration is equivalent with the two tests. **A,** Normal. (Modified from Siatkowski RM, Lam B, Anderson DR, Feuer WJ, Halikman AB: Automated suprathreshold static perimetry screening in neuro-ophthalmology, *Ophthalmology* 103:907–917, 1996. Courtesy of *Ophthalmology*.)

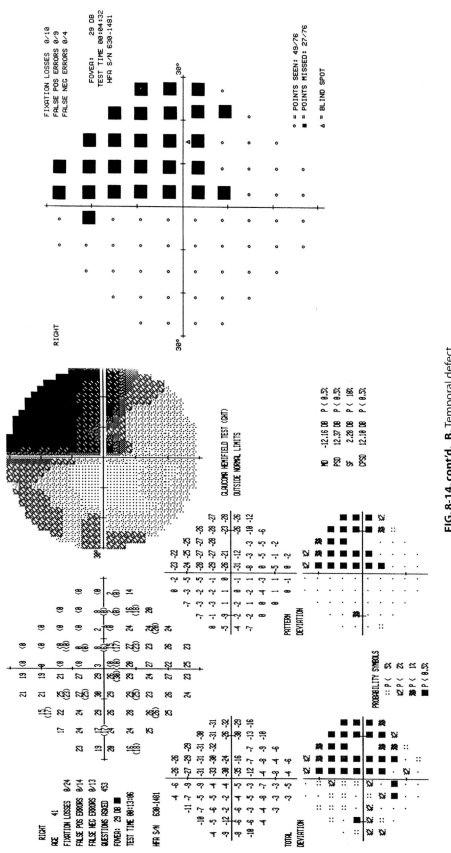

FIG. 8-14, cont'd. B, Temporal defect.

223

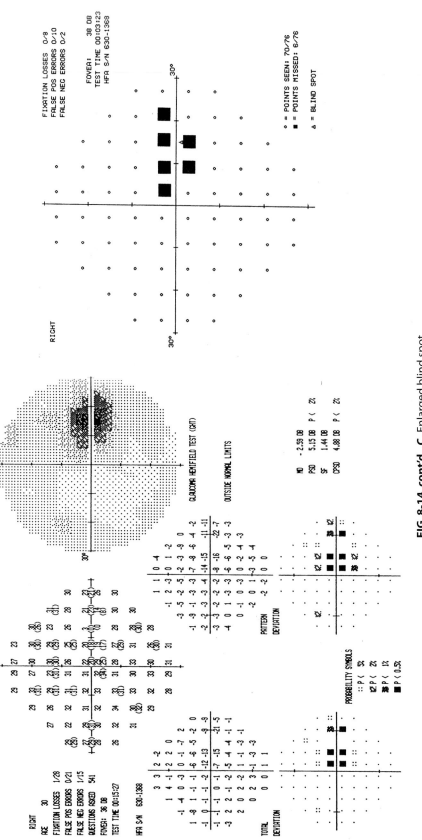

FIG. 8-14, cont'd. C, Enlarged blind spot.

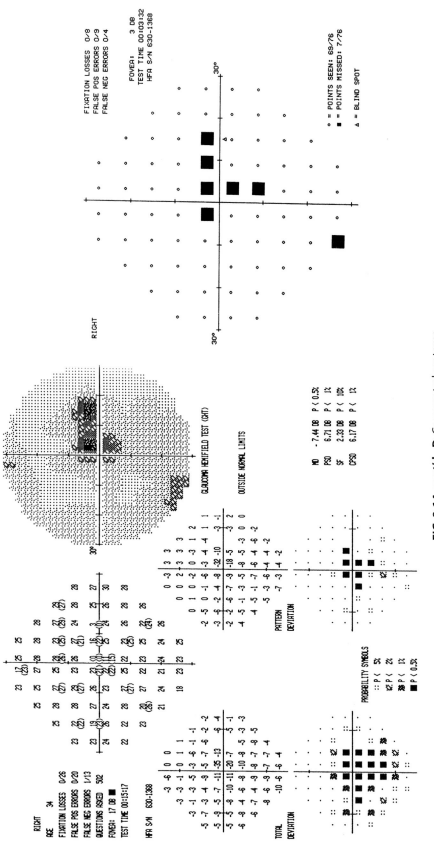

FIG. 8-14, cont'd. D, Cecocentral scotoma.

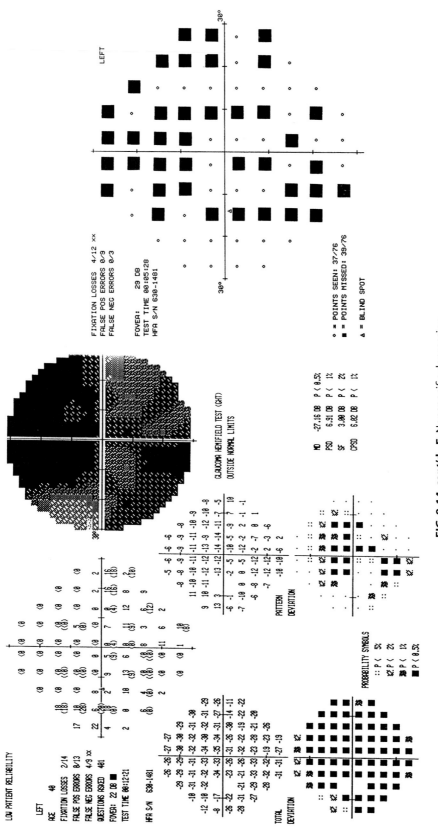

FIG. 8-14, cont'd. E, Nonspecific depression.

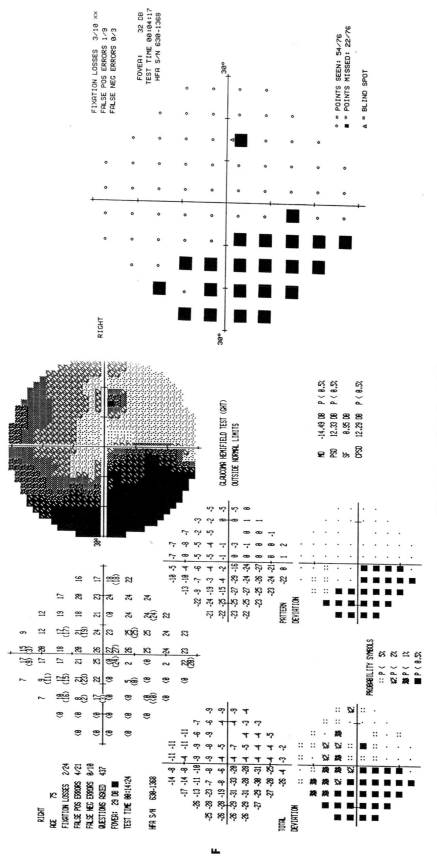
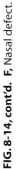

FIG. 8-14, cont'd. F, Nasal defect.

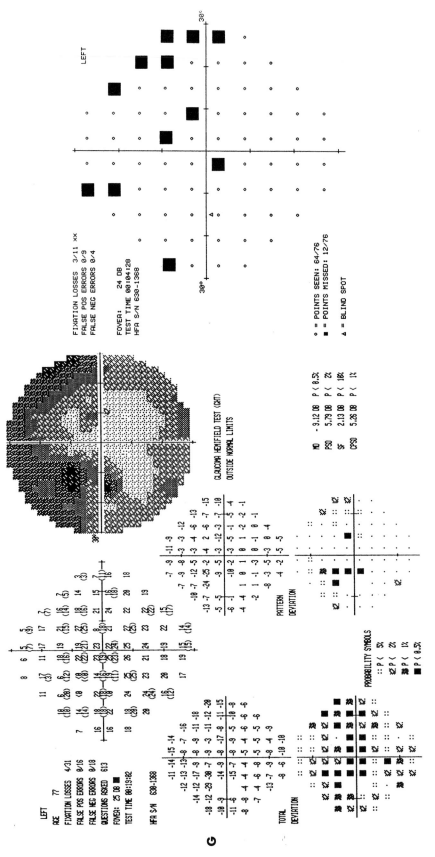

FIG. 8-14, cont'd. G, Variable responses in a nerve-fiber bundle pattern.

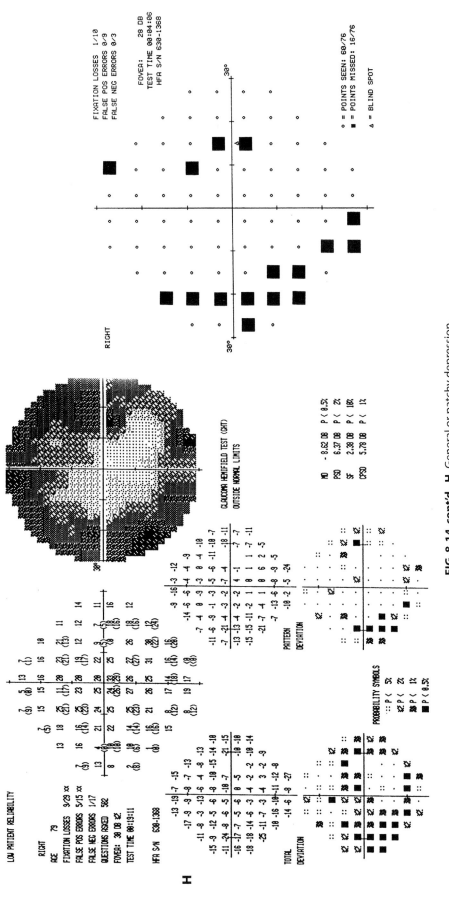

FIG. 8-14, cont'd. H, General or patchy depression.

RETINAL DISEASES

Perimetry is useful in specific retinal conditions, such as retinitis pigmentosa and toxic maculopathy, and in ruling out macular disease obscured by cataract.

There is a wide variety of retinal diseases. Ophthalmoscopy is the mainstay of diagnosis, supplemented by fluorescein angiography, electrophysiologic tests, and echography, among other diagnostic tests. Only occasionally is there a need to evaluate the visual field. When perimetry is chosen, the test is selected according to the diagnostic purpose at hand and the nature of the disease under consideration. Thus a pattern and distribution of test points are selected to cover the retinal region likely to be involved in this disease. Next, a threshold or suprathreshold screening strategy is selected according to the degree of quantification required. Three clinical examples are described to illustrate these principles, but the reader must select the test best suited for other clinical circumstances.

The first clinical setting involves a patient with visual difficulties at night and pigmentary disturbances that suggest retinitis pigmentosa. The typical field defect is in the mid-periphery; thus, the field should be tested at least to 60 degrees. Because the objective simply is to find the pattern of visual field loss to confirm the suspected diagnosis and it typically is not necessary to quantify the degree of abnormality, a screening suprathreshold strategy might be selected. A large number of test points is desirable to recognize more clearly the ring-like nature of the mid-peripheral field loss and define the limits of the area of major involvement. This might be one of the few instances in which a full-field 246-point screening strategy might be considered, although this strategy emphasizes the central region and is a lengthy test. A better alternative might be to use the central 76-point screen and the peripheral 68-point screen, which together cover 144 locations to 60 degrees of eccentricity.

Instead of looking for a ring scotoma in suspected retinitis pigmentosa, it might be better to screen the full field with a size-I stimulus at full intensity (0 dB) or at the Goldmann 4e equivalent (10 dB). If the stimulus is seen over the full extent of the field (allowing for several false responses and some normal variation in the extent of the field nasally and superiorly), no further testing is needed. However, the field virtually never is full with a small test stimulus in retinitis pigmentosa. If the field is conducted with a size-I stimulus, the test should be repeated with a larger (size-III or size-V) stimulus of the same bright intensity (0 dB or 10 dB). It would be characteristic for the field to be greatly expanded with a larger test stimulus of the same intensity in this disease.[33] To avoid a false conclusion that the mid-peripheral field is contracted, remember that the normal visual field seldom extends fully to 60 degrees in the superior and nasal quadrants (see Fig. 2-2). It should be noted that except for the difference between static and kinetic presentations, the Humphrey 10-dB size-III stimulus is the same as the Goldmann III-4e stimulus often used for disability determinations and declaration of statutory blindness.

The second clinical example relates to toxic maculopathies. Ophthalmologists and optometrists often are consulted to monitor the visual status of patients receiving chloroquine or hydroxychloroquine. Because the area of involvement is the macula and the goal is to find very subtle changes that might indicate the need to discontinue therapy, a threshold test with the 10-2 pattern is a logical selection.

Diagnostic criteria (i.e., the magnitude of depressed sensitivity compared with surround or previous status that constitutes reason for concern) have not been established, but the Statpac printout does help by providing significance limits in the normal population for the 10-2, size-III white stimuli. Use of a red test stimulus has been advocated to improve sensitivity, but no normative significance limits are available for red stimuli and no clear advantage has been demonstrated over standard testing with a white stimulus.[34]

Amsler grid screening (see Chapter 10) has been claimed to be sufficient for this purpose.[35] The truth is that maculopathy is infrequent,[34-46] especially with the use of hydroxychloroquine, and therefore the literature does not contain a sufficient assemblage of positive results among those with early, evolving maculopathy to evaluate which method is the most sensitive to early changes, the most specific, or the most cost effective for this purpose. A number of authors currently suggest that regular ophthalmic evaluation may be less important than previously believed if the patient is receiving hydroxychloroquine in recommended standard doses.[41-46]

Central scotomas are not diagnosed from the Deviation probability plots, but from threshold values lower than the surround.

A third clinical circumstance in which perimetry may be useful is with cataract that is suspected of being accompanied by macular disease (or other causes of a central scotoma). Ophthalmoscopy and confrontation methods (see Chapter 10) should most often suffice, but a central 30-2 or, preferably, a 10-2 threshold test will also show a central scotoma. The diagnostic criterion is whether the fovea and perhaps also its immediate surrounding area are less sensitive than other regions. Even with cataract, the fovea should be as sensitive or more sensitive than other parts of the field. Don't be fooled by the Pattern Deviation probability plot, such as that shown in Figure 7-19. A small deviation from normal may be more highly significant at the center, which—along with the foveal value—therefore is marked with the darkest probability symbol. In this example, however, note that the foveal threshold of 19 dB is just as high as, or higher than, almost any other location.

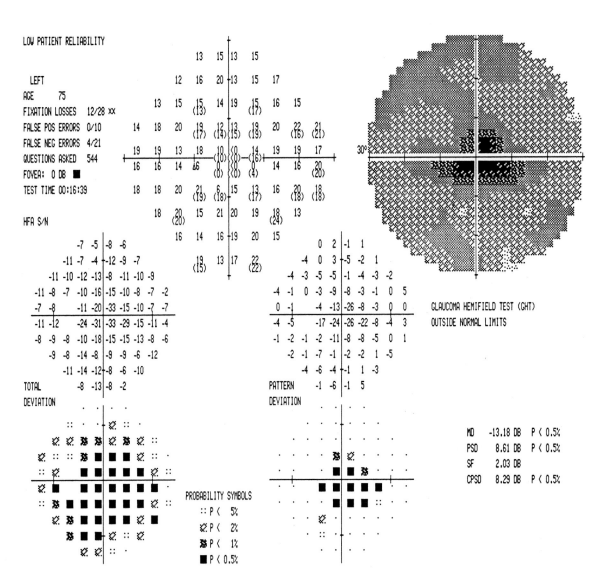

FIG. 8-15. Cataract and Macular Disease. The entire field is depressed, but sensitivity in the center is less (0 to 10 dB) than elsewhere (10 to 20 dB). Figure 3-2 shows another example of macular disease, with quite mild cataract. Compare these figures with examples of cataract alone (see Figs. 7-17 to 7-19) or a blurred image from refractive error (see Fig. 2-6), in which the reduction from normal values may be greatest at the center but actual threshold sensitivity is no worse at the center than elsewhere. Severe macular disease does produce obvious, large scotomas, as in this example; however, mild macular disease—enough to affect acuity to a mild but noticeable degree—may produce equivocal findings.

BLEPHAROPTOSIS

Perimetry frequently is used to document a visual need for blepharoplasty. Although perimetry clearly is useful,[47,48] it is not the sole basis for clinical decisions. Symptomatic restriction of the superior field might be expected if the pupil is partially covered or if the separation between the corneal reflex and the upper lid margin is less than 2.5 or 3.5 mm.[49,50] Symptoms of headache from day-long frontalis contraction to overcome ptosis may compound visual inadequacy, and cosmetic considerations may cause patients to seek correction of blepharoptosis. In any case, when using perimetry to help evaluate or document the visual effect of blepharoptosis, a few points should be noted.

First, the physician may select a test that quantifies a visual effect of blepharoptosis. From the result of this test and from other signs and reported symptoms, he may become satisfied that an impairment exists that is sufficient to indicate surgical correction apart from any cosmetic considerations. However, each third-party payer has its own specifications regarding which perimetric tests and criteria adequately document the "medical necessity" of corrective surgery, which non-perimetric evidence is required, and under what circumstances the insurance contract or government entitlements will cover the cost. Recent models of the Humphrey perimeter offer test patterns designed for assessment of superior visual field impairments, which may satisfy the requirements of many payers. If the built-in protocol does not meet local needs, the user may program suitable customized patterns for this purpose into most instruments.

Second, elderly patients without impairment or symptoms commonly show partial reduction of the superior visual field down to 30 degrees from the normal maximum of 60 degrees. The superior field usually must be less than 30 degrees for patients to be functionally disabled by their ptosis.

Third, because ptosis-induced field loss typically is absolute, it is not necessary for the patient to undergo threshold visual field tests; a single-level screening test strategy with a 10-dB (1000-asb) size-III stimulus will demonstrate any meaningful field restriction.

Fourth, there is some evidence that loss of superior field may be different in downgaze than in primary gaze. Thus, some patients may require evaluation in both postures, or at least in the posture associated with their presenting complaints.[51-53] When it is necessary to document the effect of ptosis in downgaze, the alternative fixation targets available on the perimeter are used so that the test is conducted with the gaze slightly depressed. Additional downgaze may be obtained by placing a soft spacer between the patient's forehead and the perimeter's head rest to tilt the head back slightly. As a guide to the necessity for such testing, the practitioner can compare the corneal reflex to lid distance in downgaze versus that found in primary gaze.

Finally, it is useful to explore not only whether limitation of the upper field exists and is symptomatic but also whether lifting the eyelid expands the limits of the superior visual field and relieves the visual symptoms. In fact, third-party payers may require, for example, that the field be 12 degrees taller when the test is repeated with the upper eyelid held open with tape. If the upper visual field is

> Lid-induced field loss down to 30 degrees is common in the elderly and usually not cause for concern.

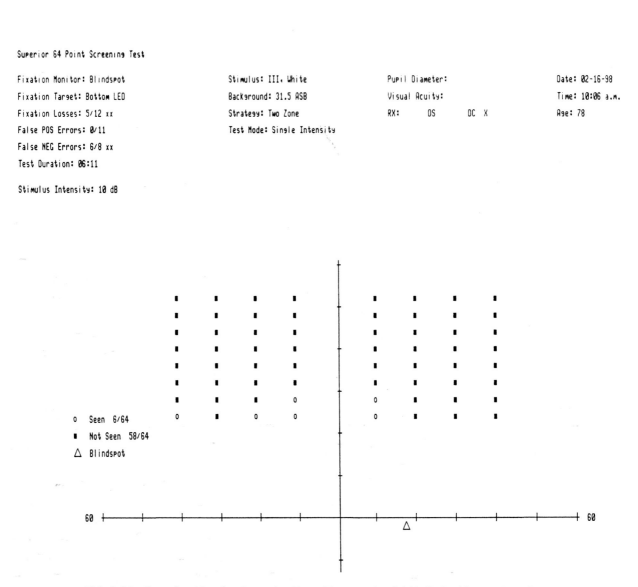

Superior 64 Point Screening Test

Fixation Monitor: Blindspot
Fixation Target: Bottom LED
Fixation Losses: 5/12 xx
False POS Errors: 0/11
False NEG Errors: 6/8 xx
Test Duration: 06:11

Stimulus Intensity: 10 dB

Stimulus: III, White
Background: 31.5 ASB
Strategy: Two Zone
Test Mode: Single Intensity

Pupil Diameter:
Visual Acuity:
RX: OS   OC X

Date: 02-16-98
Time: 10:06 a.m.
Age: 78

o Seen 6/64
■ Not Seen 58/64
△ Blindspot

60   60

FIG. 8-16. Superior 64-point Screening Test. The superior field is limited by ptosis and relieved by taping up the eyelid. Test points are 4 degrees apart vertically.

Continued

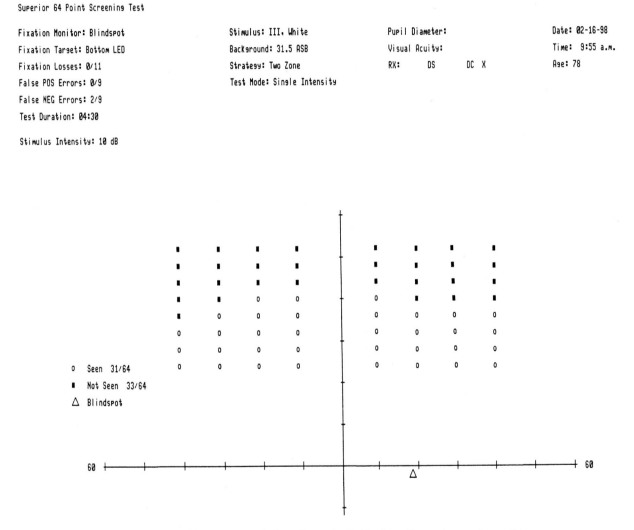

Superior 64 Point Screening Test

Fixation Monitor: Blindspot

Fixation Target: Bottom LED

Fixation Losses: 0/11

False POS Errors: 0/9

False NEG Errors: 2/9

Test Duration: 04:30

Stimulus Intensity: 10 dB

Stimulus: III, White

Background: 31.5 ASB

Strategy: Two Zone

Test Mode: Single Intensity

Pupil Diameter:

Visual Acuity:

RX: DS   DC X

Date: 02-16-98

Time: 9:55 a.m.

Age: 78

o   Seen 31/64

■   Not Seen 33/64

△   Blindspot

60

60

FIG. 8-16, cont'd.   Upper restriction of superior field relieved by taping up the eyelid.

constricted but unexpectedly is not improved when the eyelid is held up with tape, the patient probably has a visual field defect from another cause. In such circumstances, the patient may benefit from an evaluation of the retina, the optic nerve, and if necessary, the more posterior parts of the visual pathway, unless the presence of a disease affecting the visual sensory pathway already is known. If the patient is known to have a disease other than blepharoptosis that severely limits the upper field (e.g., glaucoma), raising the eyelid may produce visual improvement or symptomatic relief that is not revealed by an expansion of the visual field after taping the upper eyelid. In such cases, it becomes more difficult to produce compelling objective evidence to document the medical necessity of surgical correction.

> Look for cause if upper field fails to expand when eyelid is taped open.

DRIVING QUALIFICATION

Ophthalmologists and optometrists frequently are asked to evaluate whether a patient's peripheral vision is adequate for driving. The patient may be seeking advice, or a licensing agency may be seeking evaluation and documentation. Although reductions in peripheral function clearly are associated with increased accident rates,[54] licensing agencies differ in their definitions of acceptable limits for driving. Although practitioners must consult their own local authorities directly for licensing requirements, a few general observations may be of use when giving advice to patients.

First, after an appropriate period of adaptation to the loss, partial or even total loss of vision in one eye has minimal impact; monocular truck drivers, for example, are not necessarily disabled.[55] It also seems that even with patchy binocular loss, regions of intact vision in one eye may fill in for patches of loss in the other; for example, the monocular visual fields of patients who have undergone panretinal photocoagulation are no longer normal, but such patients do not necessarily have a visual handicap that prevents safe driving.[56,57] The pertinent characteristic may be the nature of the net binocular visual field.[54,58]

Second, driving performance depends only in part on the extent of visual field. Scanning eye movements and caution may overcome much of the impact of a visual field restriction, especially if it is not severe, so that a visual field measurement is only a partial correlate of accident risk.[59-61] Yet it is clear that profound reductions in the binocular field of vision do affect driving performance,[54,58,59] and accident-prone individuals are more likely to have field restriction than others, perhaps unknowingly.[54] Driving performance deteriorates markedly, with reductions of the binocular field to 40 degrees or less,[62] but it is not well established how much larger than 40 degrees the field of view must be to be safe. It is likely that the risk increases progressively with progressively greater field loss.

There is little evidence about how limitations of the superior or inferior fields might affect driving. Overhead tree limbs, signs, and traffic signals have a small angle of intercept when viewed from a distance; if they are 20 feet above the street, traffic signs and signals remain within 10 degrees of the horizon until one is closer than 100 feet. Therefore, it is likely appropriate that the greatest attention is given to the horizontal width of the visual field.

Third, measurements of the visual field for driving purposes are aimed at recognizing the absolute outer boundary of vision and in this way differ from clinical diagnostic tests that are designed to find and characterize regions of slight abnormality. A relative loss 45 degrees to the side may not prevent seeing a vehicle that is entering the driver's path at that angle. For this reason, the targets used for testing need not be weak stimuli meant to detect a subtle abnormality or a region of dim vision but should be stimuli that indicate where vision is profoundly affected. The stimuli may be the same as those commonly used for determining visual disability.

In the absence of more conservative guidance from local driving authorities, we suggest the following as reasonable guidelines when a patient asks whether it is safe to drive:

1. Drivers who have profound loss of vision to the right or left in both eyes are unlikely to be able to drive safely. Thus, drivers probably should have binocular fields that extend at least 50 degrees both to the right and to the left for a total span of 100 degrees.

2. Many licensing authorities require a horizontal field of view that is greater than 100 degrees (e.g., 140 degrees), and those requirements must take priority over our minimum suggested requirement.

3. Standard field evaluations for this purpose may be performed with a size-III, 10-dB (1000-asb) stimulus on a 31.6-asb background, which is the equivalent of a Goldmann III-4e stimulus, the standard used for disability evaluation; the Esterman test spans 75 degrees in each direction horizontally and might be useful for this purpose, as would other patterns that extend peripherally to the required amount. However, some agencies issuing driver's licenses may accept any reasonable demonstration of a wide field of view, including confrontation testing.

4. Periodic visual field evaluations of elderly drivers and drivers who have had several accidents may be prudent.

VISUAL IMPAIRMENT AND DISABILITY

Perimetric measurements for driving and for assessing impairment should look for areas of inadequate vision, not subtle loss.

Various agencies throughout the world have varying definitions of disability and methods for quantifying the degree of visual impairment. The visual component of permanent impairment is evaluated in terms of acuity, extent of visual field, and ocular motility or binocular diplopia. When establishing definitions, many agencies in the United States refer to the *Guide to Evaluation of Permanent Impairment,* published by the American Medical Association (the 4th edition was published in 1993; the 5th edition is due in 2000). The chapter on visual impairment is reprinted each year in the *Physicians' Desk Reference for Ophthalmology.*

The visual field element is evaluated in terms of the extent of the field over which a standard stimulus is seen. The time-honored reference is the size-III 4e stimulus of the Goldmann perimeter (0.43 degree of angular subtense at 1000 asb on a 31.6-asb background). Ignoring the difference between static and kinetic stimuli, this is the same as the size-III 10-dB (1000 asb on a 31.6-asb background) stimulus of the Humphrey Field Analyzer.

Because it is the peripheral extent of the field to this relatively strong stimulus that is of interest, trial lens correction is not used, although some protocols suggest that the patient's customary spectacles be worn in order to include their effect in the functional assessment. In the case of patients who normally wear strong spectacles because of aphakia without a lens implant or the use of a contact lens, the visibility, without correction, of a size-IV (rather than the customary size-III) stimulus is tested. The expected extent of an impaired field to the standard stimulus is given in Table 8-1.

If the visual field evaluation is performed specifically to determine impairment, the intent is not to discover subtle relative defects but to quantify the extent of the visual field over which the selected, standard, moderately strong stimulus is seen. To do so, the stimulus is presented in a suprathreshold test at a series of locations that blanket the visual field. The result sometimes is quantified by noting the outer boundary of the visual field along representative meridians; alternatively, it sometimes is quantified in terms of the percentage of tested locations at which the stimulus is seen. Most agencies accept either method.

The clinician must select the pattern (number and locations) of points to be tested with the stimulus. An increasingly popular pattern[64,65] is based on a grid of 100 unequal rectangles that divide the monocular field in accordance with functional importance, or a similar grid of 120 rectangles that cover the binocular visual field. Both grids were devised by Esterman[66-68] and give greater weight with more test points in regions at which defects are most symptomatic or disabling—for example, in the central region below fixation (see Fig. 4-8). The monocular and binocular forms of the "Esterman test" are available as an option on all Humphrey perimeters. When the Esterman test is chosen, the strategy, intensity, and size automatically are set to a suprathreshold test with a size-III, 10-dB stimulus in a pattern of locations represented by the Esterman grid. Unless the patient has diplopia, the binocular test (in which neither eye is covered) usually is the preferred test. With both eyes open, the head is positioned so that the fixation spot is approximately midway between the two eyes. Exact centration is not critical.

Table 8-1. Minimal normal extent of visual field from point of fixation.

Direction	Degrees
Temporally	85
Down temporally	85
Down	65
Down nasally	50
Nasally	60
Up nasally	55
Up	45
Up temporally	55
Total	500

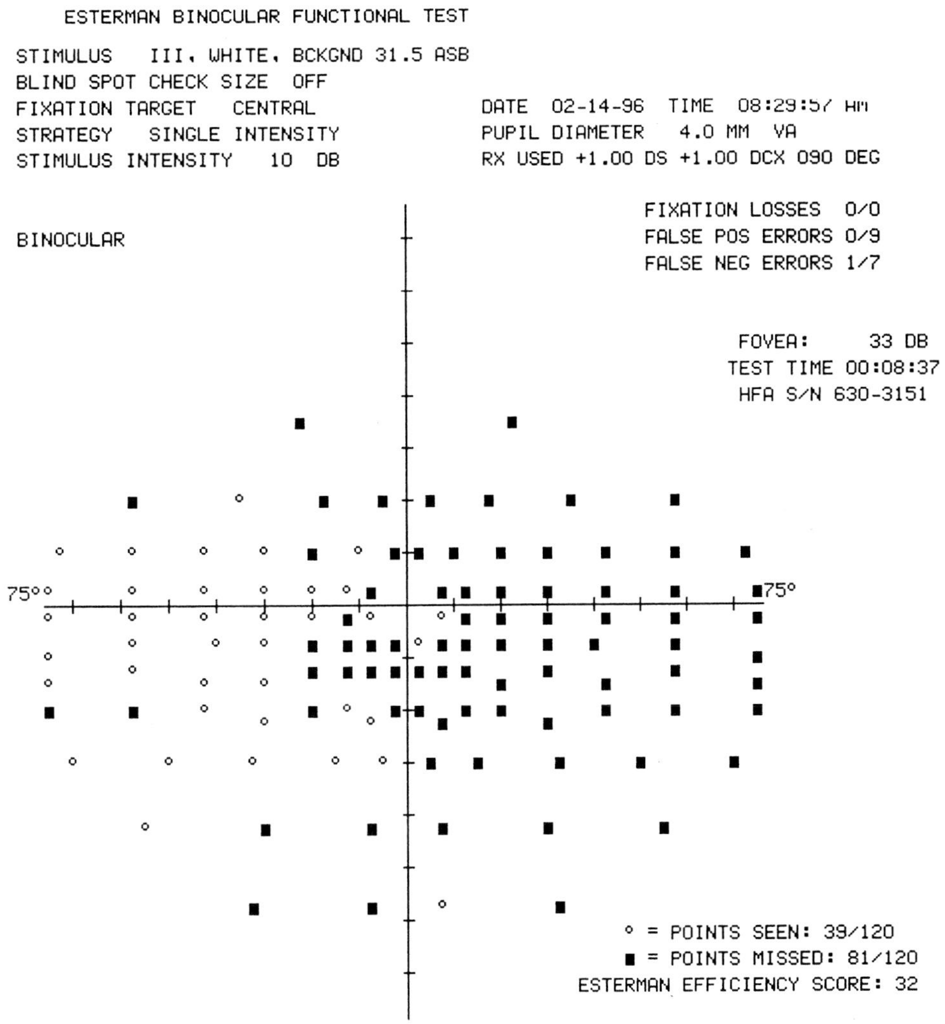

ESTERMAN BINOCULAR FUNCTIONAL TEST

STIMULUS   III, WHITE, BCKGND 31.5 ASB
BLIND SPOT CHECK SIZE OFF
FIXATION TARGET   CENTRAL
STRATEGY   SINGLE INTENSITY
STIMULUS INTENSITY   10 DB

DATE 02-14-96 TIME 08:29:57 HM
PUPIL DIAMETER   4.0 MM VA
RX USED +1.00 DS +1.00 DCX 090 DEG

BINOCULAR

FIXATION LOSSES 0/0
FALSE POS ERRORS 0/9
FALSE NEG ERRORS 1/7

FOVEA: 33 DB
TEST TIME 00:08:37
HFA S/N 630-3151

75°   75°

° = POINTS SEEN: 39/120
■ = POINTS MISSED: 81/120
ESTERMAN EFFICIENCY SCORE: 32

FIG. 8-17. Esterman Binocular Functional Test. The 10-dB stimulus was visible in 32% (39/120) of the test locations with one eye or the other. (Courtesy of Richard K. Parrish II, MD)

The full-field 135-point screening pattern available in the newer HFA-2 models tests from 50 degrees nasally to almost 90 degrees temporally and is a good option if the Esterman test has not been installed. If the 135-point pattern—or any other test except the Esterman—is used, the user must manually set the strategy to single intensity and choose a size-III, 10-dB white stimulus.

If neither of the two options mentioned is available, it is reasonable to combine a central screening pattern such as the 76-point test with the 68-point test in the periphery. This combination covers almost the entire field and leaves untested only the full inferior temporal extent of the field. The full-field 120-point screening test concentrates on the nasal side and probably gives inadequate attention to the temporal side for evaluation of field impairment. Similarly, the full-field 246-point test unnecessarily concentrates on the central field unless the patient's boundary of vision is in fact very constricted.

The patient may have had visual field examinations for diagnostic purposes—perhaps a threshold test of only the central 30 degrees. There are two circumstances in which a diagnostic test may be used for impairment evaluation so that another field test need not be performed to certify the patient's status:

1. If neither history nor findings during ocular examination suggest lesions that would affect the outer extent of the visual field, and if a 30-degree or 60-degree automated test is normal, the visual field test result may be submitted as evidence that there is no impairment; and

2. If the circumferential extent over which a standard stimulus is visible can be recognized in the diagnostic field (and it is in keeping with the history and examination), the 30-degree or 60-degree field may be used to report the extent of loss. Thus in Figures 4-20 and 4-21, for example, it is evident that the 10-dB stimulus is visible in only a very restricted region.

After the test is performed, there are two ways to quantify for each eye the percentage of loss or retained vision.

> There are two ways to quantify the percentage of loss or retained vision.

With one method, the extent of vision in each of eight directions is determined (see Table 8-1). (When the region of loss in a quadrant or hemifield is bound by a meridian, the middle extent of that meridian is used.) These numbers are added, and the sum is divided by five to give the percentage of retained visual field. This percentage is subtracted from 100 to give the percentage of loss of the visual field.

The alternate method is used to relate the percentage of loss more closely to the inability to function visually. If the Esterman test of the Humphrey perimeter is used, the percentage of points seen (or not seen) is recorded automatically. If other tests or test patterns are used with the appropriate standard stimulus, the external limit of vision is traced onto a monocular Esterman grid of 100 unequal rectangles. The number of rectangles included in the boundary are counted, and this number represents the percentage of retained visual field. Conversely, the number of rectangles excluded represents the percentage of uniocular field loss.

Similarly, if binocular function or impairment is evaluated, the extent over which the stimulus is seen binocularly is traced onto a binocular Esterman grid with 120 rectangles. The percentage of these 120 rectangles at which the stimulus is seen is determined. As with the monocular Esterman test, when the binocular Esterman test is used on the Humphrey perimeter, this analysis is performed automatically and reported on the test printout.

Once quantified, the degree of visual impairment may be used for various purposes. A certain percentage of loss or other criterion may be used, for example, to determine statutory blindness. According to the U.S. Social Security definition,* legal blindness is determined when the field is contracted to 10 degrees or less in the better eye or when the widest diameter in the better eye is 20 degrees. For some

---

*As defined in Social Security Regulations, Nos. 4 and 16, Listing of impairments, the adult listings, special senses and speech, Ophthalmology (20 CF 404.1525 and 416.925, Appendix One, Part A, para. 2.00A). Every federal, state, or local agency has its own definition, revised from time to time, and the definition may be different for each legal purpose (e.g., Internal Revenue Service or various welfare agencies).

purposes, only whether visual status is above or below some standard is determined. For other purposes, the degree of function or impairment is reported, and perhaps combined with the degree of affliction of other body systems to determine the amount of help the patient needs or how much compensation the patient should receive.

PROGRAMS THAT ARE OBSOLETE OR RARELY USED

The *central 30-1 pattern* consists of a grid of points, 6 degrees apart, with one point at the fovea and lines of points on both the horizontal and vertical meridians. The tested points lie exactly between the points that are tested in the 30-2 pattern. This pattern originally was provided as an alternative to the 30-2 pattern, or was used with the 30-2 pattern so that a total of 152 points were tested in an evenly distributed pattern over the central 30 degrees. When used in this way, the results of the two tests can be merged to make a single map of threshold values and a single greyscale. With experience, it became evident that the points along the vertical and horizontal meridians were of little use diagnostically in finding either a hemianopia or an asymmetry across the nasal horizontal meridian in glaucoma. Therefore the 30-2 pattern, which has points on either side of the horizontal and vertical meridians rather than along them, emerged as the standard. When there is a desire for more detailed information sufficient to justify doubling the testing effort, there is a difference of opinion about which is better: combining a 30-2 and 30-1 pattern to obtain a closer spatial distribution of points or repeating the 30-2 test twice to obtain more accurate threshold estimates as the average of two tests. The latter may be favored when looking for subtle differences on the two sides of the horizontal and vertical meridians. A whole region of variable sensitivity may be more characteristic of early glaucoma than the occurrence of isolated small scotomas (see Fig. 7-31). Therefore more accurate threshold determinations by duplicate 30-2 threshold tests may be equally or even more valuable for glaucoma if the clinician thinks it is necessary to expend additional effort on a second threshold test covering the same region. The rare instance in which the 30-1 pattern may be useful is to define more sharply the boundary of a defect or a very small scotoma. In this case, the closer spatial distribution achieved by combined 30-2 and 30-1 patterns may be useful.[69] It is possible to go through a professional career without ever using either the 30-1 test pattern or the pared-down 24-1 test pattern, unless the examiner has occasion to look for a possible very small but deep scotoma.

The *full threshold from prior data* strategy originally was introduced to save time in determining thresholds at individual points. (Note that prior data from an individual's previous field in this context are not the same as the statistical prior probabilities from population data used in SITA.) In this method, as the name implies, a prior test of the eye was chosen to determine for each point the stimulus intensity at which the thresholding sequence would be started. In earlier test strategies, the initial stimulus intensity for the test was based on the normal value for each location. To the extent that the patient's visual field departed significantly from normalcy, it was hoped and expected that this customized starting point

It is possible to go through a professional career without ever using the 30-1 test.

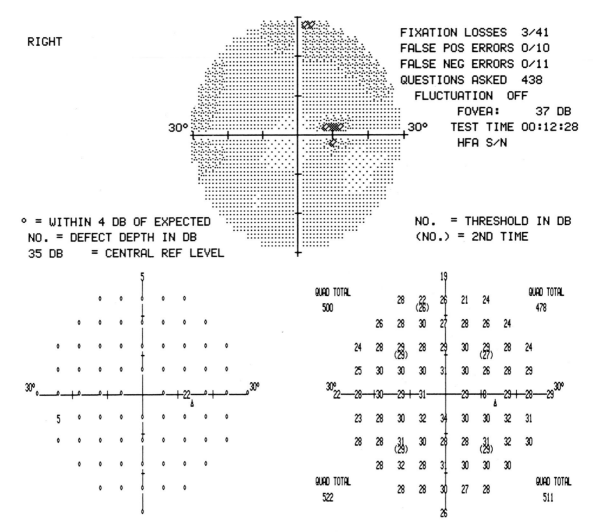

RIGHT

FIXATION LOSSES   3/41
FALSE POS ERRORS 0/10
FALSE NEG ERRORS 0/11
QUESTIONS ASKED   438
FLUCTUATION OFF
          FOVEA: 37 DB
TEST TIME 00:12:28
HFA S/N

30°   30°

° = WITHIN 4 DB OF EXPECTED
NO. = DEFECT DEPTH IN DB
35 DB   = CENTRAL REF LEVEL

NO. = THRESHOLD IN DB
(NO.) = 2ND TIME

FIG. 8-18. The Central 30-1 Threshold Test.

approach would save testing time. Unfortunately, the strategy turned out not to save time compared with the standard implemented on the HFA-1, in which the starting point for the thresholding sequence was determined from the previously tested adjacent points. Therefore, the full threshold from prior data strategy has fallen into disuse and was not even included in the software of the HFA-2.

A *"neurologic" pattern* of points was provided in the original instrument with the belief that it might be useful and efficient to determine threshold to the right and left of the vertical meridian and that this would be accurate for diagnosis without determining threshold at the many other locations in the visual field. This method has not found favor, perhaps because a tilt of the head or inability to maintain a steady head position may cause the boundary of the hemianopia to not coincide exactly with the vertical meridian of the visual field. It also appears that threshold comparison across the vertical meridian alone is not always compelling evidence of hemianopia, and judgment is more certain if adjacent points in the abnormal hemifield also are affected.

Colored stimuli and *stimuli other than size-III* have been useful for research purposes or in highly specialized clinics.[70] However, in practice, white size-III stimuli should be used to make use of present and future statistical packages as well as to facilitate comparison of test results that may be obtained in several offices. Exceptions include use of size-V stimuli or Swap under circumstances when it is agreed among clinicians that these provide advantage.

REFERENCES

1. Seamone C, LeBlanc R, Rubillowicz M et al: The value of indices in the central and peripheral visual fields for the detection of glaucoma, *Am J Ophthalmol* 106:180-185, 1988.
2. Werner EB: Peripheral nasal field defects in glaucoma, *Doc Ophthalmol Proc Ser* 19:223-228, 1979.
3. Dannheim F: Patterns of visual field alterations for liminal and supraliminal stimuli in chronic simple glaucoma, *Doc Ophthalmol Proc Ser* 26:97, 1981.
4. Caprioli J, Spaeth GL: Static threshold examination of the peripheral nasal visual field in glaucoma, *Arch Ophthalmol* 103:1150-1154, 1985.
5. Miller KN, Shields MB, Ollie AR: Automated kinetic perimetry with two peripheral isopters in glaucoma, *Arch Ophthalmol* 107:1316-1320, 1989.
6. Wirtschafter JD: Examination of the peripheral visual field, *Arch Ophthalmol* 105:761-762, 1987.
7. Johnson CA, Adams AJ, Casson EJ et al: Blue-on-yellow perimetry can predict the development of glaucomatous field loss, *Arch Ophthalmol* 111;645-650, 1993.
8. Sample PA, Taylor JDN, Martinez GA et al: Short-wavelength color visual fields in glaucoma suspects at risk, *Am J Ophthalmol* 115:225-233, 1993.
9. Johnson CA, Brandt JD, Khong AM, Adams AJ: Short-wavelength automated perimetry in low-, medium-, and high-risk ocular hypertensive eyes, *Arch Ophthalmol* 113:70-76, 1995.
10. Keltner JL, Johnson CA: Short-wavelength automated perimetry in neuro-ophthalmologic disorders, *Arch Ophthalmol* 113:475-481, 1995.
11. Johnson CA, Adams AJ, Casson EJ, Brandt JD: Progression of early glaucomatous visual field loss as detected by blue-on-yellow and standard white-on-white perimetry, *Arch Ophthalmol* 111:651-656, 1993.
12. Sample PA, Weinreb RN: Progressive color visual field loss in glaucoma, *Invest Ophthalmol Vis Sci* 33:2068-71, 1992.
13. Sample PA, Martinez GA, Weinreb RN: Short-wavelength automated perimetry without lens density testing, *Am J Ophthalmol* 18:632-641, 1994.
14. Wild JM, Moss ID, Whitaker D, O'Neill EC: The statistical interpretation of blue-on-yellow visual field loss, *Invest Ophthalmol Vis Sci* 36:7:1398-1410, 1995.
15. Wild JM, Cubbidge RP, Pacey IE, Robinson R: Statistical aspects of the normal visual field in short-wavelength automated perimetry, *Invest Ophthalmol Vis Sci* 39:54-63, 1998.
16. Mills RP, Barnebey HS, Migliazzo CV, Li Y: Does saving time using FASTPAC or suprathreshold testing reduce quality of visual fields? *Ophthalmology* 101:1596-603, 1994.
17. Boivin JF, McGregor M, Archer C: Cost effectiveness of screening for primary open angle glaucoma, *J Med Screen* 3:154-63, 1996.
18. Katz J, Tielsch JM, Quigley HA et al: Automated suprathreshold screening for glaucoma: The Baltimore Eye Survey, *Invest Ophthalmol Vis Sci* 34:3271-7, 1993.
18a. Stamper RL: Glaucoma screening, *J Glaucoma* 7:149-150, 1998.
19. Kosoko O, Sommer A, Auer C: Duration of automated suprathreshold vs. quantitative threshold field examination: Impact of age and ocular status, *Arch Ophthalmol* 104:398-401, 1986.
20. Kosoko O, Sommer A, Auer C: Screening with automated perimetry using a threshold-related three-level algorithm, *Ophthalmology* 93:882-6, 1986.
21. Johnson CA, Keltner JL: Computer analysis of visual field loss and optimization of automated perimetric test strategies, *Ophthalmology* 88:1058-65, 1981.
22. Keltner JL, Johnson CA: Screening for visual field abnormalities with automated perimetry, *Surv Ophthalmol* 28:175-183, 1983.
23. Young IM, Rait JL, Carson CA, Taylor HR: Fastpac visual field screening, *Ophthalmic Epidemiol* 2:117-21, 1995.

24. Weber J, Schultze T, Ulrich H: The visual field in advanced glaucoma, *Int Ophthalmol* 13:47-50, 1989.
25. Zalta AH: Use of a central 10-degree field and size-V stimulus to evaluate and monitor small central islands of vision in end stage glaucoma, *Br J Ophthalmol* 75:151-4, 1991.
26. Atchison DA, Lovie-Kitchin JE, Swann PG: Investigation of central visual fields in patients with age-related macular changes, *Optom Vis Sci* 67:179-83, 1990.
27. Wilensky JT, Mermelstein JR, Siegel HG: The use of different-sized stimuli in automated perimetry, *Am J Ophthalmol* 101:710-713, 1986.
28. Choplin NT, Sherwood MB, Spaeth GL: The effect of stimulus size on the measured threshold values in automated perimetry, *Ophthalmology* 97:371-374, 1990.
29. Wirtschafter JD, Hard-Boberg A-L, Coffman SM: Evaluating the usefulness in neuro-ophthalmology of visual field examinations peripheral to 30 degrees, *Trans Am Ophthalmol Soc* 82:329-357, 1984.
30. Keltner JL, Johnson CA: Automated and manual perimetry—a six-year overview: Special emphasis on neuro-ophthalmic problems, *Ophthalmology* 91:68-85, 1984.
31. Wall M, Conway MD, House PH, Allely R: Evaluation of sensitivity and specificity of spatial resolution and Humphrey automated perimetry in pseudotumor cerebri patients and normal subjects, *Invest Ophthalmol Vis Sci* 32:3306-12, 1991.
32. Siatkowski RM, Lam BL, Anderson DR et al: Automated suprathreshold static perimetry screening for detecting neuro-ophthalmologic disease, *Ophthalmology* 103:907-17, 1996.
33. Marmor MF, Aguirre G, Arden G et al: Retinitis pigmentosa, *Ophthalmology* 90:126-131, 1983.
34. Easterbrook M, Trope G: Value of Humphrey perimetry in the detection of early chloroquine retinopathy. In Lerman S, Tripathy RC, editors: *Ocular toxicology: Proceedings of First Congress of the International Society of Ocular Toxicology,* p 255, New York, 1988, Marcel Dekker. (Lens Eye Toxic Res 1989;6:255-68. ISSN:1042-6922.)
35. Easterbrook M: The use of Amsler grids in early chloroquine retinopathy, *Ophthalmology* 91:1368-1372, 1984.
36. Easterbrook M: Ocular effects and safety of antimalarial agents, *Am J Med* 85:23-29, 1988.
37. Johnson MW, Vine AK: Hydroxychloroquine therapy in massive total doses without retinal toxicity, *Am J Ophthalmol* 104:139-144, 1987.
38. Rynes RI: Ophthalmologic safety of long-term hydroxychloroquine sulfate treatment, *Am J Med* 75:35-39, 1983.
39. Mann CG, Orr AC, Rubillowicz M, LeBlanc RP: Automated static perimetry in chloroquine and hydroxychloroquine therapy. In Heijl A, editor: *Perimetry update 1988/89,* p 417, Berkeley, CA, 1989, Kugler & Ghedini.
40. Hart WM Jr, Burde RM, Johnston GP, Drews RC: Static perimetry in chloroquine retinopathy: Perifoveal patterns of visual field depression, *Arch Ophthalmol* 102:377-380, 1984.
41. Morsman CD, Livesey SJ, Richards IM et al: Screening for hydroxychloroquine retinal toxicity: Is it necessary? *Eye* 4:572-6, 1990.
42. Spalton DJ, Verdon-Roe GM, Hughes GR: Hydroxychloroquine, dosage parameters and retinopathy, *Lupus* 2:355-8, 1993.
43. Spalton DJ: Retinopathy and antimalarial drugs: The British experience, *Lupus* 5(Suppl 1):S70-2, 1996.
44. Grierson DJ: Hydroxychloroquine and visual screening in a rheumatology outpatient clinic, *Ann Rheum Dis* 56:188-90, 1997.
45. Levy GD, Munz SJ, Paschal J et al: Incidence of hydroxychloroquine retinopathy in 1,207 patients in a large multicenter outpatient practice, *Arthritis Rheum* 40:1482-6, 1997.
46. Easterbrook M: The ocular safety of hydroxychloroquine, *Semin Arthritis Rheum* 23(2 Suppl 1): 62-7, 1993.
47. Meyer DR, Stern JH, Jarvis JM, Lininger LL: Evaluating the visual field effects of blepharoptosis using automated static perimetry, *Ophthalmology* 100:651-8; discussion 658-9, 1993.
48. Klingele J, Kaiser HJ, Hatt M: Automated perimetry in ptosis and blepharochalasis, *Klin Monatsbl Augenheilkd* 206:401-4, 1995.
49. Cahill KV, Burns JA, Weber PA: The effect of blepharoptosis on the field of vision, *Ophthalmol Plast Reconstr Surg* 3:121-5, 1987.
50. Hacker HD, Hollsten DA: Investigation of automated perimetry in the evaluation of patients for upper lid blepharoplasty, *Ophthalmol Plast Reconstr Surg* 8:250-5, 1992.

51. Olson JJ, Putterman A: Loss of vertical palpebral fissure height on downgaze in acquired blepharoptosis, *Arch Ophthalmol* 114:774, 1996 [Comment].

52. Dryden RM, Kahanic DA: Worsening of blepharoptosis in downgaze, *Ophthalmol Plast Reconstr Surg* 8:126-9, 1992.

53. Patipa M: Visual field loss in primary gaze and reading gaze due to acquired blepharoptosis and visual field improvement following ptosis surgery, *Arch Ophthalmol* 110:63-7, 1992.

54. Johnson CA, Keltner JL: Incidence of visual field loss in 20,000 eyes and its relationship to driving performance, *Arch Ophthalmol* 101:371-375, 1983.

55. McKnight AJ, Shinar D, Hilburn B: The visual and driving performance of monocular and binocular heavy-duty truck drivers, *Accid Anal Prev* 23:225-37, 1991.

56. Henricsson M, Heijl A: The effect of panretinal laser photocoagulation on visual acuity, visual fields and on subjective visual impairment in preproliferative and early proliferative diabetic retinopathy, *Acta Ophthalmol* [Copenh] 72:570-5, 1994.

57. Hulbert MF, Vernon SA: Passing the DVLC field regulations following bilateral panretinal photocoagulation in diabetics, *Eye* 6:456-60, 1992.

58. Wood JM, Troutbeck R: Effect of visual impairment on driving, *Hum Factors* 36:476-87, 1994.

59. Ball K, Owsley C, Sloane ME et al: Visual attention problems as a predictor of vehicle crashes in older drivers, *Invest Ophthalmol Vis Sci* 34:3110-23, 1993.

60. Lovsund P, Hedin A, Tornros J: Effects on driving performance of visual field defects: A driving simulator study, *Accid Anal Prev* 23:331-42, 1991.

61. Wood JM, Troutbeck R: Elderly drivers and simulated visual impairment, *Optom Vis Sci* 72:115-24, 1995.

62. Wood JM, Troutbeck R: Effect of restriction of the binocular visual field on driving performance, *Ophthalmic Physiol Opt* 12:291-8, 1992.

63. Keltner JL, Johnson CA: Visual function, driving safety, and the elderly, *Ophthalmology* 94:1180-8, 1987.

64. Mills RP, Drance SM: Esterman disability rating in severe glaucoma, *Ophthalmology* 93:371-8, 1986.

65. Parrish RK II: Visual impairment, visual functioning, and quality of life assessments in patients with glaucoma, *Trans Am Ophthalmol Soc* 94:919-1028, 1996.

66. Esterman B: Grid for scoring visual fields: II. Perimeter, *Arch Ophthalmol* 79:400-406, 1968.

67. Esterman B: Grids for functional scoring of visual fields, *Doc Ophthalmol Proc Ser* 26:373-380, 1981.

68. Esterman B: Functional scoring of the binocular visual field, *Ophthalmology* 89:1226-1234, 1982.

69. Weber J, Dobek K: What is the most suitable grid for computer perimetry in glaucoma patients? *Ophthalmologica* 192:88-96, 1986.

70. Milam AH, Jacobson SG: Photoreceptor rosettes with blue cone opsin immunoreactivity in retinitis pigmentosa, *Ophthalmology* 97:1620-1631, 1990.

CHAPTER 9

Follow-up examinations

Judging whether visual function is deteriorating remains the most difficult and uncertain task in perimetry—more difficult and uncertain than the diagnostic decisions discussed in previous chapters. To illustrate the principles of monitoring the course of a disease, we use glaucoma, the most common chronically progressive condition that is monitored with serial visual field examinations.

ESTABLISHING A BASELINE

In following the visual field status of a patient in the context of glaucoma, the physician must determine whether there is continuing glaucomatous harm to the eye. Has a change occurred since observation of the initial condition? If so, how rapidly might the visual function be worsening? The baseline visual field examination(s) establishes the condition at the beginning of the follow-up period.

The first visual field examination, performed at the time of diagnosis, may not be the optimum baseline record. Lowering the intraocular pressure (IOP) may produce some immediate neurophysiologic or psychophysical changes that may alter the baseline condition. In addition, treatment may affect vascular physiology, serum electrolytes, and pupil size. Moreover, some progression in optic nerve damage may have occurred before adequate lowering of pressure was achieved. Finally, the learning effect shown by some patients may be particularly pronounced between the first and second visual field examinations.

Obtain a baseline of at least two field tests.

Therefore once management has become stable, it is wise to obtain a second visual field examination. If it matches the original examination, these two examinations together may constitute a baseline. If the second field does not match the first very well, it may be best to obtain a third visual field examination. The second and third examinations (both obtained under conditions of treatment with a stabilized IOP) then serve as a baseline. The third examination is necessary to confirm that it is the second field and not the first that is the most representative. In any event, because of the variability between examinations, it is wise not to use a single examination as the baseline for future follow-up.

Recall from Chapter 8 that sometimes there are additional reasons not to use the initial diagnostic examination as a baseline for follow-up. In particular, there may be reason to:

1. Concentrate on the central 5 or 10 degrees. With a severely contracted field, perhaps only 12 locations will have a measurable sensitivity with the central 30-2 or 24-2 threshold tests. If these locations are primarily in the central 10 degrees or at the four locations in the central 5 degrees, the 10-2 threshold test or the Macula Test (described and illustrated in the previous chapter) is better for follow-up examinations for two reasons. First, it would be a waste of time to reexamine the known blind region from 5 or 10 degrees to 30 degrees. Second, a more careful follow-up can be obtained with a closer grid of points 2 degrees apart within the precious remaining island of central vision. A 10-2 or Macula Test should be obtained on two occasions shortly after the pressure has been stabilized to act as the baseline.

2. Use a larger pattern of points. If the diagnosis was established with a 24-2 pattern and many locations are fairly abnormal, the 22 additional locations in the 30-2 pattern—especially the locations temporal to the physiologic blind spot—may be helpful in making decisions about progression. To follow the peripheral field in addition to the central 30 degrees, a rarely used option is the peripheral 68-point screen (e.g., single intensity strategy, 10 dB) to plot of the outside boundary of the remaining intact field.

3. Use a size-V stimulus. If nearly all the threshold values in a 30-2, 10-2, or macula test are less than 10 or 15 dB, it would be impossible to determine during follow-up that there had been a deterioration of sensitivity because a 0-dB sensitivity can be obtained easily just from testing variability at a point that previously had a threshold of 10 dB, or even 15 dB. In such cases, a size-V stimulus may be used instead of a size-III stimulus, with expected threshold sensitivity values rising at least 7 to 8 dB at normal locations—and even more at abnormal ones. Because test-retest variability is greater at moderately abnormal points, duplicate tests with a size-V stimulus may be even more important than with the standard parameters.

In circumstances like those described, the fundamental principle is that if the *diagnostic* test fails to provide an adequate number of points of remaining vision to permit deterioration of the condition to be recognized, it is important to try to find an optional test that will provide a baseline measure that is adequate for future comparison. The optimal time to do so is at the beginning, because it is often important to have on record a matching duplicate pair as a baseline. It may be tempting to customize the test for a particular patient, but it may be unwise to do so. Because a patient may receive care in more than one office during the course of his disease, it is wise to select test patterns and strategies that are available to other physicians. Statistical tests developed in the future also will likely apply to standard tests that are used commonly.

It is advisable to note in the patient's record which pair of visual fields will be considered the baseline for future follow-up examinations. If there is some deterioration of the visual field and more vigorous lowering of the IOP is instituted, the

Choose carefully the type of field for baseline and follow-up.

question for the future becomes whether there is any *further* deterioration. It is necessary to obtain a new baseline pair of visual field examinations to be designated as the new baseline.

The problem with obtaining duplicate consistent visual field examinations (especially if three examinations are needed to obtain a consistent pair) is that visual field examinations are time consuming and unpleasant. However, the clinician must accept the reality of this need. It is almost impossible to conclude with certainty that a field has changed by comparing the follow-up field examination with a single baseline field examination performed a year earlier. Even if a change is suspected and a second follow-up field examination is obtained immediately, which confirms a difference from the single baseline field, it still may be impossible to be confident that the first field was representative of the baseline status. The examiner must then wait another interval of time, perhaps another year, to see whether there is another increment of change at 2 years compared with the pair of visual fields 1 year after diagnosis. We thus emphasize that it is a good investment to establish a baseline with confidence, even if a trade must be made in the form of less frequent follow-up examinations (with selective repetition of any that seem to have changed from the baseline).

FOLLOW-UP VISUAL FIELD EXAMINATIONS

The judgment of disease progression is easiest if the follow-up programs and parameters (as well as the pupil size and use of optimum correction) are the same as those used for the baseline. In essence, the selection of the field type for the baseline determines the type of field examination that allows the easiest comparison during follow-up (which is why the initial selection should be made with care).

Perhaps the most frequent exception is that 24-2 and 30-2 tests can be mixed in a series of follow-up examinations, although sometimes the 22 additional edge locations of the 30-2 pattern then are not used in statistical analyses. A second exception occurs when advances in perimetric methodology occur, which is perhaps inevitable during the decades of a chronic disease. When an improved method is implemented, there may be statistical methods to compare newer test algorithms with older ones, or sometimes it is necessary to establish new baselines with the improved methods.

With regard to the Humphrey perimeters, the newer HFA-2 model has been shown to be equivalent to the HFA-1 in the central visual field.[1] Differences in test algorithms are more problematic. Even when the mean normal values of two test strategies are similar, the scaling of abnormality expressed in decibels may be different; in particular, the decibels of loss (deviation) in defective areas frequently are greater with longer tests than with shorter ones. This difference must be taken into account by the clinician judging progression, perhaps with the help of statistical calculations, such as those of deviation or change probabilities.

Comparisons between threshold and suprathreshold tests, and even more so between instruments by different manufacturers, demand even more caution. Only major changes can be judged with certainty.

A single-field examination usually is adequate for a follow-up examination, provided it is in keeping with the baseline findings (i.e., there is no evident change). However, a change nearly always must be confirmed on a second occasion before it can be concluded that there has been progression of glaucomatous damage. There are exceptions when the clinical circumstance confirms that the change likely is real; for example, when the IOP has been difficult to control, the glaucoma has not received attention for some time, or the disc shows more cupping. Even in such circumstances, a second field examination may be needed to construct a new baseline pair when the condition restabilizes.

It is a mistake to use a routine time interval for follow-up visual field tests. The traditional once-a-year timing is not frequent enough for those who may be undergoing progression, and it is too frequent for patients whose pressure is quite low compared with baseline and who have shown no hint of further change in the optic disc or visual field over 2 or 3 years. Shortly after diagnosis, especially if there is uncertainty about whether lowering of the IOP is adequate, a series of several visual field examinations in the first year or two may be needed either to reveal continued deterioration or to provide reassurance that deterioration is absent (or at least that it is too slow to detect in the short term). Conversely, a patient with undetectable visual field change for several years may need only occasional visual field examinations if the IOP and optic discs are stable.

The principles of managing glaucoma are beyond the scope of this book, except to state that the frequency with which the visual field condition needs monitoring varies with the individual patient; it depends on all clinical findings and whether the series of examinations already on record shows any trend that needs to be confirmed or denied.

AN OVERVIEW

The usual first step in evaluating a series of visual fields is to gaze at the series of fields arranged in chronological order, perhaps removing them from the patient's chart and spreading them out on a banquet-sized table. As a substitute, the Overview printout places the greyscale, threshold value table, and probability plots of Total and Pattern Deviation of each examination in a row, with the rows arranged in chronological order, making it easier to scan a series of examinations. Included, but not conspicuous, are the foveal threshold, reliability parameters, and global indices. The clinician evaluates the general trend, including the degree of any change, the nature of the change, and the consistency of any trend. The assessment is highly intuitive, based on clinical judgment built from experience, as has always been true of perimetry. The series of greyscales gives a first impression, but often an inspection of the series of Total and Pattern Deviation Probability Plots is more rewarding.

There are several visual field manifestations of continuing optic nerve damage in glaucoma.[2,3] Previously normal fields may become abnormal. If there are locations in the baseline field with moderate reductions of sensitivity (relative defects), the most frequent manner of progression is more loss of sensitivity at these locations. Defective regions may enlarge as adjacent points also become abnormal. Previously normal regions may become defective with new scotomas or depressed regions. When loss covers most of the field, the continued loss may occur everywhere, but it may be difficult to distinguish from the effects of progressive cataract. The progressive loss most often occurs continuously, shown in a series of fields with change over time that exceeds the variability of testing. Less frequently the progression may occur in recognizable episodes.

The Overview printout may provide strong evidence of progression made credible by the clinical context—for example, simultaneous progressive excavation of the optic nerve in a case of elevated pressure allowed to go without treatment (Fig. 9-1). Such cases of progression are obvious if the rate of progression is appreciable over the span of time covered by the examinations.

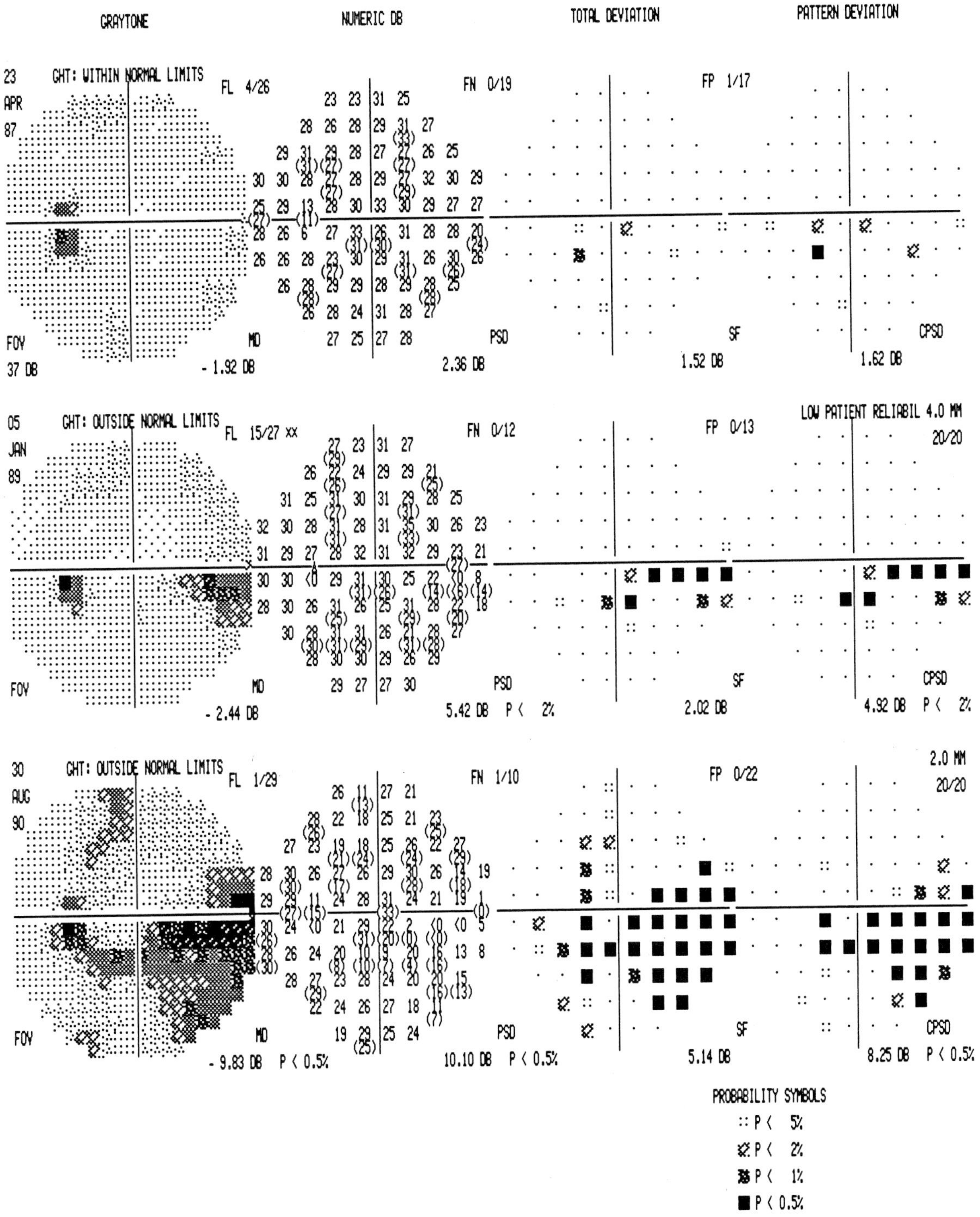

GRAYTONE	NUMERIC DB	TOTAL DEVIATION	PATTERN DEVIATION

23 APR 87   GHT: WITHIN NORMAL LIMITS   FL 4/26   FN 0/19   FP 1/17

```
        23 23 | 31 25
     28 26 28 | 29 31 27
   29 31 28 28 | 27 29 26 25
30 30 28 28 28 | 27 30 32 30 29
   28 26 6  27 | 33 31 28 28 20
   26 26 28 29 | 30 29 28 30 26
   26 26 29 29 | 28 29 28 25
        28 28 24 | 31 28 28
```

FOV 37 DB   MD -1.92 DB   PSD 2.36 DB   SF 1.52 DB   CPSD 1.62 DB

05 JAN 89   GHT: OUTSIDE NORMAL LIMITS   FL 15/27 xx   FN 0/12   FP 0/13   LOW PATIENT RELIABIL 4.0 MM   20/20

```
        27 23 | 31 27
     26 25 24 | 29 29 21
   31 25 31 30 | 31 29 28 25
32 30 28 28 | 28 31 33 30 26 23
31 29 27 28 | 32 31 32 29 23 21
30 30 30 29 | 31 30 25 22 8
28 30 26 25 | 25 31 31 25 14 18
   30 31 25 | 31 31 28 27
```

FOV   MD -2.44 DB   PSD 5.42 DB P < 2%   SF 2.02 DB   CPSD 4.92 DB P < 2%

30 AUG 90   GHT: OUTSIDE NORMAL LIMITS   FL 1/29   FN 1/10   FP 0/22   2.0 MM   20/20

```
        26 11 | 27 21
     28 22 18 | 25 21 23
   27 23 19 18 | 29 24 27
28 29 21 25 | 24 28 26 14 19
29 24 15 | 30 31 24 21 19 1
30 24 0 21 | 29 24 2 0 0 5
26 24 20 27 | 24 16 15 13 8
28 28 23 24 | 24 20 15
   29 24 26 | 27 18 16 13
        19 29 | 25 24
```

FOV   MD -9.83 DB P < 0.5%   PSD 10.10 DB P < 0.5%   SF 5.14 DB   CPSD 8.25 DB P < 0.5%

PROBABILITY SYMBOLS
:: P < 5%
▨ P < 2%
▩ P < 1%
■ P < 0.5%

FIG. 9-1. Overview. In this example, an inferior arcuate defect developed over time along with elevated intraocular pressure and progressive cupping.

A more difficult task is to discern slower progression, and especially to be certain whether a small incremental change has occurred over a short period of time (Fig. 9-2). Frequent examinations reveal the variability of testing caused by short-term and long-term fluctuations but may not help determine whether a slow genuine change also is occurring. Fortunately, the slower the rate of change, the less urgent it may be to decide whether there is change at all. Sometimes the passage of time may be more helpful than a greater number of visual field tests. With short-term follow-up, other clinical findings may have more impact on management decisions than the visual field findings.

Experience with use of an Overview provides a healthy respect for the amount of variability inherent in visual field testing. The fact that the information is displayed numerically gives the novice an exaggerated confidence in the accuracy of the threshold estimates, and he mistakenly may make a firm judgment based on an inadequate number of examinations in sequence. There must be an adequate number so that the individual's variability is evident and the physician can judge whether there is a trend that is larger than can be explained by that patient's variability. A minimum of four field examinations (two baseline and two follow-up) usually is required before evidence of progression is compelling from visual field information alone. Typically six or more examinations are required to be certain of progressive deterioration.

> Overview printouts must be analyzed for change by use of experienced judgment without statistical assistance.

FIG. 9-2. Overview. Another patient, who was watched closely for progression with seven visual field examinations during 14 months. It is difficult to be sure whether there is slow progression.

GRAYTONE   NUMERIC DB   TOTAL DEVIATION   PATTERN DEVIATION

13 JUL 89 GHT: OUTSIDE NORMAL LIMITS FL 2/25 FN 0/18 FP 0/10 20/15
FOV 36 DB MD -0.52 DB PSD 5.08 DB P< 2% SF 1.03 DB CPSD 4.94 DB P< 2%

12 OCT 89 GHT: OUTSIDE NORMAL LIMITS FL 3/25 FN 1/13 FP 0/14 4.0 MM 20/15
FOV 38 DB MD -0.27 DB PSD 4.70 DB P< 5% SF 2.88 DB P< 5% CPSD 3.37 DB P< 5%

30 NOV 89 GHT: OUTSIDE NORMAL LIMITS FL 2/26 FN 0/14 FP 0/12 4.0 MM 20/15
FOV 38 DB MD -0.54 DB PSD 7.64 DB P< 0.5% SF 1.90 DB CPSD 7.33 DB P< 0.5%

11 JAN 90 GHT: OUTSIDE NORMAL LIMITS FL 1/24 FN 0/12 FP 0/15 4.5 MM 20/15
FOV 36 DB MD -0.52 DB PSD 6.96 DB P< 1% SF 1.40 DB CPSD 6.78 DB P< 1%

24 MAY 90 GHT: OUTSIDE NORMAL LIMITS FL 1/25 FN 0/13 FP 0/15 4.5 MM 20/15
FOV 35 DB MD -1.38 DB PSD 7.66 DB P< 0.5% SF 1.44 DB CPSD 7.48 DB P< 0.5%

20 SEP 90 GHT: OUTSIDE NORMAL LIMITS FL 0/27 FN 0/15 FP 0/22 4.0 MM 20/15
FOV 37 DB MD -2.43 DB PSD 3.11 DB P< 0.5% SF 1.19 DB CPSD 3.01 DB P< 0.5%

21 OCT 90 GHT: OUTSIDE NORMAL LIMITS FL 0/25 FN 0/13 FP 0/7 4.0 MM 20/15
FOV 39 DB MD -1.08 DB PSD 3.29 DB P< 0.5% SF 1.09 DB CPSD 3.21 DB P< 0.5%

CHANGE ANALYSIS PRINTOUT

The Change Analysis printout provides a visual display of additional descriptive statistics about the visual field as a whole and includes a larger number of examinations on a single page. It quantifies certain parameters and, like the Overview printout, it can give an overall impression of a series of visual field examinations at a glance. Additional information can be assimilated quickly by a well-informed observer, but the nature of these statistical details must first be studied and understood in some detail to be helpful.

The Change Analysis display includes a boxplot panel across the top and several graphs of the global indices of the series of examinations below the panel. These graphical representations can include up to 16 visual field tests. Those that are not representative (e.g., a test that is unreliable, a test performed with the improper lens correction, or one performed with a dilated pupil after indirect ophthalmoscopy and gonioscopy) can be omitted. Information from all the selected representative visual field tests is displayed together. The display spaces the visual fields evenly in sequence without regard to the time interval between them; this must be taken into account when inferring the course of the disease.

Boxplot

In a normal visual field, it would not be expected that the threshold sensitivity estimations would be exactly the average normal values at all locations. At a few locations the estimate may be slightly better than the average normal value, and other points may be slightly worse. Experience shows that the majority are close to the mid-normal value, and the deviation (departure from normal) typically is near 0 dB for a median (50th percentile) point in a normal field. The spread is slightly smaller for the 24-2 patterns; however, for the 30-2 pattern of the normal visual field, 70% of the points range from approximately 3 dB above to 3 dB below the average normal value. All deviations, including the additional 30% of outliers, are expected to fall within the 10-dB range from 4 dB to −6 dB.

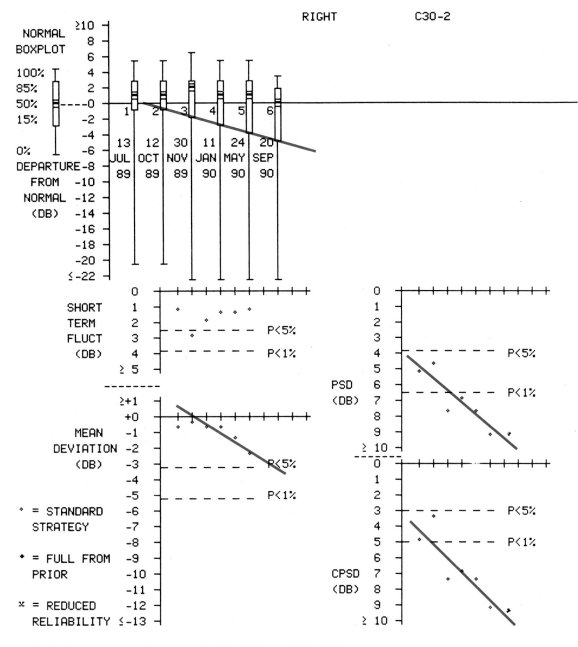

MD SLOPE = - 2.25 ± 0.82 DB/YEAR (95% CONF.)

MODIFIED MD SLOPE SIGNIFICANT (P < 1%)

FIG. 9-3. Change Analysis Printout. Progression is shown in a mild case of glaucoma, the first 6 fields shown in Figure 9-2. The boxplot shows progressive downward lengthening of the box (but the median value remains approximately the same) as the sensitivity of the 15th percentile point deteriorates. The MD index *(lower left)* as well as the CPSD index *(lower right)* show progressive deterioration. The MD in the final field is within the normal range because only a few points in the field are involved. However, the decline is statistically significant ($p < 1\%$), and the rate of 2.15 dB per year is substantial.

This "normal" expectation is represented on the change analysis display and printout by a normal reference boxplot to the left of the boxplot panel. The boxplot panel itself shows the series of visual field examinations selected.

For each examination, the deviations (differences from average normal values) are determined for each point; these are the same values that are displayed in the Total Deviation Plot of the Single Field Analysis. These deviations are ranked according to the amount of deviation. From this ranking, the boxplot shows the median deviation and the distributions of deviations. A vertical rectangle (box) represents the range of deviations for 70% of the locations. The median deviation value (not to be confused with the Mean Deviation global index) is indicated by a flanked heavy horizontal bar in the box. The extremes of deviation are shown with the extended vertical lines above and below the box, incorporating the additional 15% in each direction. The ends of the vertical lines thus indicate the total range of deviations from normal values for all points included in the analysis.*

With a 3-dB general depression of the field at all points, the boxplot retains the normal height and configuration but shifts downward by 3 dB: the median value is −3 dB, the 70% range is indicated as a box extending from 0 to −6 dB, and the total range is shown by lines reaching from +1 to −9 dB (the total width of the range is 10 dB). A composite illustration of various boxplots gives two examples of such a general depression (Fig. 9-4, A and B).

If only 10% of the points became severely depressed, the median (50th percentile) point would remain near 0 dB and the 70% range indicated by the box would remain at a 3-dB departure above and below normal. However, the lower arm would extend downward a considerable distance, indicating that at least one location (and up to 15% of locations) had more deviation than normally would be expected (Fig. 9-4, C). If 25% of the points were depressed, not only the extreme end of the range but also the lower boundary of the box would extend downward (Fig. 9-4, D); the span from the median point to the bottom of the vertical rectangle also would be longer than normal.

In this way the positions of the boxplot landmarks (the median point, the two ends of the rectangular box, and the ends of the two extensions) indicate the deviations in that examination at percentile rankings of 0, 15, 50, 85, and 100. A long box indicates that the deviation is distinctly more severe in some locations than in others, so that the 15 and 85 percentile deviations are quite dissimilar; this elongated box should be accompanied by high values of the PSD and CPSD indices. The position of the flanked dark bar in the box indicates the degree of involvement of the median point; if it is near 0 dB, it means that fewer than half of the locations in the visual field have been affected by the disease.

---

*Note that this and other multifield Statpac analyses can include a mixture of 30-2 and 24-2 fields. If they are mixed into a series for analysis, the change analysis and glaucoma change probability calculations will ignore the appropriate edge points of any 30-degree fields included, so that all calculations and displays are based only on the points that are found in the 24-degree test. The Overview printout uses for each examination the single field analyses appropriate for that individual test.

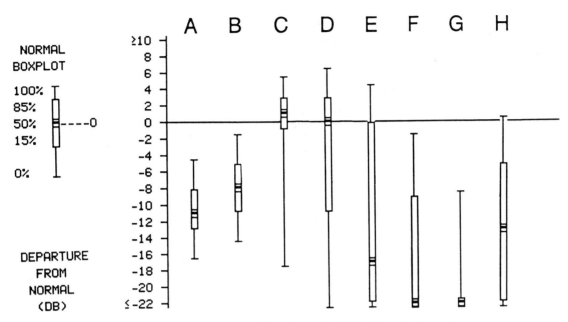

FIG. 9-4. Boxplot Examples. The normal boxplot to the left of the axis shows that an average normal field is expected to have departures (in the Total Deviation plot) ranging from 4 to 6 dB. The central box shows the 85th percentile point (11th best point of 74 locations in the 30-2 pattern) at 3 dB and the 15th percentile point (63rd ranking point of 74 locations) at −3 dB. **A,** The first example of abnormality has a short central box moved downward in position, which represents an 11-dB generalized depression caused by cataract. This field is shown in Figure 7-18. **B,** The second example is a similar 7-dB generalized depression from glaucoma (field shown in Fig. 7-20). **C,** The third example shows the boxplot of the field in Figure 7-29—a very localized abnormality. The worst point is depressed 18 dB, but fewer than 10 locations are abnormal (the 15th percentile point is normal). **D,** The fourth example shows a larger localized loss, with the worst point down more than 22 dB and the 15th percentile point down 11 dB. The median (50th percentile) point is normal at 0-dB deviation; at least 50% and as many as 84% of the locations are still normal (field shown in Fig. 7-42). **E,** The median point is depressed 17 dB. More than half the points are severely affected but the positions of the 85th and 100th percentile points show that some locations are normal (field shown in Fig. 4-18). **F,** The sixth example shows that even the 85th percentile point (11th rank of 74 locations) is depressed 9 dB, and most locations are severely affected, with the median point down more than 22 dB or more (field shown in Fig. 7-9). **G,** The seventh example shows that even the best point is down 9 dB, and 85% of the points are down 22 dB or more. The set from C through G represents localized dense field loss ranging from involvement of a few locations to the vast majority of locations. Some normal points remain except in the very late stages. **H,** The eighth example is from Figure 7-14, in which none of the points is completely normal but the degree of abnormality varies widely, so the boxplot is quite tall. Thus widespread loss, with some points much more affected than others (as is typical of glaucoma), results in the lengthened boxplot of *H,* in contrast to an equal depression of all points (characteristic of cataract), in which the boxplot remains of normal height but depressed position (*A and B*).

When a series of these boxes is plotted for a succession of fields, the change in the character of the field over time can be noted. For example:

1. A short box that remains the same height but moves progressively downward over time represents progressive generalized depression without development of local defects. This change should be reflected in an unchanged Pattern Deviation Probability Plot despite a declining MD index. It may be seen when a patient with "ocular hypertension" develops a cataract.

2. Lengthening of the box, especially the inferior arm, over time indicates the development and deepening of localized defects (Fig 9-3). The PSD index may become increasingly abnormal at the same time.

3. A long box at the initial examination that stays the same length and moves downward most often is caused by a progressive general depression superimposed on a localized defect, typically because of a change in media opacity. Less often, it may occur when glaucomatous progression affects the only remaining normal regions of the field with simultaneous deepening of pre-existing defects.

Thoughtful inspection of a series of boxplots may thus reveal a general worsening of the visual field, and also may suggest the character of the change, which should be correlated with the evolving character of the visual field diagram in the Overview printout and with changes in the global indices over time.

When a large number of points are severely depressed, the boxplot is collapsed onto the bottom rung of the graph and progression is not interpretable. Almost all methods for evaluating a change in the field have frustrating limitations when the field already is poor.

Bebie[4,5] has developed a somewhat more detailed but equivalent method to display the same information as the boxplot. Display of the "Bebie curve" is incorporated into some custom and third-party analytical software, and a comparison may help clarify the information contained in the boxplot. For both, differences (deviations) from normal are computed for each point and ranked. For the Bebie curve, the deviations are plotted in order according to rank; the resulting graph is equivalent to a cumulative frequency curve turned on its side. In a typical printout, it is compared with the normal shape of the curve and the range of normal is indicated by a shaded zone (Fig. 9-5).

If the Bebie curve has a normal shape but is displaced downward, it indicates that all the points are depressed more or less equally, and this corresponds to a downward movement (but no lengthening) of the boxplot. However, if some of the points are decidedly abnormal (Fig. 9-6), the right end of the curve dips downward, which is equivalent to a lengthening of the inferior arm in the boxplot. Changes in the Bebie curve over time correspond to equivalent changes in the boxplot: downward displacement without change in shape has the same meaning in both, and a broadening of the right-hand dip in the Bebie curve corresponds to a lengthening of the bottom segment of the boxplot.

These graphical displays assemble information across examinations to help recognize what might be missed from data that are scattered among printouts of multiple examinations. In the case of mild generalized depression, for example,

> Like an Overview plot, a series of boxplots may reveal progressive change.

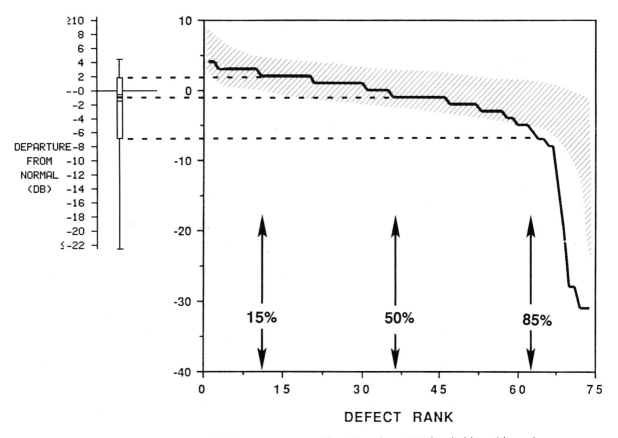

FIG. 9-5. Bebie Curve. A Bebie curve constructed for a Humphrey 30-2 threshold test (shown in Figure 9-6), compared with a boxplot of the same data. The 5% to 95% range of normal is shaded. The worst point deviates 33 dB from normal and the 15th percentile point deviates 7 dB from normal. The deviation for most of the points is within normal limits. (Courtesy of Balwantray C. Chauhan, PhD)

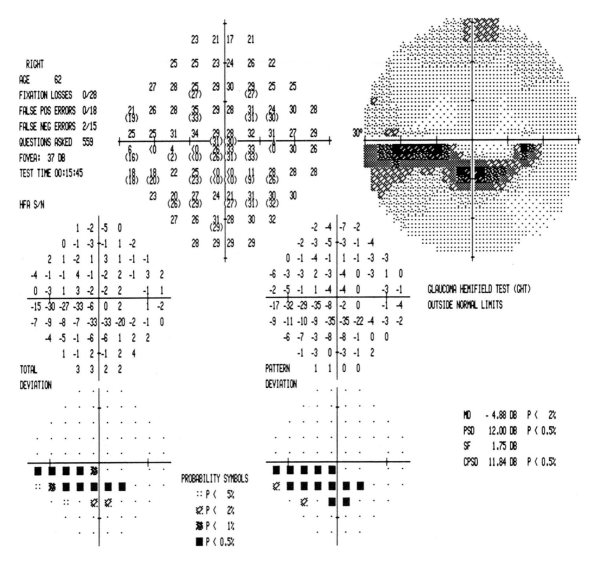

FIG. 9-6. Single Field Printout from which Curve in Figure 9-5 was Derived.

the Total Deviation values may be similar, and the Total Deviation Probability Plot may show that most points are mildly depressed ($p < 2\%$), with a scattered few at the 1% and 5% levels; the Pattern Deviation Probability Plot, corrected for the General Height, would be normal. This is equivalent to a boxplot of normal height that is slightly displaced downward, which in turn is equivalent to a Bebie curve of normal shape, displaced downward. The MD index is low, but the PSD index is normal. In contrast, a small localized defect would be represented by a lengthened bottom arm on the boxplot, which is represented in the Pattern Deviation Probability Plot by a number of points much more affected than others (and also is represented in the PSD global index). The point is that the fundamental information in these various displays and statistics is present on the Single Field Analyses; the intent of the boxplot printout is to permit the clinician to recognize a meaningful change in such parameters as a consistent trend in a series of examinations.

It should be noted, however, that when many numbers are reduced into digestible form (like the reduction of numerous pointwise threshold estimations into a boxplot or Bebie curve), some useful information is lost. In particular, the locations of the more abnormal test points are not shown. A group of points down by 10 dB at the upper edge of the 30-degree field may not be diagnostically significant, although the same threshold deviation at a group of points near the center or along one border of the nasal horizontal meridian is distinctly abnormal. The boxplot and Bebie curve do not indicate how abnormal the deviation is compared with the normal range at that location; they indicate only the number of decibels of deviation—the same magnitude of deviation may represent different degrees of abnormality at different locations.[6] There is no distinction between clustering of abnormal points in a diagnostically significant location and nonspecific scattering of abnormal points.

Like the greyscale, the boxplot therefore simply serves to call attention to markedly deviant values, the proportion of points that have marked deviation, and whether the deviations are similar or highly variant among the locations tested. In the change analysis printout, the boxplot is used to suggest at a glance the presence and nature of a change through a series of visual fields. However, the presence of abnormality and its nature, as well as the nature of the change over time, must be confirmed by reviewing the individual visual field examination results themselves in greater detail.

Deterioration of global indices

The Change Analysis printout also includes plots of each of the four global indices (SF, MD, PSD, CPSD) for the selected examinations. A plot of the Mean Deviation (MD) index over the series of examinations also is provided on the Glaucoma Change Probability Plot, and a similar plot of Mean Sensitivity (MS) is given as part of the Overview printout when there are nonstandard parameters (such as a size-V stimulus).

Mean Deviation index. The most useful first step is to glance at the plot of MD (or MS) to gain a quick impression of whether the series of field examinations shows any trend that needs closer inspection. It may be helpful to notice, for example, that the MD is much the same in each examination, which suggests that neither progressive generalized depression nor substantial progressive localized loss is occurring.

In contrast, highly variable MD values show that the examinations are not reproducible, and steady improvement of the MD index shows a progressive learning curve. If there is a steady downward trend, a systematic progressive deterioration of the visual field is evident. Both generalized and localized losses affect the MD index (or MS); therefore, when a deterioration is recognized, the character of the progressive loss and its cause must be determined.

The character of the progressive loss, whether generalized or localized, may be evident from inspection of the series of boxplots, or from the Overview display in which new localized defects (or selective deepening of previous defects) may be either present or absent. The cause is discerned in part from the nature of the progressive change, but mainly from other clinical information. The primary function of the visual field examinations is to determine whether there is a genuine change and how rapid it might be.

If there are at least five visual field examinations selected for the Change Analysis, a regression analysis of MD over time is performed. Although the display shows the examinations evenly spaced in sequence, the statistical analysis takes into account the time intervals of the examination, not simply its sequential number; the change is thus expressed as the change in MD per year, not the change in MD per field examination. The slope of the change (decibels per year) and degree of statistical significance (p value) are given. Except in the earliest release of Statpac, if the MD of the first field is lower than in subsequent fields and is inconsistent with the trend shown by the rest, the first field examination is discarded for the purpose of the analysis, based on the assumption that a learning effect had occurred after the first field and hence the first field was not a good starting point. The term "modified MD slope" is used on the printout if the first field was discarded from the statistical analysis.

The plot of MD over time does not give as complete an exposition of the field data as the boxplot, but it does permit a statistical test to be performed to see whether any trend toward deterioration is real or simply a result of test variability. Note that in a summary statistic such as a mean value, progression of a few locations is averaged with 0-dB change at the majority of locations, and a change in the mean deviation may be neither impressive in amount nor statistically significant. Therefore, the absence of a statistically significant slope does not rule out progression.[7] However, if a decline in the MD index *is* statistically significant, the deterioration probably is not a chance finding based on measurement variability. Whether the change is the result of glaucoma, cataract, learning effect, or some other cause still must be decided. In some cases, a small change may be a physiologic age change that simply differs from the *average* (approximately 0.08 dB per year) decline that is removed from consideration by the perimeter's statistical calculations (by plotting mean deviations from normal for age rather than plotting mean threshold values).

Other indices. Plots of the other global indices are less often useful but can be of help in some cases.

The PSD and CPSD indices increase as scotomas first develop,[8] but they may remain at a fixed value during most of the subsequent course of the disease. Eventually these indices decrease again when extensive areas of the visual field develop equally poor threshold sensitivity. Therefore a change in PSD or CPSD over time occasionally is helpful in recognizing the early stages of progression—as the field abnormality is first developing. However, once abnormal the lack of further change of these indices should not be taken as a sign that glaucomatous field loss is stable, or that localized glaucomatous progression is ruled out as the cause of a documented change in the MD index.

In principle, the SF should increase (because of variability at abnormal points) as a field progresses from normal to moderately defective. However, a plot of SF

> MD is slow to change, and when it does, the cause may be uncertain.

> PSD increases only in the early stages of glaucoma.

over a series of examinations rarely is useful, except occasionally to identify that one examination is less reliable than the others and therefore should be given less weight when making a judgment about progression.

POINTWISE CHANGES

Inspection of the Overview and Change Analysis printouts serves to reveal and characterize obvious changes and to give a sense of the magnitude of field-to-field variation. Such an overall perspective of global and summary descriptive statistics is invaluable; however, to discover and validate smaller increments of progressive visual field loss, a more critical evaluation of the threshold change at each point often is needed.

Compare

A change at a small cluster of points is easy to overlook when comparing two tabular displays of numerous threshold values. One way to discover a change from a baseline field is with the compare function. For this function, two field examinations are selected, the two threshold values for each location are subtracted, and a map of the differences is displayed. A cluster of locations with substantial change is easy to spot among the majority of points that show small random changes (Figs. 9-7 and 9-8). At the time of each follow-up examination, the field can be compared with the designated baseline; in most cases the comparison provides assurance that no perceptible change has occurred.

A useful variation on the HFA-1 is to combine two (or more) baseline fields into one as either an Average or a Master file that is the designated baseline. The Compare function can be applied to compare the threshold sensitivities in each follow-up examination with the mean values of the combined baseline examinations (Figs. 9-9 and 9-10).

A change in threshold from one occasion to another, noted with or without the aid of the compare printout, always must be studied in conjunction with the threshold value table of the baseline. A moderate decline in sensitivity (e.g., 5 dB) at a point may be meaningful if its initial sensitivity was normal. However, a larger decline may simply represent physiologic fluctuation if the baseline value was depressed (e.g., a 10-dB change from 15 dB to 5 dB). No conclusion can be drawn if there is no change at a point with an initial sensitivity of less than 0 dB.

The Compare function need not be used separately when the Glaucoma Change Probability analysis (see next section) is used, because it includes a map of the differences between the follow-up visual field and the chosen baseline. As in the comparison made with the Compare function, the decibel change is given for each location but is adjusted for age effects.

The amount of change that is meaningful is smaller if a comparison is made with a baseline set of field examinations instead of with a single baseline examination. Although a change from 10 dB sensitivity in a single baseline to 0 dB on a single follow-up can occur by chance, it would be unlikely that two or three

Location and degree of baseline abnormality determine the amount of change at a point that is meaningful.

Text continued on p. 268

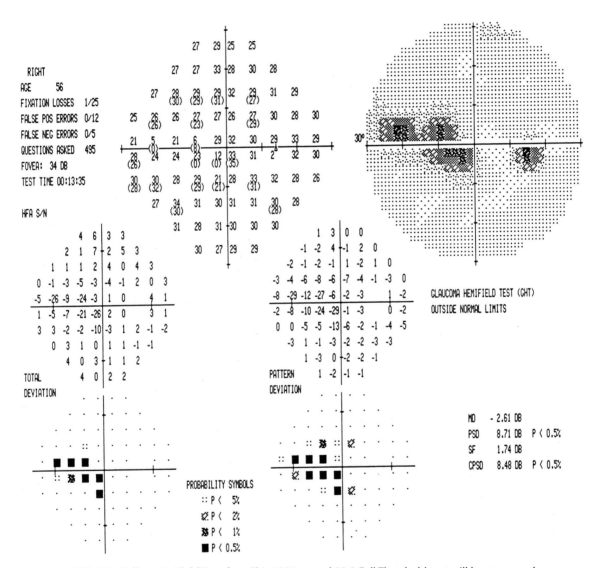

FIG. 9-7. Follow-Up Field Results. This 1988 central 30-2 Full Threshold test will be compared point by point with the baseline in 1987.

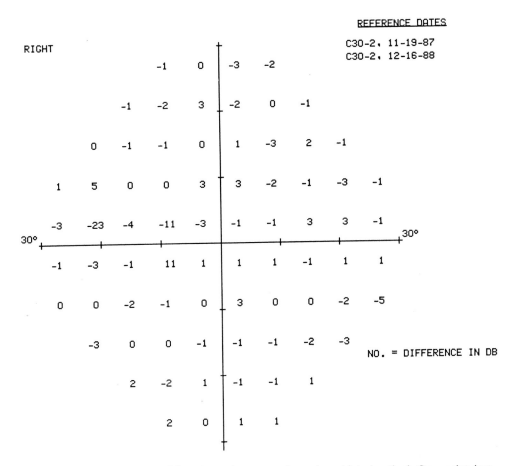

REFERENCE DATES

C30-2, 11-19-87
C30-2, 12-16-88

NO. = DIFFERENCE IN DB

FIG. 9-8. Compare. Several locations show negative values (deterioration). One point just below the horizontal nominally shows an 11-dB improvement, but inspection of that point in Figure 9-7 shows it to be variable on retesting. The first reference date is the date of the Master File (Fig. 9-10) and the second is of the current field (Fig. 9-7).

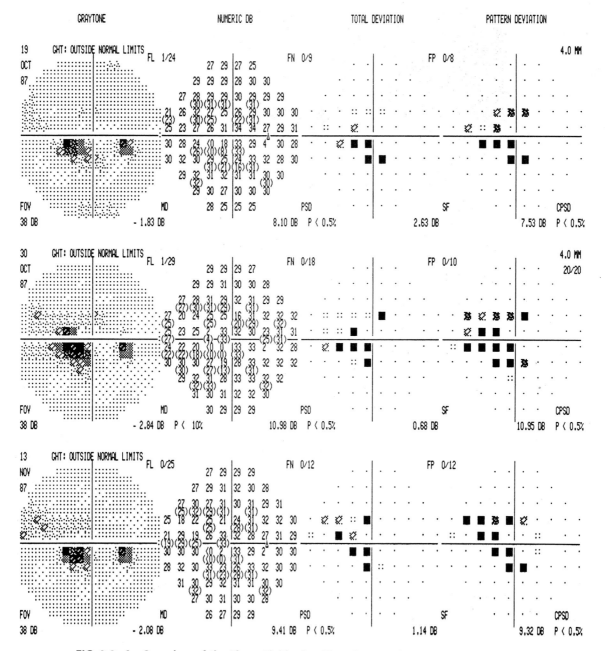

FIG. 9-9. An Overview of the Three Fields that Were Averaged to Create the Master File Shown in Figure 9-10.

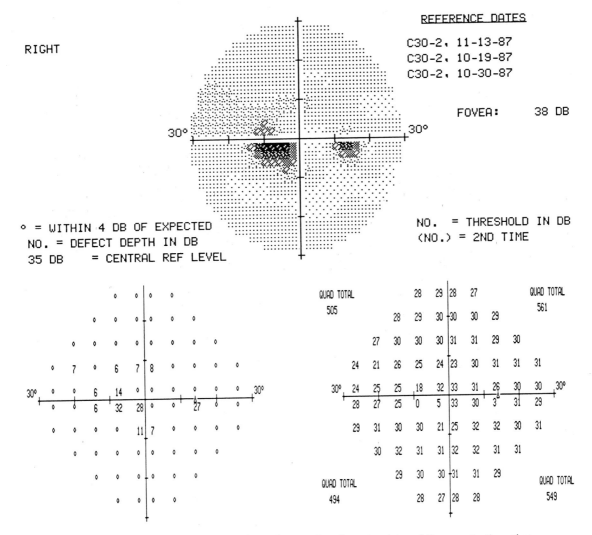

FIG. 9-10. Master File Printout. The "reference dates" are the dates of the examinations that were used to determine the average sensitivities.

baseline fields all would show measurable sensitivity initially and later that two or three fields all would show a sensitivity of less than 0 dB. To take into account the patient's individual consistency, the range of values demonstrated at a given point on the baseline fields (including all duplicate determinations) also should be considered. If the follow-up value is not outside the range exhibited during the baseline set, the conclusion cannot be made that sensitivity has declined at that location.

Glaucoma Change Probability

How much change from a baseline is meaningful? This is a complex issue. While a reproducible 5-dB change from a previously normal value at two or three adjacent points may represent a new scotoma and be meaningful, deepening of a pre-existing scotoma by the same magnitude may result from the natural variability of already abnormal locations.[9-11]

To assist with this problem, typical ranges of variability were established by repeatedly testing patients at various stages of glaucoma over a short period of time.[9] Each patient completed all testing within 1 month—a short enough time to postulate that no progression had occurred. The range of follow-up threshold values varies according to the deviation (from normal) of the initial threshold estimate. The amount by which thresholds fluctuate in the absence of progression is affected by how abnormal the test point is in the first place, the location, the overall status of the initial field as represented by the MD index, and whether the comparison is made with a single baseline field examination or with a pair of them. When these data are applied to threshold values of a follow-up field examination of a glaucoma patient compared with the baseline examination(s), it can be determined how unlikely it is that an obtained value at a given location could have occurred as a random fluctuation.

In practice, this principle is embodied in the Glaucoma Change Probability Analysis.[12,13,14] Follow-up fields are each compared with a baseline examination or with a baseline pair. The printout provides four representations: a greyscale, the Total Deviation probability, the change from baseline (Compare), and the probability that the observed change could be a chance variation (Fig. 9-11). The first two represent an analysis of the current field, and the last two a comparison with the selected baseline. The change in the MD index from baseline also is determined, along with the probability that such a change could occur by chance.

This approach can provide compelling evidence that a change of a certain magnitude is not a random finding (Fig. 9-12). The results can depend on the choice of which examinations to use as the baseline if the first several field examinations include ones affected by a learning phenomenon or an artifact. During the long course of chronic glaucoma, real changes may be statistically genuine but may be caused by media changes, other disease, long-term fluctuation, or an artifact. Judgment must be exercised, and an apparent change must be present on more than one occasion and not caused by a recognizable artifact or coexisting disease.

Text continued on p. 274

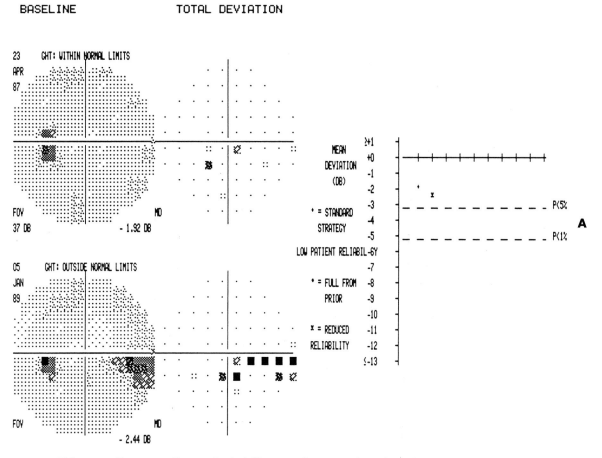

FIG. 9-11. Glaucoma Change Probability. **A,** The greyscale and Total Deviation probability plots of the first two fields in a series. They will be used as the baseline pair for the change probability calculations and are the first two field examinations shown in Figure 9-1. A plot of the MD index over time also is provided for all the fields selected for analysis. *Continued*

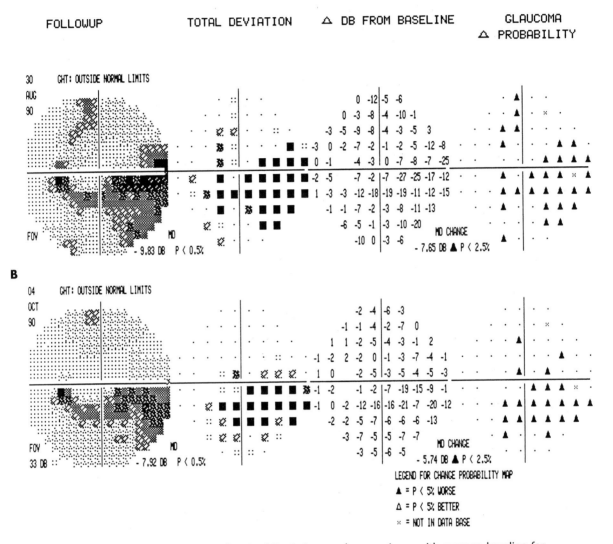

FIG. 9-11, cont'd. B, Greyscales, Total Deviations, and comparisons with average baseline for two follow-up field examinations are shown. The third field of Figure 9-1 and a subsequent confirmation field examination are shown as the two follow-up examinations. When the threshold value is unlikely to have resulted from the variability in retesting of stable glaucomatous fields ($p < 5\%$), a black triangle is printed. A point that deteriorated but was too defective in the baseline to judge progression is marked with an X. Also indicated inconspicuously is that the MD changes of -7.65 dB and -5.74 dB are larger than usual in a stable field ($p < 2.5\%$). In this illustrative example, the change is evident from the greyscale alone, without the help of statistics.

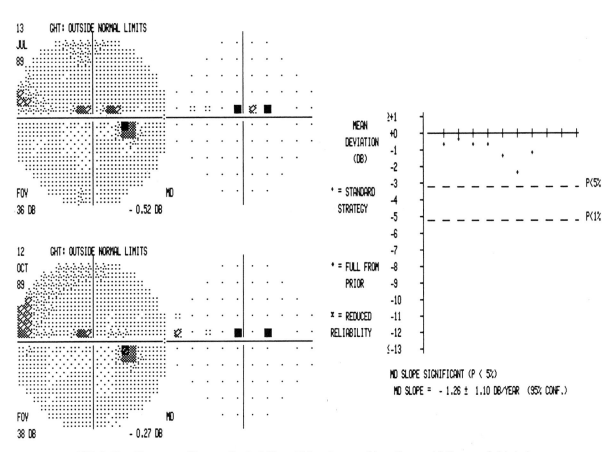

FIG. 9-12. Glaucoma Change Probability. This printout of baseline and follow-up fields helps confirm the progression above the nasal horizontal meridian in the same patient shown in Figures 9-2 and 9-3. Among the five follow-up examinations, the last two fields show a region above fixation in which several points deteriorated, even though the better parts of the field tend to be more sensitive than the baseline. *Continued*

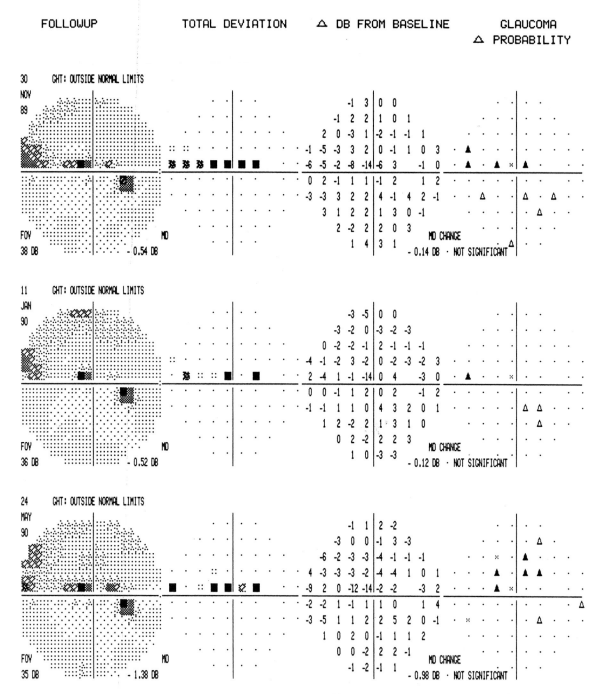

FIG. 9-12, cont'd.

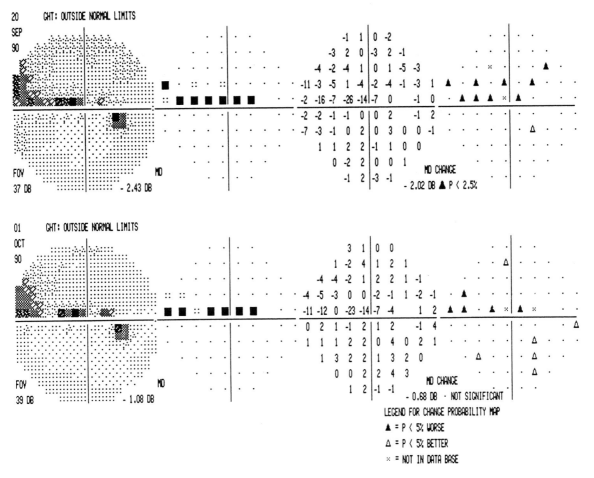

FIG. 9-12, cont'd.

273

Enhancements of the Glaucoma Change Probability Analysis should be available in late 1999. More data have been collected on both the traditional and the SITA test strategies, perhaps enough to permit designation of higher levels of significance than the currently available $p < 5\%$ for change at each test point. To reduce the impact of both transient and progressive generalized changes (e.g., those caused by learning effects, long-term fluctuation, or media change), the analysis may be performed on the Pattern Deviation values (after correction for the General Height) as shown in Figure 9-13, instead of the Total Deviation values.[15] At the time of this writing the analytical algorithms are being written, so the final form of the analysis is not fully known—nor is there experience with its use. The clinician still is required to apply some criterion, demanding a statistically significant change at a cluster of points in an expected location, that is also present on a second occasion, that is not explained by artifact or other disease and that is in keeping with other clinical circumstances.

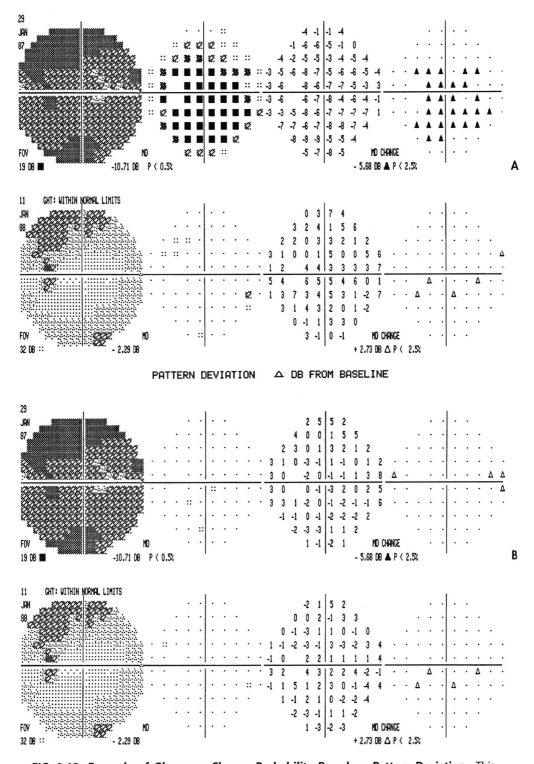

FIG. 9-13. Example of Glaucoma Change Probability Based on Pattern Deviation. This patient was examined regularly since 1976 because of elevated IOP. As cataract developed, the Glaucoma Change Probability analysis based on Total Deviation showed statistically significant changes in the upper and lower hemifields, but Glaucoma Change Probability analysis based on Pattern Deviation did not show such changes. Cataract extraction was performed in August 1987, with 20/20 visual acuity and no glaucomatous abnormality on the subsequent visual field examination. (Courtesy of Boel Bengtsson and Anders Heijl, MD)

"Fast Threshold"

Another way to detect a change at a small number of locations is with the "Fast Threshold" strategy.[16,17] This is a unique strategy that has not been used widely and was not included in the HFA-2 software. This program is not really a threshold test, but a customized suprathreshold test with selective thresholding. At each location a stimulus is presented that is 2 dB more intense than the average value found in the patient's master file (which consists of averaged baseline threshold values). If the patient responds, it is assumed that there has been no reduction in sensitivity at that location compared with the baseline, and nothing more is done. If the stimulus is not seen at a location (given two opportunities, if needed), that location undergoes a staircase thresholding procedure (Fig. 9-14).

The time-saving advantage is lost if more than three or four points are thresholded. The need for multiple thresholding may be caused by patient inconsistency or the inherent variability in fields with many locations that are moderately abnormal. Therefore the Fast Threshold strategy may be most appropriate for patients who have relatively mild defects and have shown little variability from field to field. The test should be used selectively—only for this type of patient. For the majority of such patients, most of the stimuli are seen on first (or perhaps the second) presentation, and the test is quite short. The fast threshold strategy may be slightly less sensitive in finding mild deterioration than the standard strategy because the fatigue of a longer test amplifies borderline reduction of sensitivity.[18,19] With only a few points undergoing thresholding, there is less opportunity for erroneously reduced threshold values to appear, and for that reason the test is less likely to suggest falsely that progression has occurred. However, in cases in which there are many newly abnormal points, the clinician cannot judge whether this was caused by random variability, because whether there is an equal number of points with improved threshold values is not revealed. Two rules follow: this method should not be used for patients who show highly variable threshold estimations on baseline fields (or subsequently), and any suspected progression should be confirmed with a standard test.

The Fast Threshold printout provides the initial average threshold value in the Master file. Any newly determined threshold sensitivities also are given, and the difference is apparent. The greyscale and Defect Depth table of the field is provided, based on the new thresholds of thresholded points and the baseline thresholds of all others.

In summary, the Fast Threshold strategy can be used to advantage in cases in which the fields show little variability and there is apparent stability of the disease in a series of fields and by all other clinical parameters. This test is available only on the HFA-1. With the HFA-2, the new Sita strategies challenge the speed of the Fast Threshold strategy and may be used in all types of cases.

> With the HFA-1, the Fast Threshold strategy can be useful in early cases with fields that are not highly variable.

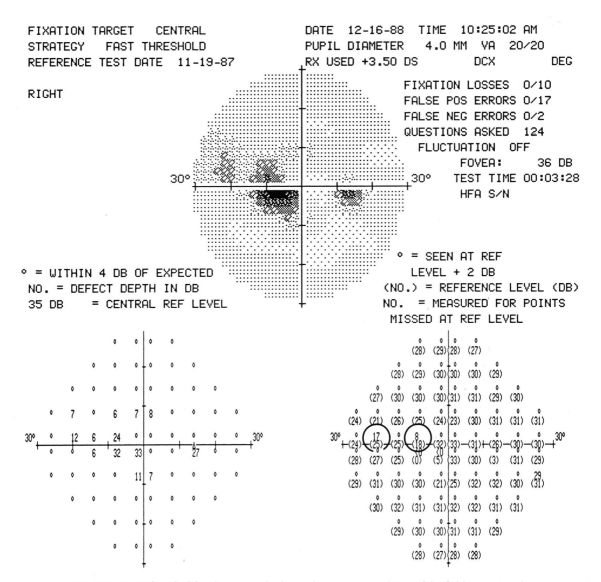

FIG. 9-14. Fast Threshold. The greyscale shows the present condition of the field, assuming the baseline average value for points that passed the suprathreshold screen and the new threshold value of points that had a new threshold value determined. On the lower left of the printout is a Defect Depth plot, the basis of which was explained in Chapter 8. The main part of the printout that deserves inspection is on the lower right. In that plot, the number in parentheses is the baseline average value, as shown in the master file printout (see Fig. 9-10). Above each point, a small circle indicates that the suprathreshold stimulus was seen, and a number at that location represents a newly determined threshold. In this example, two locations (circled) show a reduced threshold compared with baseline. This patient also had undergone a Full Threshold test on the same day (shown in Fig. 9-7), which was compared (see Fig. 9-8) with the same Master File (see Fig. 9-10) used for the test shown here. Note that the change at the two points, showing major changes in the Fast Threshold test, is not identical with the degree of change shown in the Compare printout; however, they do correspond well within the limits of testing variability.

INTERPRETATION

With the various views of data and statistical analyses available, one would think that it would be easy to judge whether progression has occurred. However, it remains a difficult task much of the time and requires attention and thought. A number of phenomena must be taken into account.

Fluctuations

The physiologic fluctuations include test-retest error (short-term fluctuation) and an actual variation in visual physiology from one time to another (long-term fluctuation). These fluctuations are transient and reversible. Long-term fluctuation occurs in both normal and abnormal fields. Long-term fluctuation is a genuine small physiologic change in visibility and is considered to be any variation that is not the result of measurement error (short-term fluctuation) or a learning effect. In normal fields, long-term fluctuation may cause threshold sensitivity to change 1 or 2 dB across the entire field (homogeneous component), and also cause a change of similar magnitude affecting some locations more than others (heterogeneous component). Both short-term and long-term fluctuations are greater in abnormal fields, especially at abnormal locations.

Loss of visual sensitivity that results from progression of disease can be recognized only when it exceeds the change that might have occurred as a result of these physiologic short-term and long-term fluctuations. It is intended that true changes— those that exceed fluctuations—are reflected in the statistical significance level of the MD slope (Change Analysis printout) and of the pointwise change in the Glaucoma Change Probability Analysis.

Manifestations of progression

Conversion from normal to abnormal. One clinical circumstance involves the patient with normal visual fields who is under observation because of an elevated IOP or for some other reason. A criterion for "progression" might be that the visual field becomes abnormal, meeting one of the diagnostic criteria for localized glaucomatous abnormality outlined in Chapter 7.

Typically the sequence of events is that slowly, over several years, there are regions of variable responses that meet a criterion for abnormality on occasion— but not reproducibly (this also can happen in nonprogressive cases). Later the defect is more persistently present and the Glaucoma Hemifield Test is repeatedly abnormal. In some of these cases, the MD index or the PSD index, or both, become abnormal. However, as shown in Figure 9-4 the field can be abnormal, and moreover detectably progress, before the MD index becomes abnormal.

When visual field examinations are repeatedly conducted for several years, a sign of abnormality may appear and require a prompt attempt at confirmation. The abnormality may not be confirmed, but if it represents the true beginning of progressive disease, it will later reappear and be consistently present. In some cases there initially may be some suspicion and uncertainty when a second examination fails to confirm a slight change, and only time will determine whether an early abnormality is real.

New defect. A new defect may appear in a normal region of an abnormal baseline field. In this situation, the Glaucoma Hemifield Test and PSD index were likely already abnormal at the time of baseline evaluation. Therefore, of the three criteria given in Chapter 7, only one can be used—that a new cluster of at least three nonedge abnormal points arises in a typical location, each with threshold sensitivities occurring in fewer than 5% of the normal population ($p < 5\%$), and with a sensitivity that occurs in fewer than 1% of the population ($p < 1\%$) at one of the points.

Worsening of a defect. The application of reasonable criteria to a pointwise numeric comparison currently is the best basis for judging follow-up visual field examinations.

When comparing point-by-point the threshold values of an examination with those of a baseline (perhaps with the help of a compare printout), a previously defective region may be judged to have worsened if three or more points in that region have deteriorated by 10 dB. A defect may be deemed widened if two or more new points are involved to this degree. If a patient has visual field examinations performed in several offices and only hard-copy printouts are available, criteria like this may be all that can be used.

However, it is far better to use the Glaucoma Change Probability information to decide whether a threshold value is out of line. A statistically significant change at one location is not sufficient to conclude that the disease has worsened, but some reasonable criterion (adjusted according to circumstances described later) must be applied, such as a statistically significant change in a cluster of three points in a typical location that is confirmed on another occasion and not otherwise explained.

Generalized change. As was true for initial diagnosis, widespread equal deterioration is not as characteristic of progression as localized deterioration. A statistically significant decline in the Mean Deviation may result from localized deterioration but if localized worsening is not evident, nonglaucomatous explanations may be more likely and must be ruled out before accepting progression of glaucomatous optic nerve damage as the cause.

Staging of disease. Another approach is based on classifying visual fields into stages of disease or degrees of abnormality. Progression is diagnosed if the field classification moves from one category to another, with much the same reasoning used when a visual field changes from normal to abnormal. These criteria serve the needs of the clinical trial for which they were devised,[20] and may permit analyses about how much progression occurred (rather than the fact that it occurred) but are cumbersome for use in clinical practice. Automated methods to stage disease show promise for the future.[21]

Effects of repeat testing

If numerous examinations are performed in the course of long-standing chronic glaucoma, or if frequent examinations are performed with the hope of detecting a very small increment of progression, the chances accumulate that somewhere along the line a statistically significant change in the threshold estimate will happen by chance alone.[22] A change that is statistically significant at the 5% level should, after all, occur about once in 20 field examinations at any one selected location; and if at least 20 locations are subjected to analysis, a statistically significant change may occur regularly at scattered locations.

Such reasoning cannot be applied exactly, because there are some correlations among locations (e.g., as the result of the homogeneous component of long-term fluctuation). Therefore, changes at a cluster of locations may occur in tandem. Such clustering may give a false sense of confidence that the change is real.

Major deterioration that is not a clinical surprise may be diagnostically compelling on a single examination. However, slight progression, especially if unexpected, should be diagnosed only if a group of points change by an amount that is unlikely by chance alone in stable fields, and if the change is confirmed on at least one more occasion. The finding is more certain (more specific*) if it is present during retesting. It is surprising how often an apparent change is not found on a repeat examination and would have constituted a false diagnosis of progression if a conclusion had been reached on the basis of the first examination.

Another way to improve the specificity of diagnosing progression is to demand a larger change when comparing the examination with the baseline (e.g., a 10-dB change rather than a 5-dB change, or at least one point with a greater significance change than $p < 5\%$). Such an approach may further reduce the detection of small increments of progression but is useful in addition to requiring a second examination whenever a small change is suspected.[22]

> A field change must be confirmed.

---

*The state of having progression from a baseline condition can be considered a clinical condition, the presence of which can be detected (or not) with various criteria that would each have some sensitivity and specificity. The statistical considerations are thereby analogous to the process of recognizing the presence of disease in the first place. If the incidence of developing new defects in the group of patients being followed is slow, the emphasis must be on specificity. Most initially positive test results are unconfirmed on repeat testing. Some of these unconfirmed changes will later reappear and persist; but most will not, and these represent the improved specificity produced by repeat testing. Those that were discounted on retesting, but later turn out to have been genuine, represent a loss of sensitivity to subtle defects, which necessarily accompanies the improved specificity.

Cataract

Cataracts have varying influence on the visual field through blur, light absorption, or light scatter. Refractive blur reduces visual acuity but may not reduce contrast or perimetric thresholds.[23] Light absorption by ocular media has surprisingly little effect on visual function,[24] which explains the frequent observation of good visual function despite cataracts that are impressively brown on biomicroscopic examination. Intraocular light scatter, however, reduces contrast in the retinal image and has considerable impact on perimetric thresholds.[25] Veiling glare from scatter may cause the symptomatic feature that the patient sees better when eyes are shaded. Back scatter accounts for whitening of the cortex or posterior subcapsular tissue on clinical examination of the lens. The forward scatter that affects the retinal image is not strongly correlated with the back scatter that makes lens opacities visible,[26] so cataracts that produce symptoms of glare and perimetric effects may not always be impressive when examined with the slit lamp, and the effect on acuity in a dark room may likewise be minimal.

Light scattering reduces visual threshold everywhere.[25,27] The threshold values all diminish, the Total Deviation values all increase, and the MD index worsens. Removal of cataract may uncover the preceding impact of cataract on normal and glaucomatous visual fields. The effect is variable, depending on the type and severity of cataract as well as the stage of the glaucomatous damage.[28-31]

Of note is that when cataract has an effect, it nearly always affects all points in the visual field more or less equally. In particular, judging from simulations[25,27] and pointwise effects of cataract removal on the visual field,[31] the cataract effect on the normal regions of the visual field is the same as on the region(s) affected by glaucoma. The obvious exception is that locations with 0-dB threshold will not be diminished further with cataract development, nor will they share in the improved threshold that might occur with cataract removal.[30] Except in the advanced stages of glaucoma, it is reasonable to assume that some region may remain unaffected by glaucoma, and that deterioration of this region represents the cataract effect. Thus, except in advanced stages of glaucoma, the foveal point, or the 85th percentile point represented by the General Height (GH) index, can be used to judge the magnitude of the cataract effect as the patient's glaucoma is being monitored.

With these fundamental effects of cataract in mind, it may be useful to consider the effect of cataract on each of the parameters typically inspected while monitoring the course of glaucoma.

Cataract is the most common reason for a progressive change in the MD index, but the MD also declines with glaucomatous progression. With care it can be recognized whether the MD decline is due to cataract or to a localized progression typical of glaucoma. For example, especially if the initial glaucomatous field defect is small and mild, the Pattern Deviation Plot may not change relative to baseline (as seen perhaps in an Overview plot) and a short boxplot symbol may move downward over time without lengthening (in a Change Analysis plot) if the cause is cataract. The clinician may also judge that the field change is consistent with an observed decline in acuity, a change in glare sensitivity, or an observed change in lens clarity and scatter.

It has been suggested[32] that ocular media changes will produce a decline in MD that is equal to the decline of GH. Eyes with a combination of progressive media changes plus progressive localized loss from glaucoma will show an MD change that is larger than the GH change. General Height changes, then, represent the portion of the field change that can be attributed to generalized loss, while the difference between MD and GH represents the effect of localized loss on the average loss for the whole field. Even without analytical tools, the clinician can note the change in threshold at the fovea and at representative locations that are not likely to be involved in the glaucomatous process. He can then judge how the change at these locations (presumptively due to media change, but not glaucoma) compares with the change at locations being monitored for glaucomatous change.

A subtle effect of a generalized reduction in threshold values is that it adds to any change that may occur from glaucomatous progression or from fluctuation. Thus if cataract produces a 3-dB decline in threshold, and if a 7-dB change at a particular location is statistically significant in the Glaucoma Change Probability calculation, then the criterion might be met by a random 4-dB change at that location. The calculation correctly reveals that the change is not entirely the result of random fluctuation, but the presence of cataract enhances the opportunity for fluctuations to cause the criterion to be met without progression of glaucoma. It is anticipated that in a future software revision, a GH correction will be incorporated into the Glaucoma Change Probability Analysis, so that the criteria can be applied to the Pattern Deviation values instead of the Total Deviation values.[15] Such a GH correction would remove effects not only of cataract, but also other causes of generalized changes, including homogenous long-term fluctuation and perhaps, to some extent, learning effects. However, there is not yet clinical documentation of the effectiveness of applying this concept.

The PSD index is useful for monitoring glaucoma only in the earliest stages of glaucoma. Cataract should not worsen the PSD in such cases, and in those circumstances a stable PSD is reassuring. As fields progress to moderate levels of glaucomatous loss, PSD peaks, may be stable with further progression, and then starts to decline; thus PSD is an unreliable indication of loss in moderate disease. In very advanced stages, when many locations have 0-dB sensitivities, the PSD may decline as either glaucoma or cataract reduces the threshold of the locations with remaining measurable thresholds. Thus, if the PSD index worsens in a case of early glaucoma, it is a useful sign; but otherwise, it is not very helpful to monitor the PSD index.[30]

Other disease

Cataract and other diseases may cause field change in a patient being monitored for glaucomatous change.

Patients with glaucoma are in an age group that may develop macular disease, branch retinal vessel occlusions, and cerebrovascular disease. These conditions may produce localized changes in the visual field that more closely resemble glaucoma than do the changes produced by cataract. The unwary clinician may be fooled into thinking that the glaucomatous optic nerve damage has worsened. Others may find a branch retinal vessel occlusion, or (if the field change is hemianopic and bilateral) evidence of an otherwise silent occipital lobe infarct.

Learning effect

Patients frequently fail to give consistent and reliable permetric responses in the first tests they undergo.[33,34] Sometimes the first field is not as reliable as subsequent examinations, and has the features of inexperience (see Chapter 7, Figs. 7-43 through 7-48). Typically the initial field has a slightly reduced overall sensitivity, reflected in the MD index, but if the first field had a high FP rate, it may have a higher MD index than subsequent fields. It is for this reason that a second baseline field examination is always advised.

A learning effect that spans a series of several examinations (Figs. 9-15 through 9-17) makes interpretation difficult. Usually the clinician concludes that the improvement is a result of learning and is pleased by the assumption that there is not a simultaneous slow worsening of the disease that has been overwhelmed by the learning effect. In such cases, it is frustrating that progression cannot be judged until the patient has finished learning and produces a stable baseline series.

Long-term fluctuation

Some patients are much more highly variable on repeat testing than others. To be detected, deterioration must exceed the variability of the individual (Fig. 9-18). If the MD slope over time is statistically significant, the change in MD must have exceeded the long-term fluctuation of that patient; however, the long-term fluctuation may make it difficult for a meaningful decline to be detected and determined to be statistically significant. The Glaucoma Change Probability may give variable and anomalous results in an individual with uncommonly large fluctuations. Corrections of these statistics for the General Height index could make a glaucoma-caused decline in MD easier to appreciate and reduce the variable results of the Glaucoma Change Probability Analysis, but there is not yet enough clinical experience with a GH correction to validate this hopeful expectation.

The isolated poor field

There are many causes other than physiologic fluctuations and statistical variation that may produce an occasional field examination that is out of line with the baseline (Figs. 9-19 and 9-20).

Text continued on p. 290

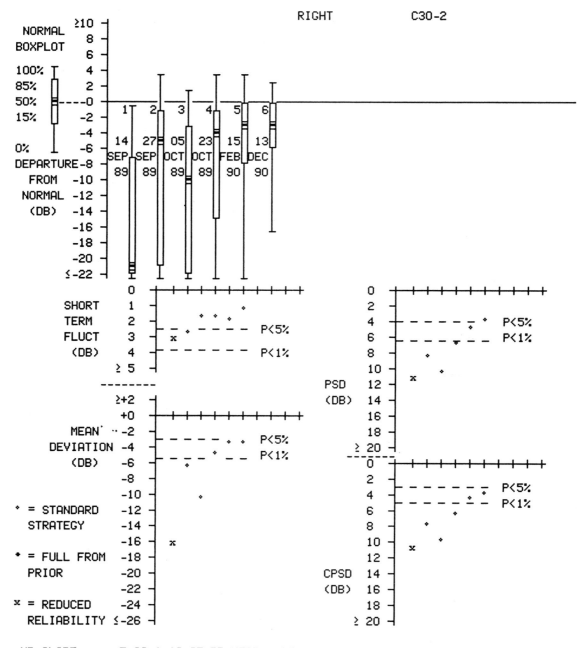

MD SLOPE = + 5.89 ± 12.05 DB/YEAR (95% CONF.)

MD SLOPE NOT SIGNIFICANT (P ≥ 5%)

FIG. 9-15. Progressive Learning Effect Over Several Examinations (Change Analysis). Any progressive deterioration is difficult to judge until a stable baseline is accomplished.

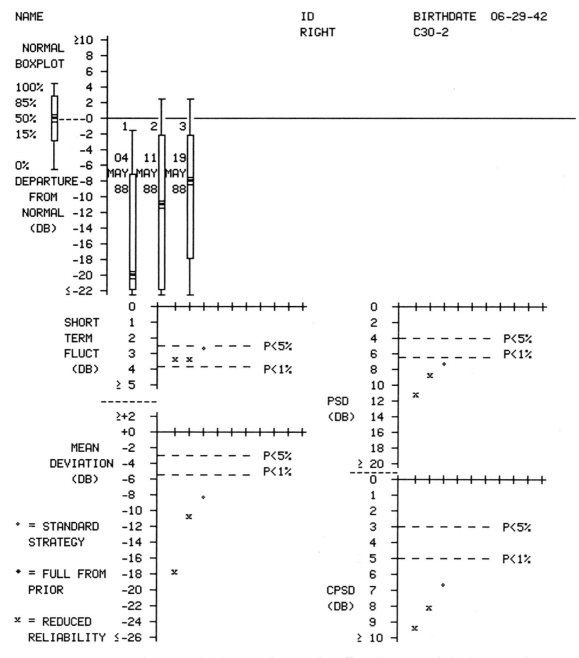

FIG. 9-16. Another Example of Progressive Learning Effect (Change Analysis). (Courtesy of Anders Heijl, MD)

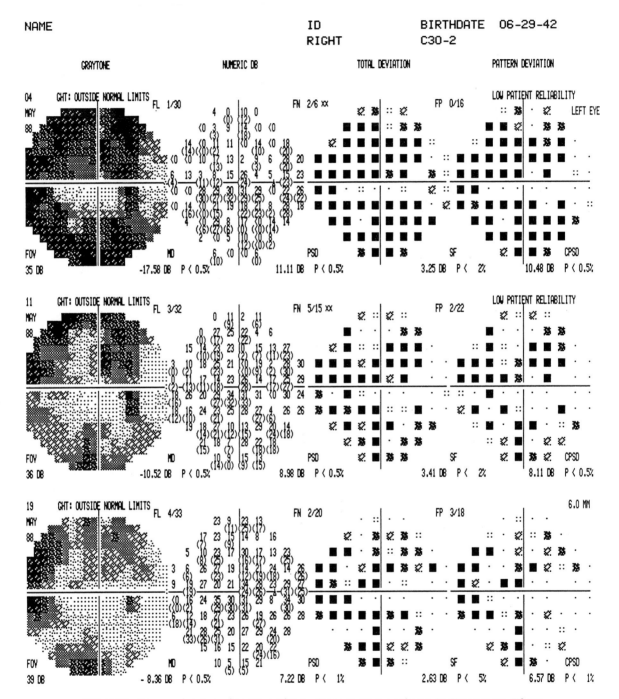

FIG. 9-17. Progressive Learning (Overview). Same patient as shown in Figure 9-16. Fifteen days elapsed between the first and the third fields. (Courtesy of Anders Heijl, MD)

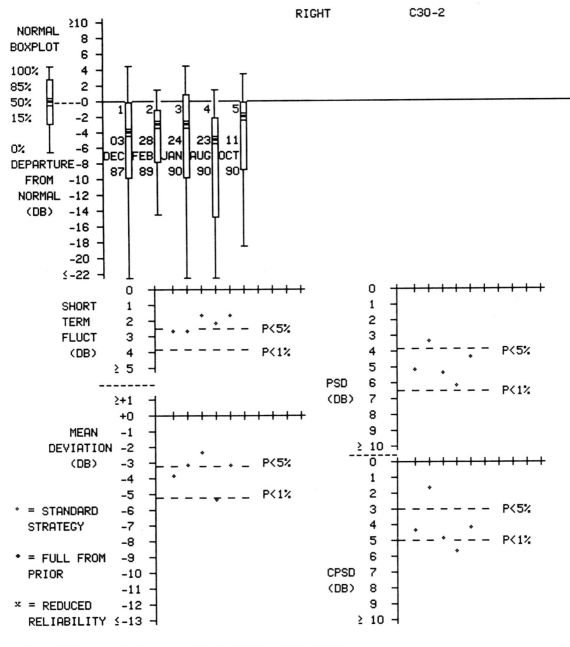

MD SLOPE = - 0.04 ± 1.68 DB/YEAR (95% CONF.)

MD SLOPE NOT SIGNIFICANT (P ≥ 5%)

FIG. 9-18. Variability (Long-Term Fluctuation) in Mildly Abnormal Field. All fields in this series have acceptable reliability parameters. The boxplot and graphs of global indices over time are highly variable.

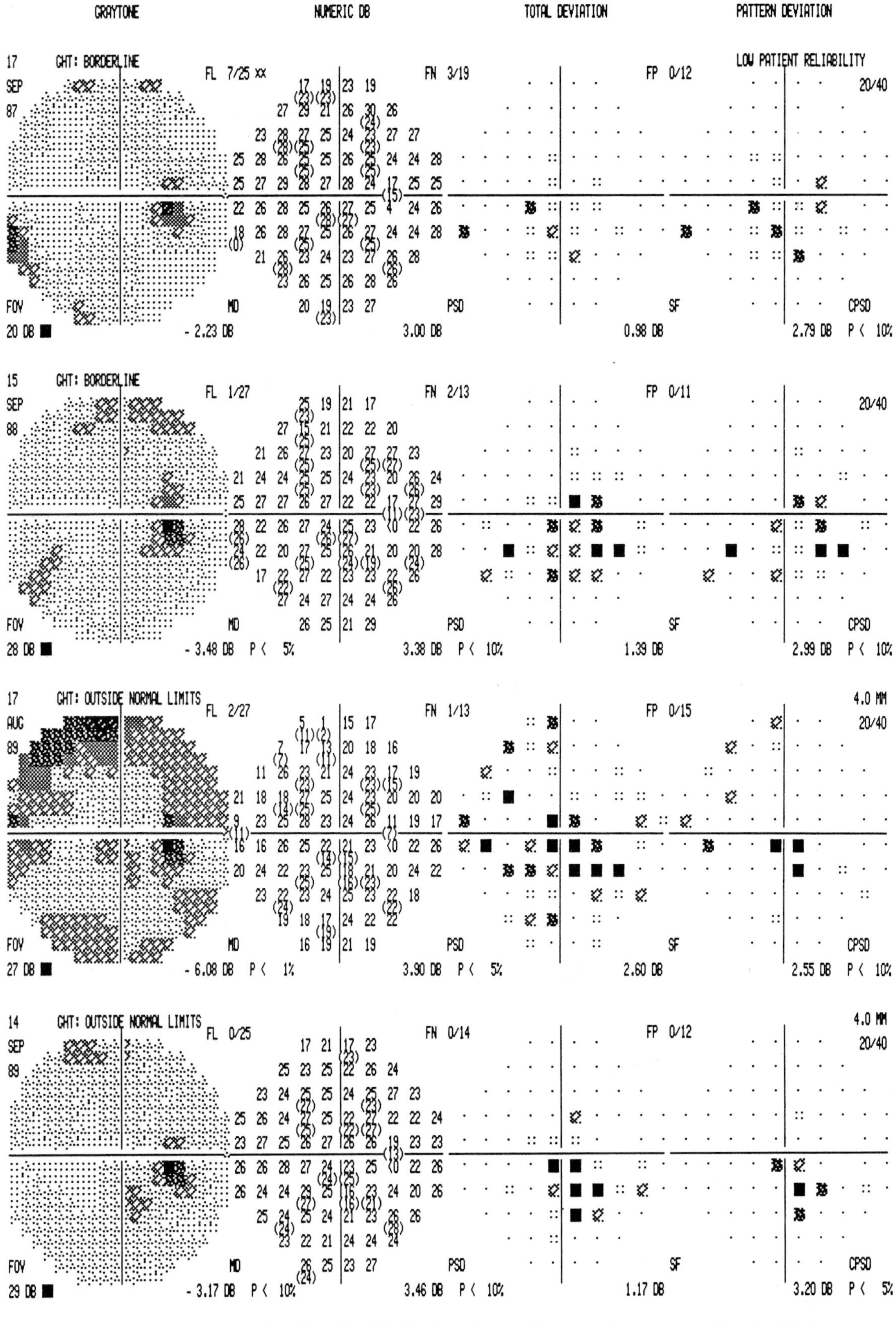

GRAYTONE NUMERIC DB TOTAL DEVIATION PATTERN DEVIATION

FIG. 9-19. Unexplained Isolated Bad Field (Overview). The worsening suggested by the third
annual field examination is not confirmed a month later.

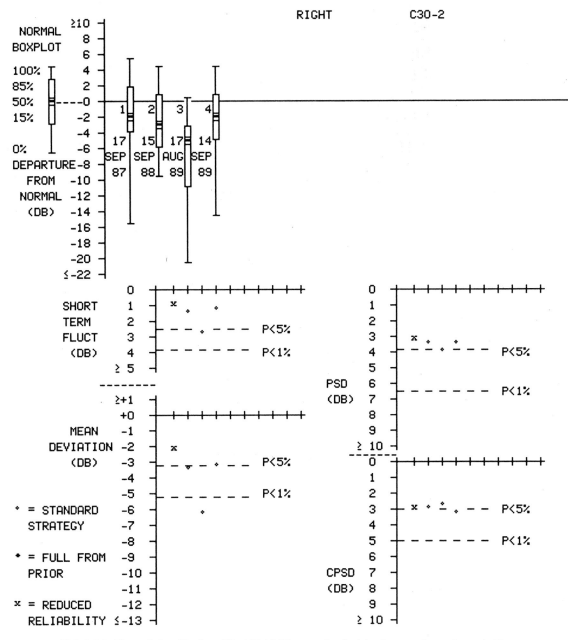

FIG. 9-20. Unexplained Isolated Bad Field (Change Analysis). Same series as shown in Figure 9-19.

Sometimes the cause is evident, such as a lens rim or eyebrow artifact. A poor field may be caused by a constricted pupil, or interestingly, by a dilated pupil.[35,36] Improper refraction (e.g., the inadvertent use of a plus lens instead of a minus lens) affects the result. Sometimes the patient is tired or distracted by noise in the office environment.

Sometimes the cause is not apparent and never is discovered. Unexplained changes are common enough that all suspected changes must be confirmed (Figs. 9-19 through 9-21). The effect of pupil size must be kept in mind (Figs. 9-22 and 9-23).

The already poor field

> It is difficult to monitor the late stages of glaucoma.

If the field is poor initially, it is more difficult to judge progression. Even with use of a size-V stimulus in a 10-2 or macula pattern there may be many locations with absolute loss (0-dB stimulus not seen), leaving only a few points at which to judge progression. If these remaining points are abnormal, they will be highly variable from one occasion to another. There is no easy solution to this problem. A pattern must be found that tests as many locations as possible with threshold values high enough to permit detection of change. An accurately observant patient may be able to state whether vision is worsening in his daily experience, apart from formal visual field testing.

Change in perimeter

Difficulties are compounded if the baseline field is on one type of perimeter and the follow-up on another. However, it is desirable to make use of any available baseline when possible. For the Goldmann perimeter, the III-4e stimulus is identical with the 10-dB size-III stimulus of the Humphrey Field Analyzer. Well-quantified differences from normal may be helpful but threshold estimates vary according to strategy and test conditions, and stimuli equivalence established at normal locations may not apply to abnormal locations. Thus, although examples are shown here (Figs. 9-24 and 9-25) in which progression or stability can be reasonably certain when comparing perimeters, it usually is impossible to make convincing comparisons. See Appendix C concerning comparison of HFA-1 and HFA-2.

Text continued on p. 298

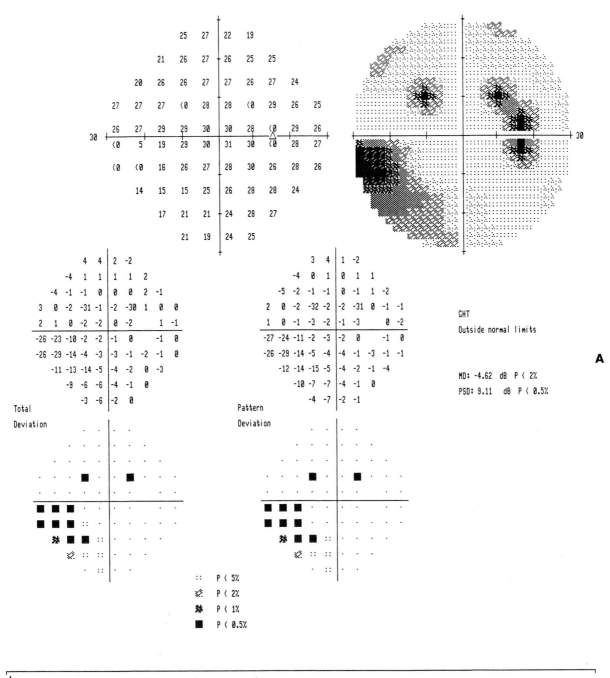

			25	27	22	19			
		21	26	27	26	25	25		
	20	26	26	27	27	26	27	24	
27	27	27	<0	28	28	<0	29	26	25
26	27	29	29	30	30	28	<0	29	26
<0	5	19	29	30	31	30	<0	28	27
<0	<0	16	26	27	28	30	26	28	26
	14	15	15	25	26	28	28	24	
		17	21	21	24	28	27		
			21	19	24	25			

30 △

30

Total Deviation

		4	4	2	-2		
	-4	1	1	1	1	2	
-4	-1	-1	0	0	0	2	-1
3	0	-2	-31	-1	-2	-30	1	0	0
2	1	0	-2	-2	0	-2		1	-1
-26	-23	-10	-2	-2	-1	0		-1	0
-26	-29	-14	-4	-3	-3	-1	-2	-1	0
-11	-13	-14	-5	-4	-2	0	-3		
-9	-6	-6	-4	-1	0				
-3	-6	-2	0						

Pattern Deviation

		3	4	1	-2		
	-4	0	1	0	1	1	
-5	-2	-1	-1	0	-1	1	-2
2	0	-2	-32	-2	-2	-31	0	-1	-1
1	0	-1	-3	-2	-1	-3		0	-2
-27	-24	-11	-2	-3	-2	0		-1	0
-26	-29	-14	-5	-4	-4	-1	-3	-1	-1
-12	-14	-15	-5	-4	-2	-1	-4		
-10	-7	-7	-4	-1	0				
-4	-7	-2	-1						

GHT
Outside normal limits

MD: -4.62 dB P < 2%
PSD: 9.11 dB P < 0.5%

A

```
::  P < 5%
⬚  P < 2%
⬚  P < 1%
■  P < 0.5%
```

FIG. 9-21. Importance of Confirming Test Results. The visual field in **A** (this page) shows striking paracentral defects in the upper arcuate region. They were not confirmed on any of three other tests performed in the same month (one of which is shown in **B**, p. 292) and were likely a test artifact, perhaps from patient inattention at the beginning of the test when the primary points were tested.

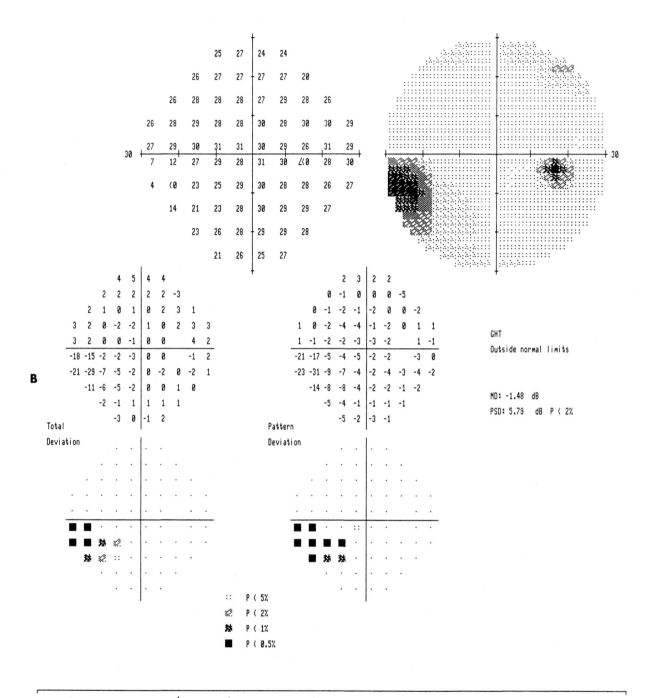

B

Total
Deviation

Pattern
Deviation

GHT
Outside normal limits

MD: -1.48 dB
PSD: 5.79 dB P < 2%

:: P < 5%
⊠ P < 2%
✸ P < 1%
■ P < 0.5%

FIG. 9-21, cont'd.

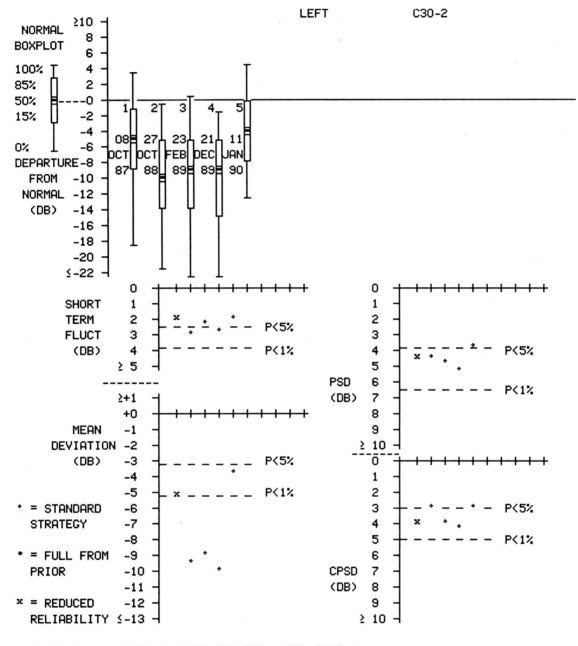

MD SLOPE = - 0.34 ± 5.56 DB/YEAR (95% CONF.)

MD SLOPE NOT SIGNIFICANT (P ≥ 5%)

FIG. 9-22. Effect of Small Pupil (Change Analysis). Reduced sensitivity in examinations 2, 3, and 4 was caused by pilocarpine treatment and was reversed by pharmacologic pupil dilation for examination 5.

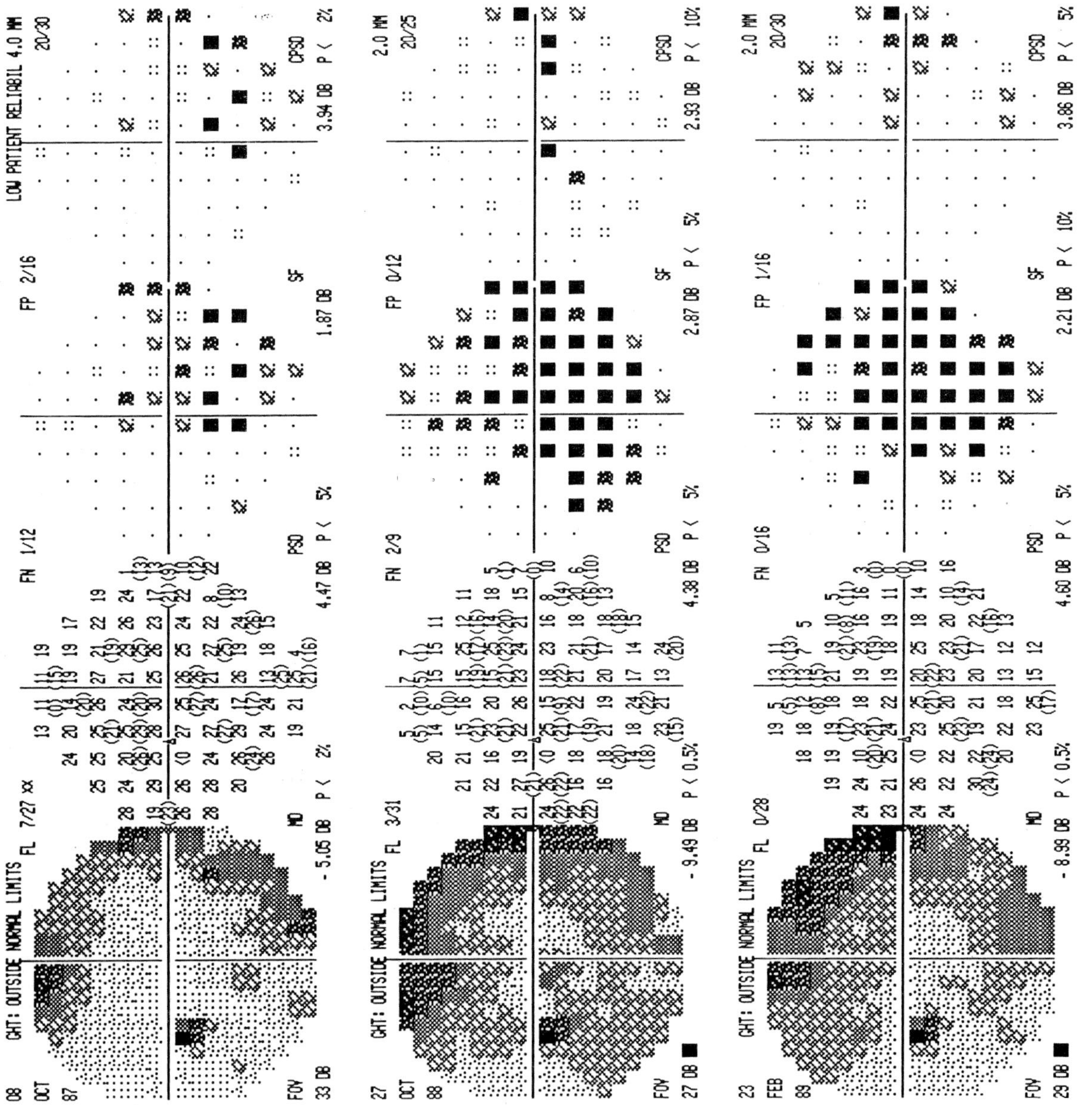
GRAYTONE
NUMERIC DB
TOTAL DEVIATION
PATTERN DEVIATION

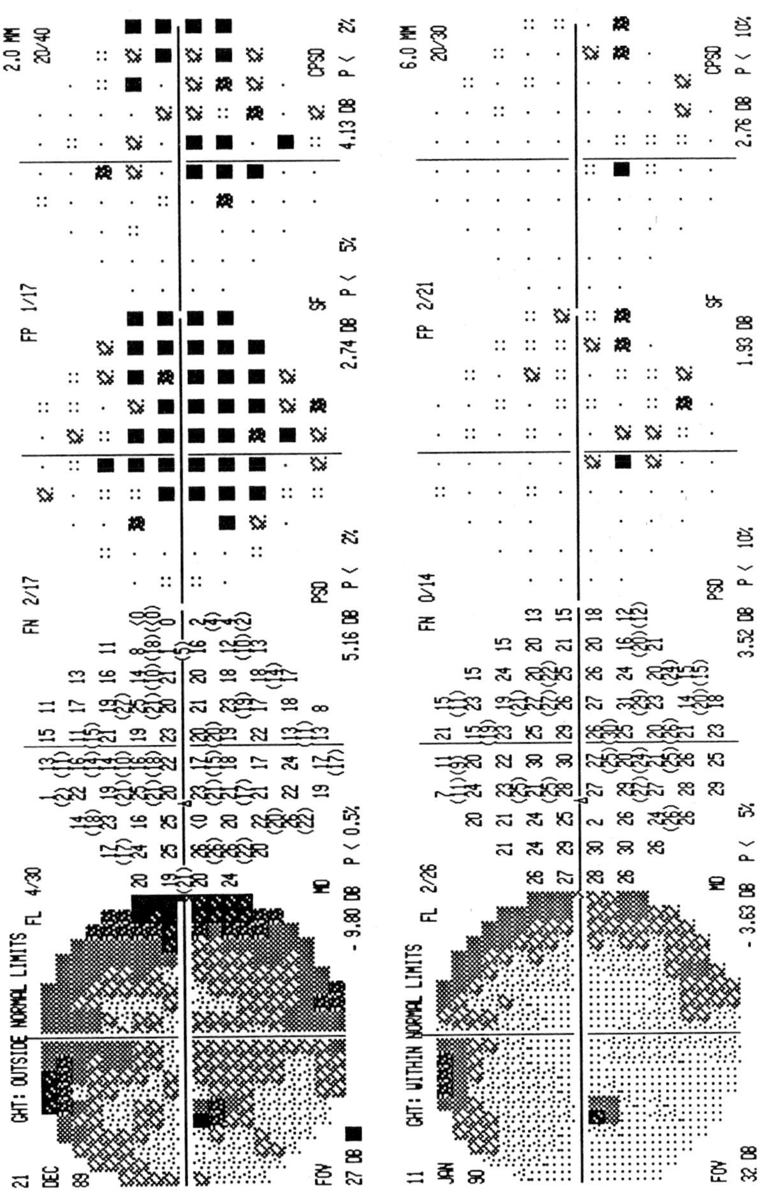

FIG. 9-23. Effect of Small Pupil (Overview).
Same series as seen in Figure 9-22.

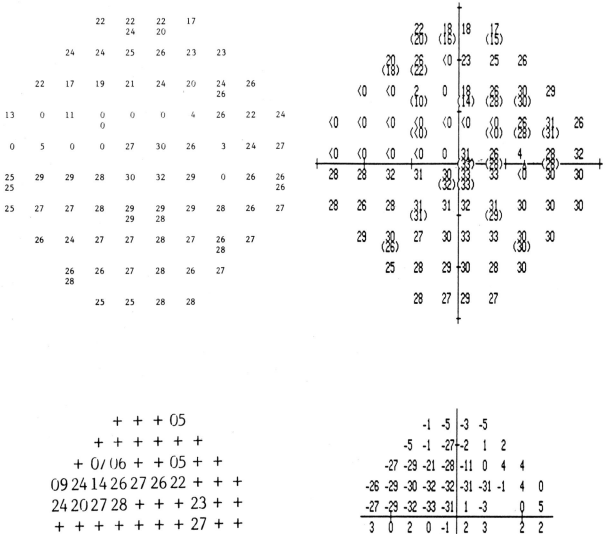

FIG. 9-24. Apparent Progression Shown Between Octopus Program 32 in 1987 *(left)* **and Humphrey 30-2 Full Threshold Test in 1991** *(right).* The upper panels show the actual threshold values and the lower panels show the difference from normal values (positive integers signify reduced sensitivity for the Octopus; negative integers signify the same for the Humphrey. In most areas there is no deterioration and the Humphrey numeric values are the expected 2 to 3 dB higher than the Octopus values. However, points in the third row and one point in the fourth row above the horizontal meridian do not match. The absolute arcuate scotoma seems to have widened. As always the final judgment depends on comparing a baseline of two or more fields with more than one follow-up field. Such replicate information was available and confirmed the change in this case.

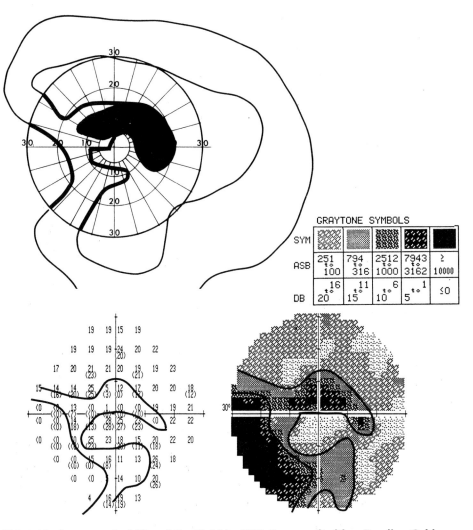

FIG. 9-25. Apparent Stability of the Field in 1991 Compared with a Baseline Goldmann Kinetic Examination in 1986. The Goldmann isopters plotted were III-3e (equivalent to the size-III, 15-dB stimulus of the Humphrey Field Analyzer) and IV-4e (approximately equivalent to a 6- or 7-dB size-III stimulus of the Humphrey Field Analyzer). On the greyscale plot of the Humphrey field examination, the 0-dB and 15-dB isopters have been drawn in. The 15-dB isopter is the boundary between the 11- to 15-dB grey level and the 16- to 20-dB grey level and is equivalent to the Goldmann III-3e.

CONCLUSION

From several printouts of visual field data, the statistical analyses constitute but one element in the determination of glaucomatous progression; not every statistically significant change represents progression of glaucoma. Not every case of continued glaucomatous damage is manifest by recognizable or verifiable visual field change. The data displays and statistical analyses serve at least three purposes: (1) to call attention to subtle changes that might otherwise be overlooked; (2) to give confidence that small, suspicious changes are real; and (3) to show in some cases that an impressive change is nonetheless within a statistically expected range of variability, given the starting condition, and therefore ought be discounted—at least temporarily.

Even with such help, the clinician uses intuitive criteria about how many points in what kind of location and grouping would constitute reasonably certain evidence of disease progression. The criteria may be chosen partly based on how small a degree (or rate) of progression one is anxious to detect, or is willing to overlook for the time being. Whatever criteria are selected to be worthy of attention, there are bound to be examinations that falsely suggest progression and make a confirming examination necessary.

Criteria may vary. It is common sense to accept minor changes in visual threshold when progression is suspected on the basis of other clinical information, but to demand firmer numeric evidence when other clinical evidence suggests the condition is stable. The chance that a new defect might be real is influenced by the clinical setting; for example, the change is likely genuine if there is simultaneously a disc hemorrhage, enlargement of the optic nerve head excavation, or uncertain control of the IOP. In the absence of such reasons to suspect progression, a false result may be suspected, especially if there is evidence of fatigue or artifact; the clinician constantly must be alert to other diseases that may arise and produce a new defect.

It is statistically sound to use such clinical judgment; the other clinical findings represent the *a priori* probability of progression. Sometimes it is sound to accept that there may be residual uncertainty. In such cases, the passage of time may best determine whether a test result represents an emerging minimal change just peeking through or is a transient fluctuation. Clinical findings also indicate the *cause* of statistically significant changes—whether they are caused by glaucoma, artifact, or another concurrent disease.

Finally, the most relevant clinical question usually is not whether vision is deteriorating but at what rate increments of visual loss are occurring. More to the point, a projected future course and final outcome might be estimated, given the patient's longest reasonable life expectancy (not the patient's *average* life expectancy). Experienced clinicians take this into account, but only informally, because a meaningful measure of satisfactory vision has not been developed. Rate is presently represented, but only crudely, by the slope of MD loss in decibels per year. Such measures—if we only knew how to translate them into symptoms and function—are as important as whether the decline is real (i.e., statistically significant). Perhaps the future will bring us measures and criteria more pertinent to visual contentment and means to quantify the rate or risk of its ultimate loss.

Rate of visual loss also can help determine when the next field examination should be conducted. If the finding of progression over 5 years is uncertain, it means that the rate is small if not zero. A prompt reexamination of the visual field may help decide whether it is small or zero, but need be undertaken only if a slow, genuine deterioration would alter clinical management. However, if a case has been monitored for a short time, an apparent rate of deterioration, even if not statistically different from zero, is at risk of being over- or underestimated; testing inherently is variable and only a short interval separates the tests. Recognizing the uncertainty of the present estimation of the rate of change, the wise clinician obtains an examination at a time that would reveal the worst rate estimate from available data, expecting that on the average the rate would be better than the worst estimate but knowing that sometimes the worst estimate will turn out to be correct.

REFERENCES

1. Johnson CA, Cioffi GA, Drance SM et al: A multicenter comparison study of the Humphrey Field Analyzer I and the Humphrey Field Analyzer II, *Ophthalmology* 104:1910-1917, 1997.
2. Mikelberg FS, Drance SM: The mode of progression of visual field defects in glaucoma, *Am J Ophthalmol* 98:443-445, 1984.
3. Mikelberg FS, Schulzer M, Drance SM, Lau W: The rate of progression of scotomas in glaucoma, *Am J Ophthalmol* 101:1-6, 1986.
4. Bebie H, Flammer J, Bebie TH: The cumulative defect curve: Separation of local and diffuse components of visual field damage, *Graefes Arch Clin Exp Ophthalmol* 227:9-12, 1989.
5. Bebie H: Computer-assisted evaluation of visual fields, *Graefes Arch Clin Exp Ophthalmol* 228:242-245, 1990.
6. Asman P, Olsson J: Physiology of cumulative defect curves: Consequences in glaucoma perimetry, *Acta Ophthalmol Scand* 73:197-201, 1995.
7. Chauhan BC, Drance SM, Douglas GR: The use of visual field indices in detecting changes in the visual field in glaucoma, *Invest Ophthalmol Vis Sci* 31:512-520, 1990.
8. Pearson PA, Baltwin LB, Smith TJ: The relationship of mean defect to corrected loss variance in glaucoma and ocular hypertension, *Ophthalmologica* 200:16-21, 1990.
9. Heijl A, Lindgren A, Lindgren G: Test-retest variability in glaucomatous visual fields, *Am J Ophthalmol* 108:130-135, 1989.
10. Holmin C, Krakau CET: Variability of glaucomatous visual field defects in computerized perimetry, *Graefes Arch Clin Exp Ophthalmol* 210:235-250, 1979.
11. Werner EB, Petrig B, Krupin T, Bishop KI: Variability of automated visual fields in clinically stable glaucoma patients, *Invest Ophthalmol Vis Sci* 30:1083-1089, 1989.
12. Heijl A, Lindgren G, Lindgren A et al: Extended empirical statistical package for evaluation of single and multiple field in glaucoma: Statpac 2. In Mills RP, Heijl A, editors: *Perimetry update 1990/91*, p 303, New York, 1991, Kugler Publications.
13. Heijl A, Lindgren A, Lindgren G: Reply, *Am J Ophthalmol* 109:110, 1990.
14. Morgan RK, Feuer WJ, Anderson DR: Statpac 2 glaucoma change probability, *Arch Ophthalmol* 109:1690-1692, 1991.
15. Bengtsson B, Lindgren A, Heijl A et al: Perimetric probability maps to separate change caused by glaucoma from that caused by cataract, *Acta Ophthalmologica Scand* 75:184-188, 1997.
16. Heijl A: The Humphrey Field Analyzer: Concepts and clinical results, *Doc Ophthalmol Proc Ser* 43:55-64, 1985.
17. Araujo ML, Feuer WJ, Anderson DR: Evaluation of baseline-related suprathreshold testing for quick determination of visual field nonprogression, *Arch Ophthalmol* 111:365-369, 1993.
18. Heijl, A: Time changes of contrast thresholds during automatic perimetry, *Acta Ophthalmol* (KBH) 55:696-708, 1977.
19. Heijl A, Drance SM: Changes in differential threshold in patients with glaucoma during prolonged perimetry, *Br J Ophthalmol* 67:512-516, 1983.

20. The Advanced Glaucoma Intervention Study Investigators: Advanced glaucoma intervention study. II. Visual field test scoring and reliability, *Ophthalmology* 101:1445-1455, 1994.

21. Henson D, Spenceley S, Bull D: Package for the spatial classification of glaucomatous field defects. In Wall M, Heijl A, editors: *Perimetry update 1996/1997. Proceedings of the XIIth International Perimetric Society Meeting, 1996,* p 289, Amsterdam/New York, 1997, Kugler Publications.

22. Schulzer M, The Normal-Tension Glaucoma Study Group: Errors in the diagnosis of visual field progression in normal-tension glaucoma, *Ophthalmology* 101:1589-1595, 1994.

23. Heuer DK, Anderson DR, Feuer WJ, Gressel MG: The influence of refraction accuracy on automated perimetric threshold measurements, *Ophthalmology* 94:1550-1553, 1987.

24. Heuer DK, Anderson DR, Feuer WJ, Gressel MG: The influence of decreased retinal illumination on automatic perimetric threshold, *Am J Ophthalmol* 108;643-650, 1989.

25. Heuer DK, Anderson DR, Knighton RW et al: The influence of simulated light scattering on automated perimetric threshold measurements, *Arch Ophthalmol* 106:1247-1251, 1988.

26. Dengler-Harles M, Wild JM, Searle AET, Crews SJ: The relationship between backward and forward intraocular light scatter. In Mills RP, Heijl A, editors: *Perimetry update 1990/91, Proceedings of the Ixth International Perimetric Society Meeting, 1990,* pp 577-582, Amsterdam/New York, 1990, Kugler Publications.

27. Budenz DL, Feuer WJ, Anderson DR: The effect of simulated cataract on the glaucomatous visual field, *Ophthalmology* 100:511-517, 1993.

28. Lam BL, Alward WLM, Kolder HE: Effect of cataract on automated perimetry, *Ophthalmology* 98:1066-1070, 1991.

29. Stewart WC, Rogers GM, Crinkley CMC, Carlson AN: Effect of cataract extraction on automated fields in chronic open-angle glaucoma, *Arch Ophthalmol* 113:875-879, 1995.

30. Smith SD, Katz J, Quigley H: Effect of cataract extraction on the results of automated perimetry in glaucoma, *Arch Ophthalmol* 115:1515-1519, 1997.

31. Chen P, Budenz DL: Effect of cataract extraction on the glaucomatous visual field, *Am J Ophthalmol* 125:325-333, 1998.

32. Åsman P, Bengtsson B, Heijl A: Linear regression analysis in glaucoma: Separation of local and diffuse visual field deterioration, *Invest Ophthalmol Vis Sci* 36(4):S170, 1995.

33. Heijl A, Bengtsson B: The effect of perimetric experience in patients with glaucoma, *Arch Ophthalmol* 114:19-22, 1996.

34. Wild JM, Dengler-Harles M, Searle AE et al: The influence of the learning effect on automated perimetry in patients with suspected glaucoma, *Acta Ophthalmol (Copenh)* 69:210-216, 1991.

35. Lindenmuth KA, Skuta GL, Rabbani R, Musch DC: Effects of pupillary constriction on automated perimetry in normal eyes, *Ophthalmology* 96:1298-1301, 1989.

36. Lindenmuth KA, Skuta GL, Rabbani R et al: Effects of pupillary dilation on automated perimetry in normal patients, *Ophthalmology* 97:367-370, 1990.

CHAPTER 10

Alternate and supplemental techniques*

    A number of methods have been used to test visual function throughout the visual field (e.g., to test visual function away from the point of fixation). This chapter presents an overview of the techniques commonly used. Some techniques have features that make them particularly more suitable for specific clinical purposes. Every practitioner should have several methods available to use in different clinical situations.

---

*Drawings in this chapter are by Leona M. Allison.

AMSLER GRID

The Amsler grid is a method of testing the inner 10 degrees of the central visual field.[1,2] The standard chart consists of a grid of white lines on black paper. The size of each square is 5 mm, which occupies 1 degree of the field when held at a reading distance of 28 to 30 cm. The complete set of Amsler grids has six other patterns useful in special situations in which the standard chart does not suffice.* The patient is asked to look at a fixation point in the center of a grid of squares and describe the areas where the lines are either missing or distorted. It is a qualitative test but one that is quite useful in detecting central or paracentral scotomas and areas where the vision is distorted even if there is no reduction in light sensitivity. Distortion (as opposed to absence) of the grid squares, called metamorphopsia, suggests a retinal lesion. Central or paracentral scotomas may be caused by macular disease or an optic nerve lesion.

Because of its ease, rapidity, and sensitivity the Amsler grid is useful in settings in which the clinician does not want quantitative information but simply wants to know quickly and accurately whether a central scotoma is present.

---

*For more details on the Amsler grid, consult Amsler.[1,2]

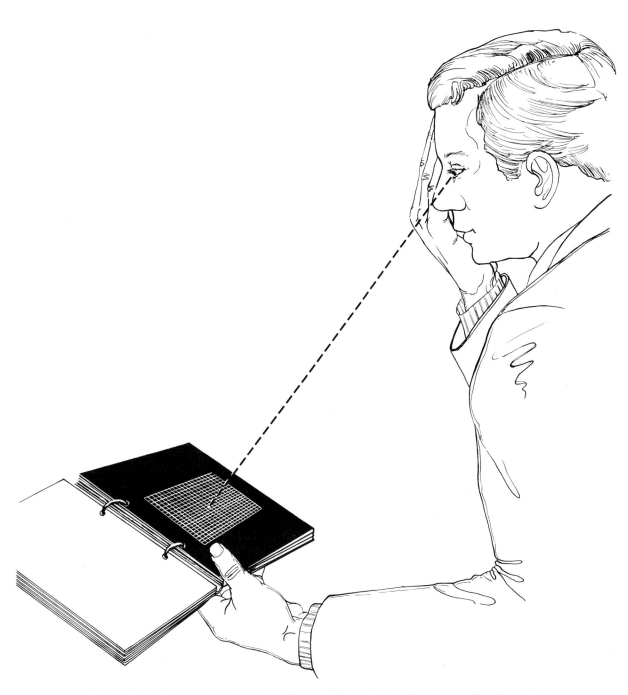

FIG. 10-1. The Standard Amsler Grid. The patient is asked whether he sees the white dot at the center. While the patient continues to stare at the dot, he is asked whether all four corners of the grid are visible, whether there are absent areas in the pattern, and whether the squares are distorted or blurred.

CONFRONTATION TECHNIQUES

Confrontation techniques for evaluating the visual field can be useful in a variety of situations:

1. To screen for the presence of unsuspected field defects as part of a routine eye examination that would not ordinarily include formal field testing (we include a quick confrontation finger-counting field in every complete eye examination but of course do not perform formal perimetry on every patient);
2. To educate the patient about field testing before performing perimetry (see Instructing the Patient about the Test, Chapter 11);
3. To determine approximately the type and extent of a field defect to be expected on perimetry;
4. To confirm or deny perimetric findings (e.g., extreme contraction of the field detectable by perimetry may or may not be present on confrontation and the perimetry may be wrong; likewise, confrontation comparison tests may either suggest a hemianopia not discovered by perimetry or confirm the perimetric findings); and
5. As the only type of field examination that is feasible for some patients. (The examiner should not underestimate the amount of valuable information obtainable by a careful confrontation method, even for patients who cannot perform well on the perimeter.)

The basic confrontation techniques to be described in the following pages are the finger-counting method and the comparison method.

Finger-counting method of screening

The finger-counting method of screening originally was described by Welsh.[3] As with most field testing, each eye is tested separately. The patient should use the palm, not the fingers, to occlude the other eye. The palm is used to ensure that the patient does not peek between fingers and does not exert pressure on the covered eye, which would cause residual blurring of vision and make subsequent testing of this eye difficult. There should be no glare; the examiner's back ideally should be toward a blank, evenly illuminated wall without windows or other bright sources of light.

The patient is asked to fixate on the examiner's face (traditionally the nose) and to report how many fingers the examiner holds up in the peripheral field. Each quadrant is tested separately by placing the hand 3 or 4 feet away from the patient, approximately 45 degrees from fixation. A person with a normal pupil size and without opacity in the media or other visual abnormality should be able to count fingers 3 to 4 feet away at 45 degrees if the visual field is normal.

The examiner can hold up either one finger or two and the patient can report how many fingers he sees. The examiner also can present four fingers or a whole hand so that the patient has a choice of one, two, or all. A closed fist (no fingers) also can be used. Three fingers never should be used because three is exceedingly difficult to differentiate from two or four.

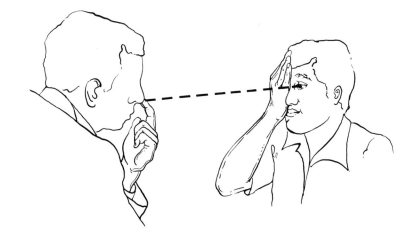

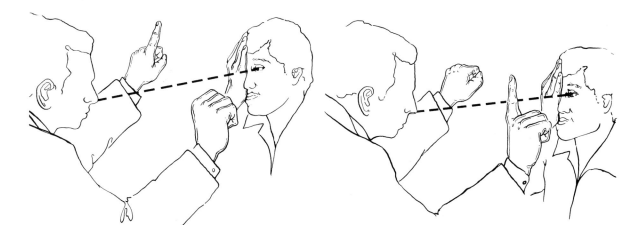

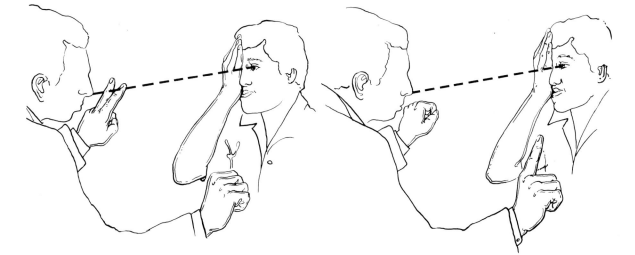

FIG. 10-2. Finger-Counting Confrontation Field.

The clinician can hold up both fists in a manner that will not allow the patient to tell which hand will be used, especially if the patient is having trouble fixating. Next, one, two, or four fingers of one hand or the other can be elevated and lowered again before the patient shifts his fixation to look directly at them.

Finger-counting method: quantitation

If the fingers cannot be counted in a given quadrant at 45 degrees, two maneuvers, shown in Figure 10-3, are helpful.

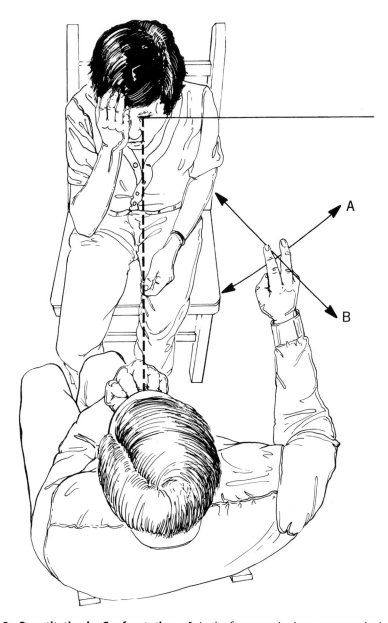

FIG. 10-3. Quantitation by Confrontation. A, In the first quantitative maneuver the hand with upheld fingers can be moved transversely in an arc toward fixation, remaining 2 to 3 feet from the patient. The procedure resembles kinetic perimetry, and the idea is to determine how close to fixation the hand must be before the fingers can be counted. Similar to the technique used when plotting an isopter, the direction of movement need not be toward fixation. If, for example, there is a marked difference between two quadrants, it may be possible to confirm dramatically the presence of a hemianopia or a nasal step if the patient is suddenly able to count the fingers as the hand crosses the vertical meridian or the horizontal meridian nasally. **B,** In the second quantification maneuver the hand is moved toward the patient, along the line 45 degrees from fixation, until the fingers can be counted (or beginning from 6 feet away and moved backward until the fingers cannot be counted), and the minimum closeness required to count fingers is compared among the four quadrants. This maneuver resembles static perimetry. In the segments of the field where fingers cannot be counted, whether the patient can distinguish wiggling fingers from fingers held still should be determined. If the patient cannot make that distinction, it should be determined whether with correct projection he can detect the presence or absence of a light. This will help make the distinction between a severe depression and a contraction of the field, which is an absolute defect.

When visual sensation is so poor that the clinician is looking for the presence or absence of light perception in different areas of the field, it is important to note whether the patient can determine accurately where the light is located; only then can the examiner be certain that this area of the field is intact to light perception. Suppose, for example, that a patient has a contracted field with only a temporal island of vision remaining from glaucoma and also has a cataract (which diffuses light within the eye). When a light is placed in the nasal field, the patient may be able to state correctly that the light is on as a result of scatter of the light by the cataract onto the seeing retina. The patient also may determine either that he sees light temporally or sees the light but is not sure where it is located. However, with the light on the temporal side, the patient may be able to recognize where the light is located and report that he sees it more brightly than when the light was on the nasal side.

Sometimes it is quite striking that, as the light is moved, the patient suddenly can localize the light accurately, letting the clinician know that he has crossed the boundary into the seeing portion of the field. It may be encouraging when a patient with cataract and glaucoma can project light not only on the temporal side but in a region around fixation as well, even though he cannot accurately localize light seen in the nasal quadrant. The finding of accurate projection around fixation suggests that there is an intact central island of vision, perhaps with the potential of good acuity when a cataract is removed. The outlook is not so good if accurate light projection exists only in the temporal field, or if the patient reports that the light is dimmer at fixation than it is in the temporal field.

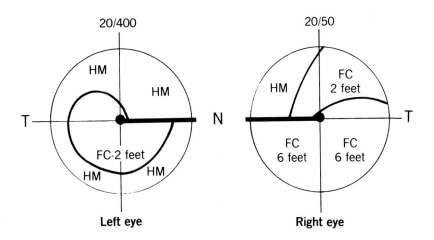

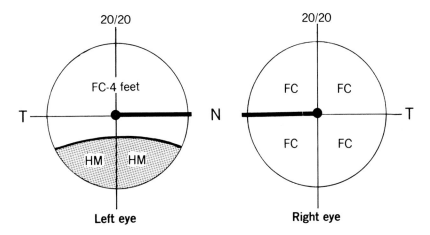

FIG. 10-4. Diagram of Hypothetical Visual Fields by Confrontation. In the first example, as might occur in a patient with both glaucoma and cataract, generalized depression and reduced acuity are seen, especially in the left eye. A localized depression also is noted in the upper nasal quadrant. In the second example, as might occur in the presence of retinal detachment, there is very localized visual loss. *HM*, Region where vision is limited to the detection of hand movements; *FC*, region where fingers can be counted at the indicated distance.

Diagramming confrontation fields

The conventional method of diagramming all visual fields is "as the patient sees it" (i.e., the right eye to the right; the left eye to the left; the nasal side of the field toward the center; and the temporal side toward the edge). This diagramming is easy to accomplish with a technique such as the tangent screen and the perimeter; however, with confrontation methods the examiner must invert right and left from his perspective so that it is finalized on the paper "as the patient sees it." In so doing, it is a good idea to label the diagram with an "N" between the two eyes and a "T" on the two edges, marking the right and left eyes so that there is no ambiguity. This is particularly important because some experienced individuals intentionally diagram their confrontation findings in the unconventional manner, "as the examiner sees it."

Considerable qualitative and even semi-quantitative information can be obtained from a carefully performed finger-counting confrontation field with quantification of abnormal areas. With care, the examiner may be able to determine whether there is a central scotoma or whether a patient with glaucoma has a central island of vision remaining or only a temporal island. This can be determined even when the vision is so poor (because of cataracts) or fixation is so poor (because of reduced vision) that an adequate examination with a perimeter cannot be accomplished. For such occasions, the clinician must be experienced in performing confrontation fields.

It also is useful to perform confrontation field testing routinely in conjunction with perimetry to confirm or deny the perimetric findings when there may be a fault in perimetric technique, as well as to learn through experience how to perform a better perimetric examination. If, for example, the confrontation technique does not reveal a defect and the perimetric examination shows a reasonably dense defect in one quadrant, the confrontation field should be repeated, both to corroborate the presence of a defect and to learn why the defect was missed initially by confrontation. With such experience, the routine use of confrontation fields with patients seen in the office becomes a quick but reasonably accurate technique.

Confrontation fields are useful on every patient, either to screen for abnormality or to confirm defects found on perimetry.

Comparison techniques

With each of the techniques previously described, the patient should be asked whether he is able to see a certain stimulus (e.g., a light or wiggling fingers). Even with the finger-counting technique, the examiner is basically asking whether the patient is able to see the fingers; asking the patient to state how many fingers are up simply confirms that he can see them.

With a comparison technique, the patient is asked to perform a fundamentally different task: to compare a stimulus in two locations and to state whether they are the same or different. The usefulness of the technique depends on the fact that if visual sensation is reduced because of a change in visual threshold, all stimuli are subjectively less bright in that region (see Chapter 2).

For many individuals it seems easier to appreciate differences in color saturation than to distinguish differences in brightness; thus, a colored object often is used in comparison testing by confrontation. A red object, for example, may seem maroon to the right and bright red to the left of fixation. To detect this difference, the examiner may use a red object of reasonable size, one-half to 2 inches in diameter (such as the cap from a cycloplegic bottle), have the patient fixate on the examiner's nose, and ask him or her whether the red object has the exact same color 3 to 6 inches to the right of fixation as it does 3 to 6 inches to the left. This can be done somewhat above fixation and again somewhat below fixation.

The clinician should place the greatest emphasis on the patient's first response. The color difference should be instantly obvious to the patient. If he has to think about it, the patient may be reporting some subtle lighting difference or other phenomenon, and thus the test is unreliable.

The patient can be asked to compare the two sides with the red object shown in sequence, as seen in Figure 10-5, or two red objects can be held up simultaneously, one on each side.

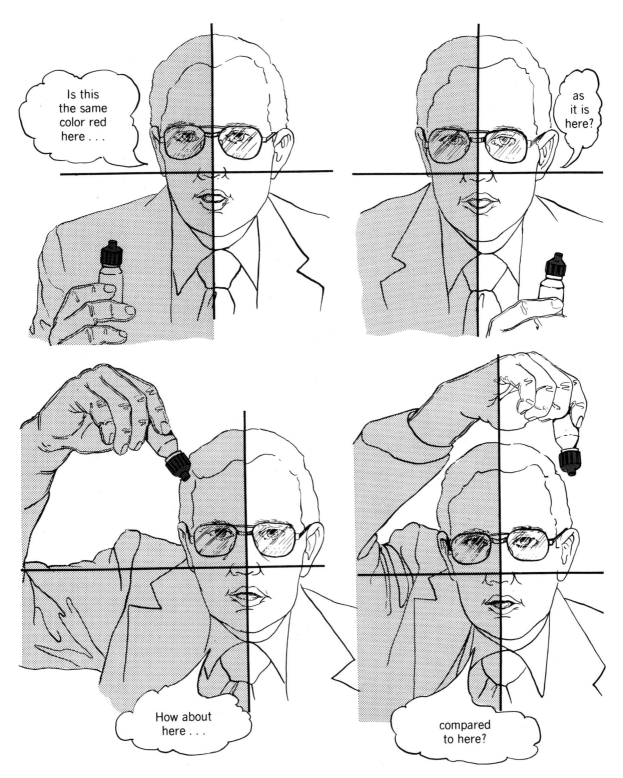

FIG. 10-5. Searching for Quadrant Differences in Color Saturation.

In experienced hands, comparison by confrontation can be exquisitely accurate for hemianopias and central scotomas.

If the patient reports that the color is different (or, to confirm in the clinician's mind that there is no difference), the object should be moved horizontally and the patient should be asked to state when it changes color as the object is moved across the vertical midline above fixation and then repeated below fixation (Fig. 10-6).

Comparison tests are good because they are quite sensitive in detecting hemianopias: if an alert patient is certain that there is no difference in visibility on the two sides of the vertical meridian, it is unlikely that a hemianopia is present. Conversely, a convincing difference of visibility across the vertical meridian is rather specific evidence that a hemianopia is indeed present.

Because important neurosurgical diagnostic decisions may be based in part on the field examination, it is usual to have corroborating evidence of a hemianopia by one of the other methods of field testing, especially if the patient responded with uncertainty when tested by confrontation comparison methods. Nonetheless, the color comparison by confrontation is so accurate, despite its simplicity, that it may be used routinely both to detect a hemianopia and to double-check the findings of other perimetric methods.* These may be clinical circumstances in which other clinical tests already establish a diagnosis and confirmation of a field defect is sufficient without formal perimetry.

The practice of having the patient compare the two sides of the vertical meridian also can be used to compare the clarity with which the patient can see two palms held on the two sides of fixation. He may be able to report that the two palms seem different after being asked whether they appear equally bright and equally distant.

Comparison methods also can be used to check for central scotomas (Fig. 10-7). The patient may find that the red object has a duller color at fixation than it does to the side. In a normal field, color, brightness, and acuity are greatest at fixation.

---

*Additional information about confrontation testing can be found in Frisen[4] and Glaser.[5]

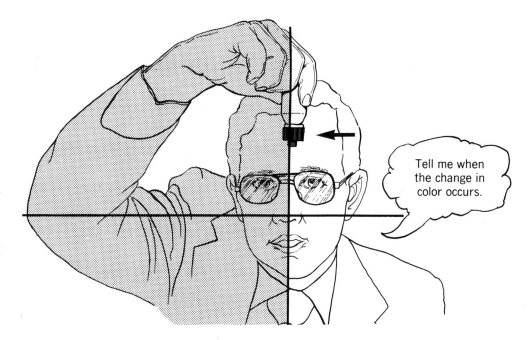

FIG. 10-6. Confirming a Hemianopia. If the patient reports that the object changes color exactly at the vertical midline, there is strong evidence that a hemianopia is present. A definite absence of color difference is strong evidence that there is no hemianopia. This test is so sensitive that it should be performed whenever a visual field examination is conducted in search of a hemianopia, even if the perimetric or tangent screen examination has not revealed a hemianopia. If a hemianopia is not revealed by perimetry but is found by a color comparison test, the perimetric testing should be performed again.

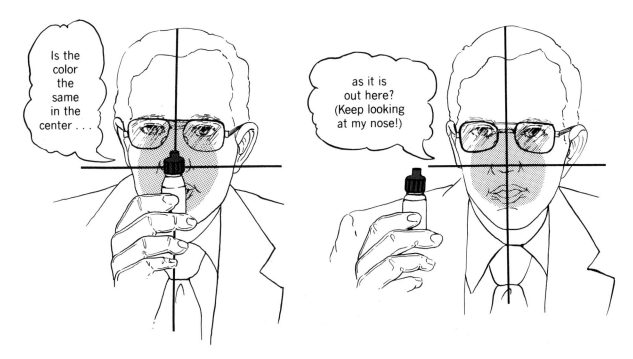

FIG. 10-7. Checking for a Central Scotoma by Color Comparison Techniques. A central scotoma is present if the patient reports that the color is brighter away from fixation than at fixation.

315

REFERENCES

1. Amsler M: L'Examen qualitatif de la fonction maculaire, *Ophthalmologica* 114:248-261, 1947.
2. Amsler M: Quantitative and qualitative vision, *Trans Ophthalmol Soc UK* 69:397-410, 1949.
3. Welsh RC: Finger counting in the four quadrants as a method of visual field gross screening, *Arch Ophthalmol* 66:678-679, 1961.
4. Frisén L: A versatile color confrontation test for the central visual field: A comparison with quantitative perimetry, *Arch Ophthalmol* 89:3-9, 1973.
5. Glaser JS, editor: *Neuro-Ophthalmology,* p 25, ed 2, Philadelphia, 1990, JB Lippincott.

CHAPTER 11

Administering the visual field test

PATIENT'S PERCEPTION OF THE TEST

Automated static threshold perimetry is a different experience for the patient from kinetic perimetry, for example with a Goldmann perimeter. It is not just that the automated static test is longer, and not just that the stimulus is moving in kinetic perimetry whereas it is stationary in static perimetry. Patients also have the perception in static perimetry that everything is dimmer, that it is more difficult, and that somehow it is more stressful.

To understand this, consider the patient's perception during kinetic perimetry. A stimulus comes in from the side. There comes a time when the patient suspects that he sees something, but it is dim and he is not sure. He doesn't push the button yet, and the stimulus continues to move in. As it moves in closer to the fovea it becomes more easily visible. The perception is that it becomes brighter, so that he is more certain he sees it. (Brightness is a subjective sensation. In fact, the light did not change its intensity at all.) A point occurs when he is absolutely convinced he sees the stimulus, so he pushes the button. After he has responded, the light goes off and he waits for another.

Contrast that experience with the perception of the static stimulus with automated perimetry. A certain intensity is presented as a brief flash for one-fifth of a second. The patient may think he sees it, but is not quite sure. The stimulus does not progressively become brighter until he is certain, but he must decide about the stimuli that are barely visible and uncertain. When he reports that the lights are much dimmer on this automated perimeter, he means that there are some presentations that he thinks he saw, but he didn't have a chance to confirm it in his mind by waiting for it to become brighter.

Another difference is that the light never goes off in kinetic perimetry until the patient pushes the button. The stimulus moves in and stays on until he pushes the button. Only then does the light go off. The perimetrist moves the light to another position, and the process starts again. To the patient the test consists of this sequence: the light comes on, it gets brighter, he pushes the button, the light goes off,

The patient should understand what is expected: *after* he sees a brief stimulus, he should respond promptly but not in haste.

and then he waits for another visible stimulus. With the automated perimeter, the light goes on, it stays on for 0.2 second, and it goes off, whether or not he sees it and responds. If he did see it, it goes off before he has a chance to respond. That short stimulus may give the patient the sense that he has missed his chance to respond, especially if he previously underwent kinetic perimetry and always responded while the light was still on. Because the light went off, he may have the feeling that now he shouldn't push the button, because it's too late. He may wait for the next one, and now may try to respond too quickly, sometimes pushing the button when there was no stimulus (false-positive response).

Once the examiner considers the patient's experience, it is easier to give instructions. If the patient has undergone kinetic perimetry before, for example with the Goldmann perimeter, the instruction may be: "You have had a field examination before, but we are now using a new instrument. You need to understand a couple of things about it. First, the stimulus will not be moving. Second, it might be dim and stay on only for a flash. You have to be sure you see it. Don't respond if you are not sure, but if you are sure it was there, go ahead and push the button. You can take your time to be sure you saw it, because you don't have to push the button while the light is still on. The machine will present the stimulus as a flash, and then wait for a second or two for you to respond. You can push the button any time after the flash, at a comfortable speed."

The patient should be told that the machine will adjust its pace according to his own actual response time. If the examiner notices that the patient is making false-positive responses, the patient should be reminded to "slow down, the machine will wait for your response. Be sure you see it before you respond." Some patients also may feel rushed because the stimulus seems to come too quickly after they push the button (or, more accurately, after they release the button).

For patients who find the test too rapid in this second sense, there is a Slow Mode, which can be selected from the change parameter option on the menu. It increases the length of time before the next stimulus is presented, so that the patient has a chance to breathe; but it very rarely is used. If the machine is put in the Slow Mode for a person who is a quick responder, he will get bored because there is too much time between stimuli. Moreover, the test takes longer—thus, the Slow Mode should not be used indiscriminately. The Slow Mode also should not be used if the patient feels the test is too fast because he believes he must respond while the light is still on. To apply the appropriate solution, the perimetrist must determine what the patient means when he senses the test is proceeding too quickly.

PERIMETRIST'S TASK

The patient should be greeted warmly, not only because the perimetrist should reflect a caring attitude on behalf of the clinical office but also to set the patient at ease for the upcoming task. Many patients have learned to hate perimetry. It is in fact a demanding task for them, requiring attentiveness and an effort to give the "correct answer," perhaps unconsciously recreating the stress experienced in earlier days when taking a school examination. Patients must know that the "field

The perimetrist's job is to enhance the patient's ability to respond accurately.

test" is not a test of their intellectual, artistic, or physical abilities, but is a determination of their visual function in the sense of a medical test. Only the patient can say what he can or cannot see, therefore the technician's task goes beyond sitting the patient at the perimeter and turning on the machine. The perimetrist must enhance the ability of the patient to report accurately which stimuli are seen. This includes placing the patient at ease, making him physically comfortable in position at the perimeter, and ensuring that he understands the task.

With a kindly and encouraging perimetrist, most of the hateful elements of perimetry disappear, except that the patient must concentrate on the task for its duration.

INSTRUCTING THE PATIENT ABOUT THE TEST

Preliminary confrontation testing achieves two purposes.

The patient must understand that the test asks him to report what he sees peripherally while his gaze is fixed straight ahead. Sometimes all that is needed is an explicit instruction to look straight ahead at the fixation target and push the button when a light is seen anywhere within the field of view. Especially for a patient who has not experienced field testing before, it is helpful to begin with a confrontation test (see Chapter 10), in which the patient practices reporting what is seen with his peripheral vision (Fig. 11-1). At the same time, the examiner receives clues about any major field defect that may be present. This information is helpful in deciding which eye to test first at the perimeter and in selecting appropriate tests to use on an automated perimeter.

FIG. 11-1. Educating the Patient by Confrontation Testing. Initially it does not matter whether the patient has one eye covered or not. The patient can be asked to look at the examiner's nose. Holding up his arms 1 foot to each side of the line of sight, the examiner can instruct the patient to say which hand is wiggling. The patient cannot look at both hands while waiting to see which one moves; he can look only at one point of fixation (the examiner's nose) and describe what is happening at the sides without actually looking. Next, the examiner can have the patient cover one eye (if this has not already been done) and ask him to count fingers in the four quadrants (see Chapter 10) until the patient seems able to hold fixation and report what is seen and until the examiner can estimate how severe any existing field defect may be.

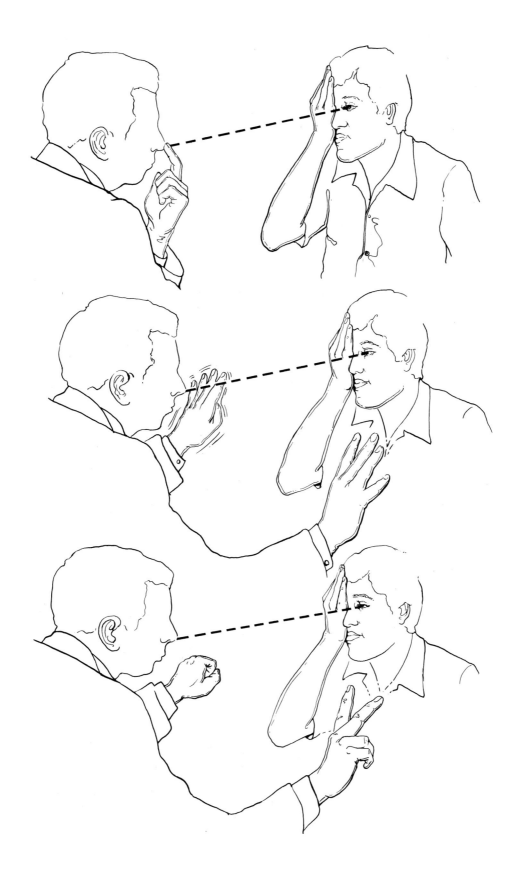

After the demonstration by confrontation, additional instruction usually can be brief because the patient usually understands immediately the nature of the test at the perimeter. Before actually starting the test, the examiner can use the "demo" function to present two or three stimuli and be sure that the patient is responding correctly. The examiner may wish to explain that the patient can pause the test by holding the button down when giving a response, and that the test will not continue until he has released the button. Tell the patient that he should tell the examiner whether the test is going too fast. Then the examiner can evaluate if the complaint is that the next stimulus comes too soon and use the Slow Mode, as appropriate. Usually, however, the patient simply needs reassurance that he isn't expected to respond immediately but should simply make prompt, but not hasty, responses.

In summary, special instructions are needed for automated perimetry, especially if the patient has undergone manual perimetry previously. The patient must be told that in automated perimetry the light will be a brief flash, after which there will be an interval when the machine waits for a response. The patient needs to know that it is all right to respond after the light goes off and that he should not feel frustrated or inadequate upon realizing that it is impossible to respond while the light is still on. The machine will wait a short time for a reasoned response. Thus, after the flash, the patient should answer quickly, but not so quickly as to respond in error. The patient also should be told that most stimuli will be quite dim, and in fact more than half of the stimulus presentations will be too dim to see. He should be told to respond to the presentations that are seen, but only when the patient is sure, because there may be times when the machine will pretend to present stimuli (catch trials). Finally, the patient also should be told to do his best, but not to worry about occasional mistakes.

POSITIONING THE PATIENT AT THE PERIMETER

Alignment of the eye is important.

It is best to test a patient's better seeing eye first, especially if the patient has not undergone perimetry before. The perimetrist can learn from the patient's history, by testing visual acuity, or from the confrontation field test which eye is better. When neither eye is drastically worse, the right eye traditionally is tested first.

The eye not being tested is covered. For comfort and to avoid pressure, the patch ideally should form a slightly concave cup over the eye and allow the eye to be open beneath it. An eye pad taped over the closed eye or a patch that puts pressure on the eye should be avoided. If it is necessary to close the eye with a pad and tape, it should not be tight. The edge of the patch should fit the face snugly to prevent the covered eye from seeing stimuli in the peripheral field.

Goldmann advocated the use of a white translucent cover that maintains light adaptation of the covered eye (which is tested next). However, it is now recognized that if an opaque patch is used, the eye light-adapts quickly when uncovered, so a black or white opaque patch is more commonly used. Because of retinal rivalry of the bright background from the uncovered eye and the darkness in the eye covered with an opaque patch, the patient may complain that the background seems to fade in and out. This is natural, and the patient should be reassured that it is a normal phenomenon that will not affect the test result.

The eye to be tested is centered squarely in front of the trial lens holder. The face may be turned slightly to the left when testing the right eye, and slightly to the right when testing the left eye, so that the nose does not obstruct the nasal periphery of the field.

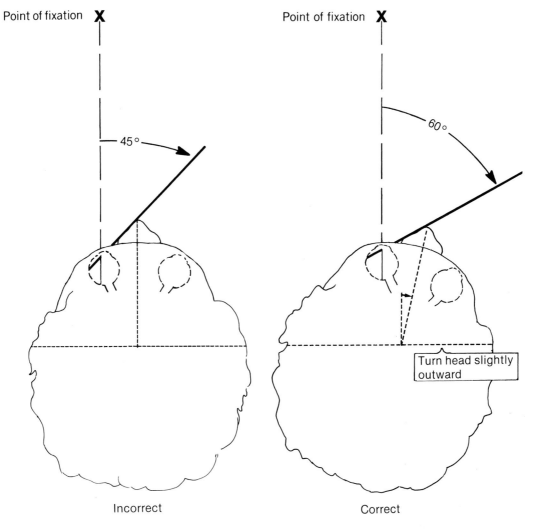

Point of fixation **X**   45°   Incorrect

Point of fixation **X**   60°   Turn head slightly outward   Correct

FIG. 11-2. Face Turn During Perimetry. The turn should be very slight. A straight-ahead position usually is quite acceptable. The main reason for a slight turn away from the eye being tested is to ensure that the face does not shade the peripheral field if the head drifts slightly during the test. Remember: the patient may be uncomfortable if the head position is awkward.

Similarly, the chin should be positioned so that the plane of the face is directed straight ahead or slightly upward (thus putting the eye in slight down gaze to see the fixation target) to reduce interference from the eyebrows and upper eyelids. The side turn and upward tilt of the face should be slight, neither exaggerated nor uncomfortable. A modest downward and temporal gaze position is preferred only to ensure that the eye is not in nasal or upgaze position, which would cause facial structures to shade the peripheral field.

FIG. 11-3. Effect of Tilting the Face. If the patient's face is tilted forward (forehead against the rest but chin not fully forward), the eye will be in slight upward gaze when looking at the point of fixation. The patient's eyelid and eyebrow may interfere with the upper portion of the visual field. However, with his face straight, or perhaps slightly tilted backward (chin forward), interference from the eyelid and eyebrow is reduced. These greyscales are from an automated static threshold test performed on one of the authors, with his head in the correct and incorrect positions. There is no ptosis of the eyelid, only an incorrect head position.

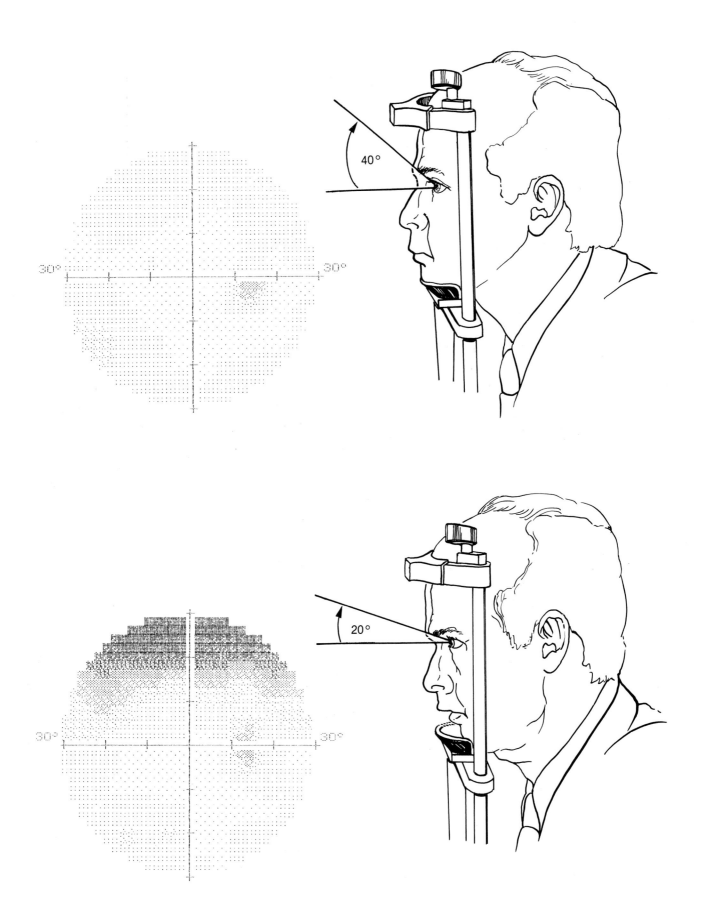

Care in positioning the head also overcomes the additional problem that with improper downward tilt of the head, the correcting lens cannot be positioned close to the eye. The upper edge may touch the eyebrow, but the lower edge will be distant from the cheek and block some of the inferior visual field. Thus the upper edge of the field is shaded by the eyebrow, and the lower edge is shaded by the correcting lens (and the lens holder).

The height of the instrument must be adjusted so that the patient is comfortable and able to concentrate on the task of responding to the visual stimuli. He should not have to bend or stretch to reach the chin rest. An uncomfortable patient will tire quickly, and fatigue is a leading cause of inaccurate test results.

Aside from the considerations of comfort, if the patient must stretch to reach the chin rest (because the instrument is too high or the chair is too low), relaxing during the test will cause the patient's forehead to drift backward, with the eye too far behind the correcting lens (see Fig. 11-7, later in chapter). Consequently, a lens rim artifact results when points near the edge of the 30-degree central field are tested. If the instrument is too low (or the chair too high) the patient's neck may be flexed and his chin slightly backward when the forehead touches the forehead bar. This causes the eyebrows and eyelids to impinge on the upper part of the field.

The distance of the chair from the instrument should be coordinated with the height of the instrument so the patient leans slightly forward (Fig. 11-4, *A*).

If the chair is too far away or the perimeter is too low, the patient will be bent uncomfortably forward during the test. His face may be tilted forward and, once again, the eyelids and eyebrows may be in a position where they will interfere with testing of the upper visual field (Fig. 11-4, *B* and *C*). If the patient is heavyset, he may have to lean forward more than is optimal so that his head reaches beyond the anterior protuberance of the body (Fig. 11-4, *D*). In such cases the examiner must be particularly careful to set the chin forward in the chin rest, even though hyperextension of the neck may be uncomfortable and difficult to maintain.

If the chair is too close or the perimeter is too high (Fig. 11-4, *E* and *F*) the patient may be off balance and continually strain to maintain his position at the perimeter. If the patient feels the need to prop himself or herself with arms back or to hold onto the instrument to keep from falling backward, the instrument may be too close and may need to be adjusted (Fig. 11-4, *E*).

> Comfort reduces fatigue and helps maintain eye alignment. Both affect the test result.

FIG. 11-4. Influence of Chair and Instrument Positions on the Patient's Comfort and Face Position. A, The correct position, leaning slightly forward. **B,** The instrument is too low, which not only makes the patient uncomfortably hunched but also causes his face to tilt forward so that his chin moves backward in the chin rest. **C,** The patient is leaning uncomfortably forward. **D,** The heavyset patient may have to lean forward so that his face will reach the instrument. **E,** The instrument is too close. The patient must sit perfectly straight instead of comfortably leaning slightly forward. **F,** The instrument is too high, causing the forehead to drift back from the forehead rest (and the eye back from any correcting lens in place). This position also is uncomfortable because the patient must stretch upward in a vain effort to keep the forehead in place.

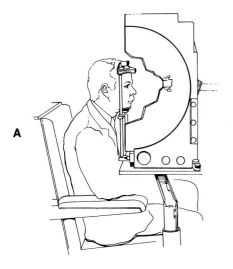

A

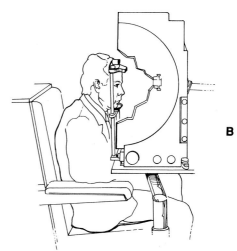

B

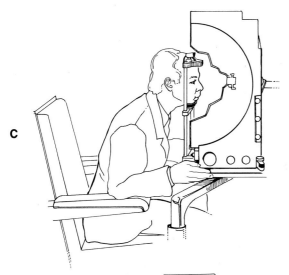

C

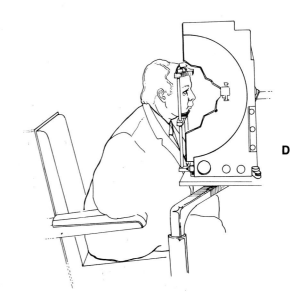

D

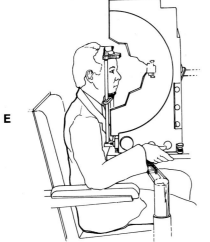

E

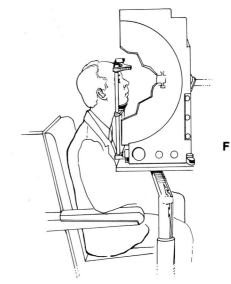

F

CORRECTIVE LENSES
General principles

Test stimuli must be in focus on the retina for optimum visualization. Therefore the patient may need corrective lenses to obtain an optimum visual field examination with consistent responses. Optical correction for the entire visual field would be ideal; however, as a practical matter, the lens holder and the rim of the lens are obstructive and therefore a lens cannot be used in front of the eye to test the field outside 30 degrees. Fortunately, there is less need for a sharply focused retinal image in the peripheral field than in the central field. It is also fortunate that with the size-III stimulus in standard use in static perimetry, focus is less critical than it was when a small size-I stimulus was the standard (for kinetic Goldmann perimetry).

To determine the appropriate lenses, the examiner must consider (1) the refractive error of the patient at a distance (distance correction); (2) the total amount of added adjustment (or "near add" that must be provided by accommodation, a lens, or a combination of these) needed for the patient to see the test stimuli, which is +3.00 diopters (D) for the HFA-1 Humphrey perimeter and +3.25 D for the HFA-2 Humphrey perimeter; and (3) the amount of this perimetric near add that can be provided comfortably by the patient's accommodative ability, which reduces the amount needed from the lenses. The patient's accommodative ability is determined by age, but is 0 D, no matter what the age, if the eye is aphakic, psuedophakic, or under the influence of a cycloplegic drug.

Choosing the appropriate lens power

The first step in choosing the appropriate lens power is to determine the best distance correction for the patient. This can be done by means of a complete refraction, or by establishing the power of the patient's present distance glasses and determining the visual acuity at a distance. If the visual acuity is 20/20, or if it is less but cannot be improved with a pinhole, the present glasses probably have the best distance correction. If a pinhole improves the vision, plus or minus spheres can be placed over the present glasses to see whether the vision is improved to a satisfactory level; if it is, the combination of the spheres and the present glasses can be considered close enough to the best distance correction. As a general rule, +0.50 and −0.50 D spheres should be tried over the glasses if the vision is in the range of 20/50. Similarly, +1.00 and −1.00 D spheres should be tried if the vision is 20/100.

Once the distance correction is known, the perimetrist can enter the information with the patient data, and the perimeter will calculate the lens power to use for perimetry. Whether determined by the perimetrist or by the perimeter, the basis for the calculation follows.

If a cylinder correction is included in the "best distance correction," it should be ignored if it is 0.25 D or less. If the power of the cylinder is 0.50 to 1.00 D, no cylindrical correction is used for the visual field tests, but the distance sphere is adjusted by 0.25 or 0.50 D, as required to maintain spherical equivalence. However,

Table 11-1. Add (to the best distance correction) for perimetry with a 30- to 33-cm bowl radius with intact accommodation*

Age (yrs) 30 cm	Add (diopters)
30 to 40	+1.00
40 to 45	+1.50
45 to 50	+2.00
50 to 55	+2.50
55 to 60	+3.00
60 to 65	+3.25

*Maximum is +3.00 D for 33-cm bowl and +3.25 D for 30-cm bowl.

if the power of the cylinder is more than 1.00 D, the cylindrical lens is used for the visual field test. Be sure that the lens is placed in the lens holder at the correct axis.

The spherical lens used for visual field testing is the "best distance sphere correction" combined with an add according to the patient's age. Table 11-1 gives the add recommended for the Humphrey perimeters.* These are generous adds; thus, the patient uses some of his accommodation but is not fatigued by having to use all or most of it. Note that the selection of the add for perimetry is not determined by the patient's reading glasses. Note also that *the full add* (+3.00 D for the HFA-I with a 33-cm radius of the bowl or +3.25 D for the HFA-II with a 30-cm radius bowl) *is used in four circumstances:* (1) for patients over 60 years old; (2) at any age if the eye has undergone cataract surgery; (3) after cycloplegia; and (4) in patients who are more than 3.00 D myopic.

The reason for not choosing the full add for all individuals, requiring some to use their own accommodation, is to minimize the prismatic and other effects of the lenses. The principle is to use the weakest lens possible but to provide a generous enough add that the patient is comfortable, not having to use all of his accommodative reserve. However, more add than the table recommends may be used if the increased add would result in the use of a weaker minus lens—provided the maximum 3.00- or 3.25-D add is not exceeded.

In summary, the lenses used for perimetry are (1) the cylindrical lens, as required by the patient for distance if it is 1.00 D or more; and (2) the spherical lens. The calculated required power of the spherical lens is the patient's own distance correction adjusted by 0.25 or 0.50 D if the distance correction includes a 0.50- to 1.00-D cylinder that is not being used for perimetry. The spherical lens power is adjusted further according to the patient's accommodative ability (i.e., depending on age and other factors). If the calculated spherical lens requirement is less than 1 D, no spherical lens is needed, especially for a size-III or larger stimulus, and is best avoided to reduce the risk of a lens rim artifact.

Four circumstances that require a full add for perimetry.

*The add depends on the distance from the eye for the fixation target and therefore is different for various perimeters. It is between 3.25 and plano for instruments with a bowl radius of 30 cm, between 3.00 and plano for instruments with a 33-cm bowl radius, between 2.50 and plano for instruments with a bowl radius of 42.5 cm, and between 2.00 and plano for instruments with a bowl radius of 50 cm.

Perhaps the simplest and most error-free method of determining the trial lens correction is to let the perimeter make the calculation. Only the patient's date of birth and distance refraction must be entered; the Humphrey perimeter makes the calculation automatically.

Positioning the cylinder axis

It is easy to place cylindrical lenses incorrectly. The standard notation for the axis of the cylinder is consistent with standard mathematical coordinates when the examiner looks at the patient's face (Fig. 11-5). Thus 45 degrees is toward the upper nasal quadrant of the right eye or the upper temporal quadrant of the left eye.

An important difference between perimeters, however, must be observed when placing lenses in the lens holder. With some perimeters, the perimetrist inserts the lens while looking at the lens holder from the side that will be toward the perimetric bowl. With others, including the Humphrey perimeters, the perimetrist inserts the lens while looking at the side that will be against the patient's face (Fig. 11-6). It is important to pay attention to this difference when placing lenses.

Three other important considerations pertain when positioning the lenses:

1. When placing a lens in the lens holder, the spherical lens must be in the slot that will be nearest to the patient's face and the cylindrical lens must be positioned with the front toward the bowl. If two spherical lenses are used (to achieve the total add required), the stronger one is placed closer to the eye.
2. Use a full-aperture lens with a narrow metal rim around the glass, not a lens with a broad rim around a smaller glass.
3. Be careful to notice whether the patient's correction is expressed in plus or minus cylinders and use the appropriate type. They are not the same. If the cylindrical lenses available for perimetry are not of the same type as the refraction record, the spherocylinder expression must be transposed before determining which lenses to use for perimetry.

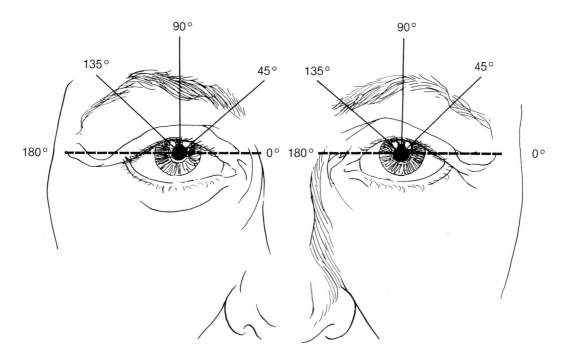

FIG. 11-5. Axis of the Cylindrical Lenses Used for Astigmatism.

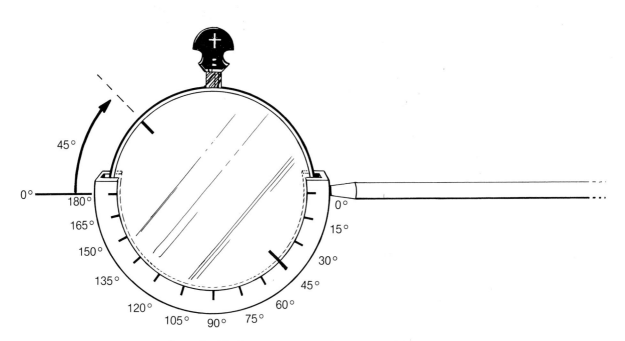

FIG. 11-6. Angle for Cylindrical Lens Placement in a Lens Holder Viewed from the Patient Side when Placing a Lens.

Assuring the proper corrective lens position

It is important that the corrective lens be close to the face, almost touching the eyelashes. Otherwise, its edge will impinge on the edge of the 30-degree field to be tested.

In addition, the eye must be centered with respect to the corrective lens. For the lens to be centered over the pupil, it must be positioned snugly against the bridge of the nose. No patient can hold perfectly still during the course of a perimetric examination, and it is easy for the patient's head to drift away from the correct position. Both the lens-to-cornea vertex distance and the centration of the eye in the lens must be monitored continually lest the patient's head shift during the course of the test; these must be monitored in addition to fixation.

In a test of the central 30 degrees, the 3.00- or 3.25-D lens used for a presbyopic, emmetropic patient will begin to produce an edge artifact if the eye is decentered by more than 5 mm at a vertex distance of 15 mm. As much as 8 mm of decentration can be permitted, with a closer vertex distance of 10 mm (Fig. 11-9). The permitted decentration decreases with higher plus power lenses. Allowable decentration also is reduced for lenses with optical regions that occupy less than the full 37-mm diameter of the standard trial lens.

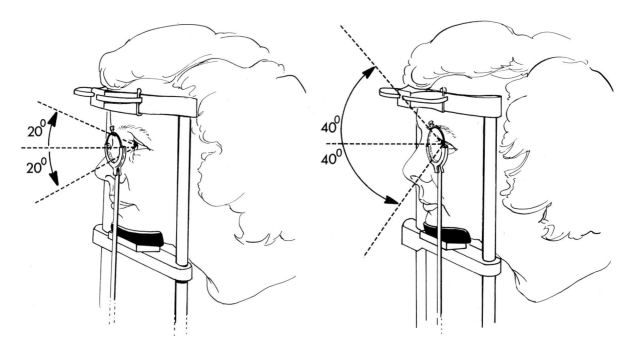

FIG. 11-7. Effect of Lens Distance on the Limits of the Field that Can Be Tested. See Figures 7-33 to 7-38 for examples of the artifacts that can result.

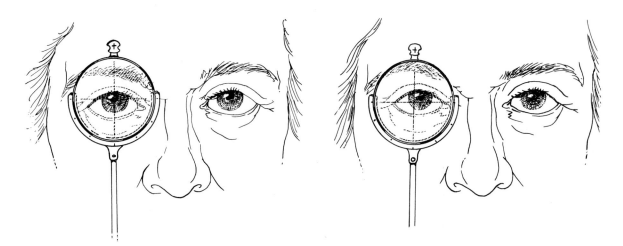

FIG. 11-8. Correctly Centered Lens *(left)* **and Incorrectly Centered Lens** *(right).* In the incorrect position, the upper nasal portion of the field is blocked by the lens rim. Stimuli presented in that quadrant may not be seen, simulating visual field loss. Even the slight misalignment shown here can cause a false field defect, an example of which appears in Figure 7-34. An improper head tilt (see Fig. 11-3) causes the lower edge of the lens to be far from the eye (blocking the lower part of the field), even if the upper part of the lens is as close as possible to the eyebrow.

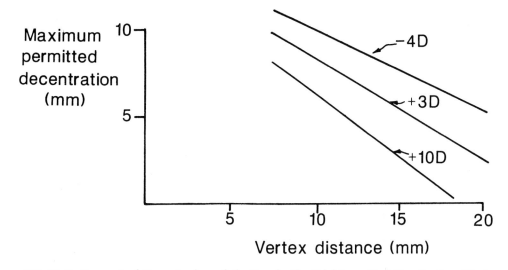

FIG. 11-9. Amount of Decentration of the Eye in the Trial Lens that Can Be Permitted without Partially Blocking a Light Stimulus 30 Degrees from Fixation. Calculations for these graphs for 4-, 3-, and 10-D lenses are based on a trial lens diameter of 37 mm, pupil radius of 5 mm, and an entrance pupil of the eye located 3.5 mm behind the corneal apex. The vertex distance (x-axis) is the distance from the cornea to the corrective trial lens. The formula for permitted decentration is $R - r - (x + E)(\tan 30° RP/1000 - R/B)$, where R is the radius of the corrective trial lens, r is the radius of the pupil, E is the distance of plane of the "apparent pupil" behind the cornea, P is the power of the corrective trial lens, B is the perimeter bowl radius, and x is the cornea-to-trial lens vertex distance, with P in diopters and all other measurements in millimeters. (Courtesy of Alan Kirschbaum)

Contact lenses

> If the patient wears contacts lenses, the "distance refraction" is plano or the distance refraction over the contact lens.

If the patient wears contact lenses with his proper distance correction, the contact lenses are left in for the entire field examination (for both central and peripheral fields). The contact lens alone is used for the peripheral field; when testing the central 30 degrees of the field, however, the required add for perimetry is provided by using a loose trial lens along with the contact lens. In essence, the patient who wears only distance contact lenses is considered to have no refractive error at distance; however, an add is needed for perimetry in the central 30 degrees according to the patient's accommodative ability. If he wears glasses over the contact lenses for distance, the spectacle correction is considered the distance refractive error to be used as the starting point in determining the near correction for perimetry. If the patient uses the "monovision" contact lens method to achieve crisp near vision in one eye, the minus lens needed to refract the eye to optimal distance acuity with the lens in place is the "distance refraction" to use when determining the add needed for perimetry of that eye.

Cycloplegia

If a patient has been given cycloplegic drops to dilate the pupil or for refraction, the full add of +3.00 or +3.25 D is required for any age because the cycloplegic drug will have eliminated almost all accommodative ability. This is one circumstance in which the perimeter's calculation of lens power, based on the patient's age, may not be appropriate. Another circumstance involves patients who have had cataracts removed (see next section).

Aphakia and pseudophakia

After cataract extraction a patient no longer has accommodation and requires a full add regardless of his age. If the patient has a lens implant or wears contact lenses, a +3.00- or +3.25-D add combined with any distance overcorrection in spectacles is needed for the central 30 degrees. The contact lens or lens implant alone is adequate for the peripheral field outside 30 degrees.

If the patient has no implant and does not wear contact lenses, the necessary distance spectacle correction plus the full add for perimetry will be strong. This circumstance is encountered very infrequently now, so it is easy to forget that there are major problems with the use of such strong lenses for perimetry. First, their magnification effects cause the central field to be miniaturized on the field diagram—with the blind spot migrating toward fixation and the apparent limit of the field produced by the lens edge moving inside 30 degrees. Second, the vertex distance (from the lens to the cornea) is critical with strong lenses and it is difficult to maintain the proper vertex distance during the entire field examination, especially for elderly patients.

A solution, when feasible, is to use contact lenses for the visual field examination in patients with aphakia, even if they do not usually wear contact lenses. Soft contact lenses are useful, because they are comfortable, fit a wide range of eyes, and have large optical zones. Contact lenses that provide both the distance correction and the full add for perimetry can be used for both central and peripheral field examinations. Using contact lenses for testing the peripheral field provides the additional theoretical advantage of allowing stimuli to be adequately focused on the retina, which seems to improve the peripheral field examination when there is a strong refractive error (as with aphakia), even though corrective lenses are not extremely important for testing the peripheral field in the presence of the more frequent lesser degree of refractive error.

Hard contact lenses also may be used, with greater success than might be expected. A hard contact lens with a 10-mm diameter and a steep base curve (7.60 mm) is used to reduce lens movement, which would be disturbing to a patient not accustomed to wearing contact lenses. A steep immobile lens is tolerated by the cornea for the duration of the examination, although it would not be suitable for regular wear. Additional comfort may be provided by instilling topical anesthetic before putting the lens in place.

A selection of four hard lenses may be kept on hand for use in perimetry (13.00, 16.50, 19.00, and 21.00 D). To select the proper lens, the examiner determines the spectacle correction, adding (1) the sphere; (2) the cylinder expressed in plus form (the minus cylinder is ignored); and (3) the 3.00-D add for perimetry. The vertex distance of the spectacle is calculated and the total required correction (sphere, cylinder, and 3.00-D add) is converted to a vertex distance of zero. Next, the strength closest to this result is selected from among the four standard lenses; often this is the 16.50-D lens.

The use of contact lenses rarely is perfect. Plus and minus spheres can be used over the contact lens, and the patient may be asked which superimposed trial lens best brings the fixation spot into focus. Any additional lenses that are required can be used in combination with the contact lens for the central 30 degrees but the contact lens alone is used for the peripheral field. The same lenses can be used for all subsequent field examinations without going through the process of determining the best lens each time.

High myopia

The high power lenses required for the correction of axial myopia occasionally produce some of the problems that occur with aphakia. However, it is fortunate that many such patients wear contact lenses and require only the use of an add for age. If contact lenses are not worn, the power of the trial lens is reduced by using the full 3.00- or 3.25-D add for all ages. If such a lens is still strong enough to present a problem, a temporary contact lens can be used, in the same manner that temporary lenses can be used for aphakia, as described earlier. The power of the lens is the patient's distance refraction with a full +3.00- or +3.25-D add for perimetry, adjusted for vertex distance. However, the use of a temporary contact lens is not an optimal solution, and is best reserved for unusual needs determined by the clinician. Axial myopia often presents the additional problem of refraction scotoma as an artifact (see Chapter 7).

Refinements and application

Ideally, lens thickness should be minimized to avoid distortions and prismatic effects. For this reason, as already noted, it is best not to use the full add routinely on all patients. To lessen the need for unnecessarily strong lenses, the strength of minus spheres should be reduced as long as the patient is using any accommodation. This offers the double advantage of reducing the strength of the minus sphere while simultaneously reducing the need for the patient to accommodate.

To implement these principles, the perimetrist should start with the distance spectacle refraction of the patient expressed in the plus cylinder form, adjust it to maintain spherical equivalence if the patient's refraction includes a cylindrical lens that will not be used for perimetry, and apply the following rules:

1. If the distance sphere component is a plus lens, the spherocylinder combination calculated by providing the usual add for age (see Table 11-1) should be used.
2. If the distance sphere component is between plano and -3.00 D (HFA-1) or -3.25 D (HFA-2), the age correction to calculate the required near spherical correction for perimetry should be used as follows:
   A. If the calculated spherical correction for near is plus, it should be used along with any cylinder that is needed.
   B. If the calculated spherical correction for near is minus, no sphere should be used but only the cylinder that is needed.
3. If the sphere component of the distance correction represents more than 3 D of myopia, the near correction for perimetry should be calculated by using the full add.

This refinement is included in the automatic calculation of the lens power available in the perimeter's software.

MONITORING AND MODIFYING THE TEST

A common misconception is that with automated perimetry the machine conducts the test by itself once it is set into motion. However, it is the perimetrist who conducts the test, using the machine as a tool. The perimetrist can conduct a good test or a poor test with the machine, and his attentiveness to the task has a profound influence on the validity of the results for many patients.

> Pay attention to the patient during the test.

The perimetrist should understand the general nature of field testing and the sequence of stimulus presentations in the test (see Chapters 1 and 5). The progress of the test requires constant monitoring. After the foveal threshold has been tested, the patient is instructed to look at the central fixation target, and the perimetrist should observe whether the patient understood the instruction and complied. The patient may need to be instructed again. It is sometimes helpful to point at the fixation target (without touching the bowl and making a smudge).

After central fixation is achieved and the test resumes, the third presentation is in the presumed location of the blind spot if the Heijl-Krakau fixation loss method (blind spot technique) is used. If the patient responds to this presentation or to the next one in the blind spot, a subroutine follows in which stimuli are presented first in a horizontal array and then in a vertical array to find the center of the true location of the blind spot. If the patient does not respond to the third stimulus, the blind spot is assumed to encompass this location and the subroutine to locate its exact center is not undertaken, unless the perimetrist pauses the test and specifically selects to have the blind spot relocated. This should be done if there is doubt about the validity of the patient's lack of response to the blind spot stimulus—for example, if the perimetrist notices that the patient has not yet settled into a state of readiness to respond, which may be manifest by a failure to respond to the preceding stimuli.

Some Humphrey perimeters include a gaze tracker that makes the blind spot fixation checks unnecessary, although both can be done. Instead, the perimetrist monitors the record of the gaze tracker and watches the image of the eye on the screen. If the gaze tracker is giving false information by recording fixation loss of a steady eye, the perimetrist should pause the test and reinitialize the gaze tracker.

The perimetrist should watch the patient's eye position and movements, in addition to the reported fixation loss rate from blind spot checks or the tracing of the gaze tracker throughout the test. If fixation is wandering, or the patient is searching for upcoming stimuli, he should be gently reminded and encouraged. The perimetrist must be understanding and recognize that many patients find it difficult to overcome the natural, involuntary movement of the eye to look at something when it is seen. All day long, without thinking about it, we look at whatever catches our attention in the side vision. It is not a serious problem during perimetry if the patient looks at each light he sees, provided the patient looks back at the fixation target when waiting for the next stimulus.

As the test proceeds, threshold values are displayed on the screen as they are determined. It is a good practice to evaluate the results as they unfold so that the test selection can be modified if necessary. If, for example, the first four points tested (the primary points) have threshold values that are quite low (e.g., 10 dB) it might be best to stop the test and restart it with a size-V stimulus.

Also displayed are the catch trial results, including fixation losses, false-positive responses, and false-negative responses.

The "fixation loss" frequency is determined as the test proceeds by presenting the stimulus in the location of the physiologic blind spot from time to time. If the patient responds, it is reported as a "fixation loss." The patient will see the stimulus if indeed his gaze wandered so that the light did not fall within the boundary of the physiologic blind spot. However, the patient also may see the light, without losing accurate positioning of the eye, if the light is not being presented at the blind spot but in a seeing part of this person's retina. This "pseudoloss of fixation" occurs if the localization of the blind spot early in the test was faulty or if the head tilt shifted slightly after the localization.

To overcome this problem, fixation should be evaluated while the test is being conducted. As the test proceeds, the fixation loss rate is presented on the screen and should be monitored. The fixation loss trials (presentations in the blind spot) are particularly frequent near the beginning of the test; thus, the attentive perimetrist can undertake any necessary corrective action early in the test.

If the perimetrist recognizes that fixation is steady, but the first two tests of fixation are reported as fixation losses on the screen, the test should be immediately paused. The "relocate blind spot" menu should be chosen and the test continued. After this point there should be no further reports of fixation loss unless the patient changes the tilt of his head, in which case the blind spot again can be relocated. If this becomes too bothersome, it can be specified on the printout that fixation was steady despite reported fixation losses, so that those who look at the field diagram will know that the field test should not be considered unreliable just because of a reported high rate of fixation loss. Alternatively, the fixation monitoring can be turned off (change parameter menu), but these two methods to bypass the automatic fixation monitoring should be avoided whenever possible.

The gaze tracker in the HFA-2 eliminates the need for use of the blind spot technique to check the frequency of fixation loss. It also may give false reports of fixation loss but the attentive perimetrist should notice this, pause the test, and reinitialize the gaze tracker.

During the test, "false-positive responses" also should be monitored. Sometimes the patient pushes the button when in fact no stimulus is presented. He may push the button simply because it seems to be time for another stimulus, or because he heard a noise made by the machinery. The patient is trying to do his best during the test, guessing at the correct answer as during cognitive examinations in school. The patient pushes the button if he thinks the light is on, even if it is not seen. This may happen when a stimulus is presented in the physiologic blind spot, leading to a reported high frequency of fixation loss even though the patient's fixation was steady. Another way to recognize the occurrence of false-positive responses is to observe that the measured threshold values displayed on the video screen are exceedingly high (e.g., 38 dB). Such stimuli are almost impossible to see and higher threshold values must be the result of a high false-positive rate.

False-positive responses can greatly invalidate test results. If the perimetrist realizes that the patient is giving false-positive responses, it is necessary to pause the test and explain to the patient that the purpose of the test is not to report when he thinks the light might be on, but to report when in fact it is actually seen. The patient should expect to see the light only half of the time. Also, the patient should know that the machine is trying to keep him honest by sometimes not shining a light in the bowl at a time when it would seem that there ought to be a light. Remind the patient that it is not necessary to respond within the two tenths of a second that the light is on. After the light has been shown, the machine waits a second or two for a response, so the patient need not feel pressured into pushing the button rapidly—and perhaps by mistake.

False-negative responses are reported when the patient fails to respond after a stimulus that should be seen has been presented. Such stimuli are presented in locations at which threshold has already been determined, and a stimulus 9 dB more intense than threshold is presented. There are several reasons a patient can fail to respond and hence cause the presentation to be labeled a false-negative response:

1. There is a natural variability in sensation at defective points in the visual field. In a region of low sensitivity, although a threshold value has been

Fixation and false responses need monitoring during the test, to permit corrective action.

determined, a brighter stimulus may in fact not be visible when presented a moment later. Thus, false-negative responses are a natural occurrence in abnormal visual fields.

2. If the patient gives false *positive* responses, the machine believes the patient can see dim stimuli. It may select a stimulus too dim to be seen for the false negative catch trial, and the failure to respond is not really a false negative error. Thus, a high FP rate will cause a high FN rate.

3. The patient may fatigue as the test proceeds. Thus a stimulus of given intensity may have been visible at that location, but later a brighter stimulus is required for the patient to respond. When printed out, such fields have a depressed sensitivity near the edge. In extreme cases of progressive nonresponsiveness, the lighter shades have a cloverleaf shape on the greyscale printout.

4. The patient may be a variable responder, sometimes responding to a very dim stimulus that is seen but, at other times, not responding unless the stimulus is more certainly visible. It is this particular trait of the patient that the false-negative catch trials are designed to detect. This trait and the concurrent high short-term fluctuation are a guide to the degree of confidence in a given threshold value and its reproducibility.

The perimetrist cannot do anything about the fact that a visual field is abnormal and naturally leads to a high FN rate. Likewise, the perimetrist may be able to do little about a patient's innate inconsistency, except to place the patient at ease and offer encouragement. However, the perimetrist can attempt to correct any tendency for false-positive responses and also can be alert to signs of fatigue in order to give rest as needed and to keep the patient alert with a flow of conversation. **False-positive responses and fatigue are each particularly damaging to the accuracy of the test results. An attentive perimetrist can do much to help overcome these problems.**

With the SITA strategy, there are no false-positive and few false-negative catch trials; nonetheless, the perimetrist must be attentive to fatigue, inattentiveness, or hasty responses by the patient. Attention and encouragement can greatly improve the test accuracy.

The eye should be observed not only for tendency toward loss of fixation but also for its position. The eye should be well centered within the trial lens and the head should not be allowed to drift backward away from the lens. Correct centration and close position of the lens to the eye become more important near the end of the test when the edge points are being tested. The examiner therefore should be particularly careful that the patient's head and eye position do not drift from the original position with respect to the trial lens in the later stages of the test.

Likewise, the perimetrist must ensure that the patient remains comfortable and also that he stays attentive to the task. Restlessness may signify an uncomfortable position and that adjustments or a change in position are needed. Closing eyelids or a string of failed responses may be a sign for the perimetrist to say something or perhaps pause the test and give the patient a brief chance to stretch. Talking

Control patient fatigue and attentiveness.

to encourage the patient and keep him alert is increasingly important as the test proceeds. These comments should be brief and not distracting (e.g., "Keep it up," "Good!" "Keep looking at the center," "That's great!"). Do not overdo or become monotonous, and modify remarks according to the personality needs of the individual. The need for comments can be judged by watching for signs of fatigue.

Prevent distractions.

The perimetrist should be sure that there are no distractions— for example, no audible disturbances from the adjacent room. The perimetrist should not produce distractions by receiving phone calls, conversing with others, or working on something else while the test is underway. Because of the importance of monitoring the conduct of the test and correcting an impending problem, the perimetrist should become occupied with tasks or leave the patient alone. The patient should sense the perimetrist's attentive presence.

If the patient shows signs of fatigue, the test can be paused. Be sure that the head and eye are back in proper position before resuming. If the patient finds the test pace too fast, make sure he knows not to make hurried responses, and in particular that it is not necessary to respond while the light is still on. If the patient senses that the pace is too rapid because the presentation of the next stimulus comes too soon after the previous response, the "slow mode" may be helpful for a few individuals. However, the slow mode should be used sparingly because most patients find it too slow and because it adds time to the test.

All of these tasks suggest that the perimetrist should be present, and importantly also attentive, for the duration of the test. During longer tests, when performed on experienced patients known to be reliable, it is sometimes possible for the perimetrist to remain attentive to the patient while performing other tasks or even undertaking perimetry on another patient in an adjacent cubicle. With the new shorter tests, the set-up time may exceed the test time, so that little efficiency may be gained by attempting simultaneous testing of two patients. It has been shown that a large proportion of patients may provide reliable test results on their own despite divided attention of the perimetrist and perhaps even despite nearby commotion; but a sizeable minority when unattended do not do as well as they could. The elderly and those who spent less time in formal schooling are most likely to benefit from the continuous attention of the perimetrist.

AFTER THE TEST

After the first eye's test is complete, remove the patch and give the patient a short rest while the patient data are checked for completeness and the results are saved on the disk. It is wise to do this before proceeding to the second eye, so that a power failure or other accident does not cause the test results to be lost. If the patient is ready to proceed, the results can be printed later.

After the second eye's test is complete, the first job is to attend to the patient— to remove the patch, offer praise, empathize with a statement such as "I'll bet you're glad we're done!" and have the patient retire to the waiting room while you finish saving data and print the test results.

The test should be saved on a disk after verifying that the patient data are correct. In particular, if the pupil size is entered manually and is not the same for the two eyes, it must be changed before the results of the second eye are saved.

In preparation for the next test, all parameters should be changed back to standard if any nonstandard parameters were used in the test just completed. Making the change back to standard at the end of the test, in addition to checking the parameters before each test, provides double insurance that a nonstandard test will not be run unintentionally.

Evidence that the perimetrist makes a difference.

FURTHER READING

Keltner JL, Johnson CA, Beck RW, et al: Quality control functions of the Visual Field Reading Center (VFRC) for the Optic Neuritis Treatment Trial (ONTT), *Control Clin Trials* 14:143-159, 1993.

APPENDIX A

Abbreviations

Below is a list of abbreviations used in this book. More complete explanations may be found in the Glossary (Appendix B) and in the text itself.

CPSD. Corrected Pattern Standard Deviation

CRL. Central Reference Level

D. Diopter

dB. Decibel

FL. Fixation Loss rate

FN. False-Negative error rate

FOS. Frequency of Seeing

FP. False-Positive error rate

GH. General Height

GHT. Glaucoma Hemifield Test

HFA. Humphrey Field Analyzer

MD. Mean Deviation

MS. Mean Sensitivity

PSD. Pattern Standard Deviation

SF. Short-Term Fluctuation

SWAP. Short-Wavelength Automated Perimetry

SITA. Swedish Interactive Thresholding Algorithm

Glossary

Amsler grid. Method to screen the inner 10 degrees of the visual field for distortion or scotomas.

Average file. Combination of several similar threshold tests to produce an average threshold value for each test location.

Blue-yellow perimetry. See SWAP.

Boxplot. Display of the range of Total Deviation values in a visual field test, showing the extreme range along with the median, 15th percentile and 85th percentile values. Change over a series of field examinations may be discerned from a graphical display of a series of boxplots in the Change Analysis printout.

Catch trial. A period of time during perimetry during which an attempt is made to detect a loss of fixation by a blind spot check, or to tabulate a false-positive or false-negative error rate.

Central Reference Level (CRL). Hypothetical threshold sensitivity at the center of the field, ignoring the foveal peak. It may be a value projected on the basis of the normal slope of the "hill of vision" and empirically determined thresholds at 4 or 5 locations or an assigned value (by age, or as a minimal value). It is used to determine expected threshold values throughout the field to guide testing or to calculate Defect Depth.

Change analysis. A printout that displays statistical summaries of a series of field tests in the form of boxplots and graphs of the global indices.

Compare printout. Map of test point locations, showing the differences in threshold sensitivity values between field tests being compared.

Corrected Pattern Standard Deviation (CPSD). One of four global indices. The Pattern Standard Deviation is "corrected" to remove the effect of test-retest variability (or SF).

Decibel (dB). In the context of perimetry, the intensity (of a stimulus) expressed as 0.1 log-unit of attenuation of the maximal available stimulus (10,000 asb for current Humphrey perimeters).

Defect depth. Difference of threshold sensitivity at a location from the threshold expected from the assigned or calculated Central Reference Level. To be distinguished from Total Deviation.

Diopter (D). Measure of lens strength expressed as the reciprocal of the focal length measured in meters.

Esterman grid. Method to score monocular or binocular visual fields to quantify visual ability, disability, or impairment.

False-Negative (FN) rate. The frequency with which the patient fails to respond to stimuli that are expected to be visible. The basis of calculation and interpretation of the result is not identical for SITA and non-SITA strategies.

False-Positive (FP) rate. The frequency with which the patient responds to stimuli that actually could not have been seen. The manner of determining the rate differs in the SITA and non-SITA strategies, but the interpretation is the same.

Fast threshold. A follow-up suprathreshold test available on the HFA-1 in which intensity of stimulus presentations is based on threshold sensitivities in the baseline field(s), with thresholding of locations where the suprathreshold stimulus is not seen.

Fastpac. Thresholding algorithm in which stimuli are presented in 3-dB steps and the threshold value is assigned based on the first crossover from seeing to non-seeing or vice versa.

Fixation Loss (FL) rate. With the blind spot method of Heijl-Krakow, the number of times the patient responds per catch trial in which a stimulus is presented in the expected position of the physiologic blind spot.

Frequency-of-Seeing (FOS) curve. A graph of the likelihood of seeing stimuli over a range of stimulus intensities. In strict definition, the intensity at which there is a 50% probability of seeing is the threshold value. When the slope of the FOS curve is shallow, as is typical of lower visual sensitivities, the short-term fluctuation is high during perimetric testing.

Full Threshold test strategy. Algorithm used in the original HFA-1 for static threshold testing, which changes stimulus brightness in 4-dB steps until threshold is crossed, and then in 2-dB steps until threshold is crossed a second time. The starting brightness is determined from already known thresholds at other points.

General Height (GH). Total Deviation of a representative location in the most normal region of the field, which typically is the location representing the 15th percentile in rank ordering of Total Deviations. GH reflects the effects of general depression and long-term fluctuation, and is used to convert Total Deviation to

Pattern Deviations or to remove effects of long-term fluctuation and media opacities from the MD index.

Glaucoma Change Probability printout or display. Comparison of threshold data in a follow-up field to baseline, in which points are highlighted if they change by amounts that are larger than that typically seen in stable glaucoma patients. Similarly, MD values changing by more than typical amounts also are flagged.

Glaucoma Hemifield Test (GHT). Plain language analysis of a single threshold 30-2 or 24-2 test. Analysis is based on normative database and a pathological model for glaucomatous field loss.

Global indices. Single numerical values which each characterize certain aspects of the visual field; for Humphrey perimeters, MD, PSD, SF, and CPSD. MS is a substitute for MD when normative data are not available.

Greyscale. Threshold sensitivity values displayed as shades of grey, smoothed with interpolated values between actual test locations.

HFA-1. Original models (600 series) of Humphrey Field Analyzer.

HFA-2. More compact recent models (700 series) of Humphrey perimeters. It includes a gaze tracker, and a more powerful computer can run SITA. Some obsolete tests and analyses, or ones not often used with the HFA-1, were not included (see Appendix C).

Long-term fluctuation. True changes in threshold sensitivity over time, after removal of variability due to simple measurement error.

Macula Test. A pattern for threshold testing that includes the foveal point and 16 locations, 2 degrees apart, in a 4 x 4 grid centering on the point of fixation. In the HFA-1, each point is tested in triplicate, and in the HFA-1 non-SITA strategies, each point is tested twice.

Master file. A specific Average file designated as a baseline, used for the Fast Threshold test or with the Compare function to calculate change in threshold sensitivity from a baseline average.

Mean Deviation. The weighted average of the Total Deviation values in a visual field test; deviations near the center of the field are counted more heavily than those at the edge.

Mean Sensitivity. The average of the Threshold Sensitivity values in a visual field test.

Merge printout. Infrequently used method to display together the results of complementary tests of different patterns, for example the 30-1, 30-2, and 30/60-2. Both a Threshold Value map and a greyscale are obtained. To be distinguished from Average and Master files, which combine results of replicate tests of the same pattern rather than tests of complementary patterns.

Modified MD slope. Slope of a regression analysis of MD over time, in which the MD of the first field was not included because it was not in keeping with the slope determined by the regression analysis that included all the fields. Used to remove the impact of inexperience on the results of the first visual field when a learning effect is evident.

Octopus. One of the earliest perimeters capable of automated static perimetry, which with modifications has persisted to the present day. Singled out for mention because of its importance in establishing some of the now traditional patterns, test strategies, terminology, and approaches to quantitative analysis of results. Modern perimetry was also affected by principles and standards set by Goldmann on designing his perimeter, as well as the Tübingen perimeter, which emphasized static perimetry to supplement (and later to predominate over) kinetic perimetry.

Overview printout or display. Summary printout in which a whole series of test results are shown chronologically. Greyscale, threshold value map, Total Deviation probability plot, and Pattern Deviation plot for each field are displayed in a horizontal row, along with reliability parameters, global indices, acuity, and foveal threshold.

Pattern Deviation decibel and probability plots. Display of localized loss at each tested point, after removal of the effects of any generalized loss. Pattern Deviation dB values are the Total Deviation values minus the General Height. The Pattern Deviation probability map highlights locations where deviations exceed those found in fewer than 5%, 2%, 1%, or 0.5% of normal subjects.

Pattern Standard Deviation (PSD). A global index that represents the standard deviation around the mean of Total Deviations.

"Questions asked". Number of stimuli presented.

Sensitivity (statistical or diagnostic). Proportion or percentage of those with a medical condition who are correctly identified by a diagnostic test. The condition can be general ("any disease-induced visual reduction"), a particular disease ("glaucoma"), an anatomic change ("glaucoma-induced axon loss") or progression ("disease induced further reduction of visual function").

Sensitivity (visual). See Threshold Sensitivity.

Short-term Fluctuation. The test-retest variability of threshold sensitivity values obtained on repeat testing within the same test session (intratest variability). Representing measurement error, SF is expressed as the standard deviation of the distribution of repeat values obtained on replicate testing at a location in the visual field.

Short-term Fluctuation index (SF). The Short-term Fluctuation global index, SF, is an effort to represent with a single number the middle of the range of short-term fluctuations at various locations, estimated from duplicate measurements at selected locations.

Short Wavelength Automated Perimetry (SWAP).   Test that isolates the blue-sensitive portion of the visual system for testing. Also known as blue-yellow perimetry.

Single Field Analysis.   Basic Statpac display of results of a single field examination, showing threshold sensitivity values, reliability parameters, global indices, and statistical calculations to compare the results with the range of values expected from eyes with no ocular disease.

Specificity (statistical or diagnostic).   Proportion or percentage of normal individuals falsely identified by a diagnostic test as having a medical condition. Test conditions and criteria for a positive test affect both sensitivity and specificity, and thus must be tailored to the diagnostic task at hand.

Statpac.   Trademark for Humphrey software that performs a series of statistical calculations on the visual field results, with displays that include Single-Field Analysis, Change Analysis, Glaucoma Change Probability, and Overview printouts.

Suprathreshold test.   Test to determine whether threshold visual sensitivity is above or below some criterion, typically used for screening.

Suprathreshold test modes.   On the Humphrey perimeter, method by which the criterion level is determined. On the Humphrey perimeter test, modes include Single Intensity, Age-Corrected, Threshold Related, and Fast Threshold. The first three are selected within the screening test menus, and the last within the threshold test menu (HFA-1 only).

Suprathreshold test pattern.   Number and distribution of points tested. Various patterns are available, each with a different emphasis and purpose.

Suprathreshold test strategies.   Method used to determine presence and depth of abnormalities On the Humphrey perimeter includes Two-Zone, Three-Zone, and Quantify defects.

SWAPPac.   Software to perform a Statpac analysis on results of visual field test performed with SWAP.

Swedish Interactive Thresholding Algorithm (SITA).   Recently available strategy to measure threshold sensitivity and reliability parameters efficiently, to achieve optimal measurements with minimal time.

Three-in-one printout.   Traditional term for a printout that includes the greyscale, threshold value map, and a map of Defect Depth values. It predates the Statpac Single-Field Analysis now used for standard size-III threshold tests for which normative data are available. The Three-in-One printout is used to report results of tests performed using parameters (e.g., size-V stimulus) for which no normative data are available.

Threshold sensitivity.   Characteristic(s) of a stimulus that is perceived 50% of the time. In the staircase bracketing procedure used by the Humphrey perimeter, it is estimated as the weakest static stimulus intensity seen, with standard background intensity and duration of stimulus presentation, and of defined stimulus size and color.

Threshold test.   Test designed to measure threshold sensitivity; contrast with a suprathreshold test.

Threshold test patterns.   10-2, 24-2, 30-2, 60-4, 30/60-2, and Macula Test constitute the most useful selections.

Threshold test strategies.   Fastpac, Full-from-prior (obsolete), Full Threshold, SITA-Fast, SITA-Standard.

Threshold value table.   Map of the visual field with threshold values indicated at tested locations. Threshold at the foveal location is reported separately, to the side.

Total Deviation value and probability maps.   The Total Deviation decibel values are the differences between threshold sensitivity and age-corrected normal sensitivity at each tested location. The Total Deviation probability map highlights locations where deviations exceed those found in fewer than 5%, 2%, 1%, or 0.5% of normal subjects.

Characteristics and Comparison of the HFA-2 Humphrey Perimeter to the HFA-1 Model

The original HFA-1 perimeter, which is also known as the 600 series perimeter, had a hemispherical bowl with a 33-cm radius, while the newer 700 series HFA-2 perimeters are equipped with an aspherical bowl[1] having a 30-cm testing distance centrally. The aspherical design allows the perimeter to be smaller and more ergonomic.

The asphericity of the HFA-2 bowl produces less than 0.37 diopter change in accommodative distance between the center and 30 degrees eccentricity, an amount of change that likely has little or no effect on measured sensitivities in the central field. A multicenter trial found that the difference between the old and new designs was no larger than the difference commonly seen between two HFA-1 instruments.[2] Thus, both from theory and practice the two instruments produce equal results in tests performed in the central 30 degrees of the visual field.

On the other hand, the old and new instruments may produce slightly different results when testing outside the central 30 degrees. These differences are attributable to the fact that stimuli presented in the far periphery with HFA-2 will be closer to the eye than those presented with HFA-1—and thus will subtend a greater angle and be easier to see. In the extreme case—at 90 degrees eccentricity—this difference in angular subtense is roughly equivalent to 4 decibels of brightness difference.

The HFA-2 perimeter is programmed to decrease the stimulus brightness presented in peripheral field tests in order to correct for this difference in angular subtense. Of course, the correction is not exact due to the imperfect relationship between brightness and perceived size, as explained in Chapter 2, but it seems unlikely that a correction which varies only from 0 to 4 dB will be off by more than 1 or 2 dB. Given that peripheral visual field measurements are inexact at best, and that they have heretofore been performed in the absence of normative data, the corrections applied seem appropriate and adequate to the task.

Normative data for the 60-4 test of the HFA-2 have been collected for both versions of the SITA strategy, and will be released in a future software update. These normals will, of course, take implicit account of the effects of the aspherical bowl and will thus render the asphericity question moot for tests done on the HFA-2. It has not been documented how well peripheral tests on the HFA-1 correlate with those on the HFA-2, although there seems to be little need for such detailed correlative information.

REFERENCES

1. U.S. Patent 5,323,194: Perimeter with a non spherical bowl, granted to Charles E. Campbell and Vincent Michael Patella, June 21, 1994.
2. Johnson CA, Cioffi GA, Drance SM et al: A multicenter comparison study of the Humphrey Field Analyzer I and the Humphrey Field Analyzer II, *Ophthalmology* 104:1910-1917, 1997.

■ INDEX

ff = and multiple following pages